HOSPITAL MANAGEMENT SYSTEMS

Multi-Unit Organization and Delivery of Health Care

Montague Brown
Howard L. Lewis

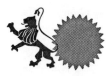

Aspen Systems Corporation
Germantown, Maryland
1976

"This publication is designed to provide accurate and authoritative information in regard to the Subject Matter covered. It is sold with the understanding that the publisher is not engaged in rendering legal, accounting, or other professional service. If legal advice or other expert assistance is required, the services of a competent professional person should be sought." From a Declaration of Principles jointly adopted by a Committee of the American Bar Association and a Committee of Publishers and Associations.

TABLE OF CONTENTS

LIST OF MAPS AND TABLES

All of the maps in this book were drawn by Jo Ann Danilovics, a free-lance artist in Wilmette, Illinois.

Foreword

Approximately ten years ago at the first Duke Forum it was my prediction that the hospital and health care industry would have to move in the direction of consolidation of facilities and resources. The reasons were clear even then. Health care was becoming increasingly a political issue, and single, autonomous, individual hospitals did not have the strength to cope with the issues which were beginning to face each of them.

Faced with increasing labor costs, increasing supply costs, new technology costs, the prospect of higher capital costs and the prospects of higher utilization of the facilities, it was equally obvious that economic pressure would force some new organizational configurations within the industry.

Additionally, it has been a social thrust in terms of additional services to the community we serve which has caused the growth of the Greenville Hospital System. It was my feeling that as part of the social fabric of the community other hospitals would assume a similar thrust.

At that time I did not foresee the growth of the investor-owned hospital chains. However, their appearance has made it even more clear that the voluntary and local governmental institutions must move to consolidate and integrate their institutional services.

The volume produced herein is dramatic evidence that a new period in our industry has arrived. Dr. Brown and Mr. Lewis are to be commended for the work they have done and for the information they have produced. This is a major contribution to the health care field. It will become a standard reference as to the point in time when it was recognized that our industry had moved from its "cottage industry" past into its corporate organizational structured future.

Robert E. Toomey
General Director

March 1976   The Greenville (S.C.) Hospital System

Preface

This book is based on a variety of personal and professional experiences by both of us during the last two decades. After meeting in 1974 we decided to collaborate our ideas.

Brown had exposure to military systems concepts when receiving electronics training from systems engineers at Massachusetts Institute of Technology during the Korean War. This training was followed by courses at the University of Chicago in corporate management of vertically and horizontally integrated companies. Research for a paper on an employee strike in a hospital led him to realize that management components of hospitals are different from those of most businesses. After graduation from Chicago, he worked to develop corporate management skills and resources with the New Jersey Hospital Association.

This experience was followed by research for a doctoral dissertation on the impact of planning on a hospital system's power structure. This research centered on the Greenville (S.C.) Hospital system and showed that a corporate management approach to a hospital system could work. These studies showed that many systems were in operation although most leaders in the health care field continued to speak and write about the industry as though there were 7,000 or so autonomous hospitals.

Robert C. Toomey, general director of the Greenville system, however, pointed to the management revolution then beginning to take hold across the United States. At the time, there were about 350 identifiable hospital systems in operation. It was clear that the industry wasn't structured the way it was—and continues to be portrayed in popular and professional reports.

In the early 1970s, Northwestern University had a major study underway on the Samaritan Health Service, Phoenix, Arizona. Other systems were not being studied. This was pointed out to the research team, and the study was expanded to include comparisons with seven not-for-profit hospital systems.

Lewis' first exposure to the health care delivery system came in the early 1960s at the West Virginia University Medical Center. Eugene L. Staples, director of University Hospital, often referred to the need to treat vertical as opposed to horizontal patients, and argued for integrated care systems. The medical center experience showed the interrelationships then existing between basic and clinical research in the fields of medicine, dentistry, pharmacy and nursing. This association also provided something of a survey course in health sciences. And there was an opportunity to see the tremendous impact of technology on the ability to provide new services and save lives.

Columbia University and *Business Week* offered opportunities to build on this experience in other ways. Classroom work stressed other systems —systems of the body, astrophysical systems, and the interrelationships between atoms, molecules and the chemical elements. Practical research and writing experience showed the interrelationships then existing between research and development institutions of all types—industrial, governmental, university and private. All of these institutions were having an impact on the development of care systems at a time when health care costs were beginning to increase at an extraordinary rate.

Further exposure to hospital systems for Lewis began in the late 1960s under Robert M. Cunningham Jr., editor of *Modern Hospital*. Over a period of six years, Lewis wrote on many facets of hospital management and operations, including the development of shared services and consortia and the impact of technology and government on the health care delivery system. It was a time when some critic coined the work "non-system." The fact is, as Cunningham has pointed out, there are many systems and partial systems in the United States. The headline on his column in the August 1972 *Modern Hospital* noted: "Everyone has a system—except those who need one."*

In 1970 *Modern Hospital* devoted a single issue to the Kaiser Health Plan.** That report by Greer Williams created much interest in the United States and won praise. And the chance to write on similar systems came along in due course.

Since 1974, our continuing dialog with the administrators and managers of hospital systems suggests several facts not well-known within the health care field. Many systems already exist; new systems are developing all the time. Systems with loose central management structures are beginning to pull their operations together into tightly-managed organizations.

---

* "Everyone has a System-Except Those Who Need One," *Modern Hospital* (August 1972), p. 7.

** G. Williams, "Kaiser: What is It? How Does It Work? Why Does It Work?" *Modern Hospital* (February 1971), p. 67.

The rush to develop hospital systems appears to be widespread, though not a generally understood phenomena. This trend stands for a pluralistic response to demands for integration that are stressed in Congressman Al Ullman's bill to set up Health Care Corporations, and in the priorities of Public Law 93-641, the National Health Planning and Resources Development Act of 1974. The response appears to be a genuine attempt by health care managers to capture economies of scale and political power to use in beneficial ways for patients.

In an industry where weak management is often cited as leading to uneconomic behavior and poor quality of health care, the development of hospital systems appears to be an important trend.

The primary purposes of this book are: to bring this trend to the attention of others, give the arguments for systems, explain the factors associated with systems development and predict some changes that appear to be inevitable.

Systems are not new—they date to 1929. There is no magic in systems —only managers, physicians, trustees and consumers can bring them about and make them work. But systems are here to stay. And it appears that the health care industry is rapidly evolving into a provider field that one day will be dominated by hospital systems.

Montague Brown

Howard L. Lewis

Evanston, Illinois
August 1976

Chapter 1
Forces for Change

Between fiscal years 1970 and 1975, the United States federal budget grew from $196.6 billion to $358.9 billion. In each of the fiscal years, about one-third of the money went to finance activities and programs of the Department of Health, Education and Welfare. Before he resigned as Secretary of HEW in July 1975 Caspar W. Weinberger told the Commonwealth Club of San Francisco: "If social programs continue growing for the next two decades at the same pace they have in the last two, we will spend more than half of our whole Gross National Product for domestic social programs alone by the year 2000. Should that day ever come, half of the American people will be working to support the other half."[1]

Weinberger added that "federal spending has shifted away from traditional federal functions such as defense and toward programs that reduce the remaining freedom of individuals and lessen the power of other levels of government. This shift in federal spending has transformed the task of aiding life's victims from a private concern to a public obligation. There are benefits and burdens in this . . . ". He went on, saying that the United States has "built an edifice of law and regulation that is clumsy, inefficient, and inequitable. Worst of all, the unplanned, uncoordinated, spasmodic nature of our response to these needs—some very real, some only perceived—is quite literally threatening to bring us to national insolvency."[2]

Weinberger, an attorney, first came to the attention of hospitals in his budget-slashing activities as head of the Office of Management and Budget. He was always a tough critic of hospitals and often touched sensitive nerves by complaining about the cost of care and overbedding.

But in this last major speech he was not overstating the central problem facing the federal government and hospitals alike. How can budgets be balanced? How can costs be contained? How can the rate of inflation be mediated? How can natural and human resources be used more effectively? How can productivity be increased? How can institutions survive so that they can meet human needs?

Private problems have become public problems. Federal programs now pay for about 40 percent of all hospital care in the United States. The government's presence is pervasive—through plans, programs, laws and regulations. The ability to allocate and spend more money means that power and control are becoming vested more in the federal government. The balance of power has tipped in favor of the legislative branch, Congress, and the executive branch, the Administration and its vast network of departments, agencies and regulatory authorities. Big government is getting bigger, more powerful every day. The federal government now has about 2,896,952 employees, including 147,125 in HEW.

Congress and the administration have identified in the area of medical and health care what they see as major issues facing the nation in the 1970s. The central problem is the rising cost of health care at a time when the federal budget is rising out of sight. Other issues include roadblocks to accessibility, inner city and rural health care needs, the increasing dependence on high-cost technology, increasing numbers of medical specialists when most patients need generalists, maldistribution of paraprofessional and professional manpower, and a lack of coordination between providers, leading to overcapacity in some areas of the United States and duplication in others.

Two hundred years after the United States declared its independence, there are 7,174 hospitals of all types with 1,513,000 beds. About one-third of these beds, 401,012, can be placed in the psychiatric-mental category. In round numbers, today's hospitals have 35.5 million admissions a year, an average daily census of 1.16 million patients, and 250 million outpatient visits a year. There are more than 3 million births a year in hospitals. Hospitals employ 2.9 million persons. The employee to patient ratio is 2.5:1. Total expenses of all hospitals are $41.4 billion a year—almost 3 percent of the Gross National Product. Average cost of a day of care in all hospitals is $97.23. The total assets of hospitals are $51.7 billion.[3]

Hospitals today are the focal point of the health care delivery system and the medical health services industry. They are an important force, and some believe, a big drag on the economy. This industry had a total income of more than $41 billion in 1973. The U.S. health care delivery system is part of a huge political arena. Congress, federal and state governments are demanding do more with less. Patients are saying they want more services at lower cost with quality and compassionate care. Physicians are calling for better facilities and higher levels of technology.

The conditions that federal and state officials say they want to improve are comparable to a disease. Policymakers see the problems as population shifts and a lack of accessible care; lags in the development of manpower and a poor distribution of physicians; unwise use of expensive technological devices and machines; the lack of comprehensive, quality care; the need for more services and less duplication. The underlying problem, the real cause of the disease, however, is the organization of the system; its principal poison is rising cost. In fiscal year 1974-75, the United States spent an estimated 8.3 percent of its Gross National Product on medical and health care—about $116 billion. The rising cost of acute, inpatient care has been recognized by policymakers as the obvious culprit. The general governmental criticism is that hospitals are both expensive and inefficient, based in large part on the views of the consumers of hospital services.

An urban area that is completely stable is a rare thing. In the last twenty-five years, signals coming from the environment are sharp and clear. Patients, doctors and tax dollars continue to move out of inner cities to the suburbs. A 1975 demographic source points out that the central cities of metropolitan areas have lost population since 1970. This loss is accounted for primarily by declines in the white population. The population of black and other minority groups has decreased in nonmetropolitan areas and increased in metropolitan areas since 1970. The increase among black and other minorities in central cities is 1.9 percent per year since 1970, a lower annual increase than in the 1960s, however ... only 26 percent of the metropolitan population of black and other minorities lived outside the central cities in 1974, compared with 62 percent of their white counterparts.[4]

Those who have moved to urban fringe and suburban areas want to be near shopping centers and divided highways. The interstate highway system, in particular, has a great impact on the nation's hospitals. Business and industry have followed the highways—and so have patients and hospitals.

Inner city areas are occupied primarily by blacks, other ethnic minorities and poor whites; many of these people are old and impoverished. Many city hospitals have watched this migration and seen their neighborhoods change drastically as paying patients flee and doctors follow. Urban hospitals are left with mostly Medicare and Medicaid case loads—the sickest patients who need the most expensive, long-stay care. They concentrate in neighborhoods and areas once occupied by wealthy and middle-class groups who supported and maintained many of the older urban hospitals. Often this influx is due to migration, as in New York City and Miami, where Spanish-speaking populations have settled in increasing numbers. This population shift is often one of abandonment; the older poor can't afford to move to the suburbs after their children have left home.

As a result, inner-city hospitals face many pressures—to move, to build satellites and to change their service roles more in keeping with changing demography. As cities wither, suburbs prosper. Along with this prosperity, suburban hospitals grow. Their services become more complex; they no longer have any real need to refer patients into cities for specialized work.

At the same time with population shifts in recent years, average gross revenue per patient day in community hospitals has risen from $68.82 in 1969 to $118.54 in 1974.[5] Most of this increased cost is due to inflation, labor costs and new technology. Real consumer buying power has decreased though incomes are up. Average length of stay has gone down nationally. Over this ten years, the cost of all other goods and services has increased greatly for homes, cars, furniture, food, and clothes. But unlike a new sedan or new sport coat, a day of care in a 1975 hospital is not something anyone might choose to buy, if he had an option.

The fact is that consumers of medical and health care want more, not less treatment. Their expectations are rising with their standard of living; they believe more is better; they are not yet tuned into self-help, healthy modes of living that could save them expensive hospital bills. Consumers have little understanding of staffing levels, labor contracts, malpractice costs, new technology, cost of money, government regulations and third-party relationships.

New strains on the free-standing institution come from high cost, economy of scale considerations, capital equipment obsolescence, cost containment directives and changes in reimbursement programs. High volume laboratory equipment, such as automated analyzers, highly specialized diagnostic and therapeutic equipment, computer systems and other technological innovations often need large scale operations to make them economically possible. Quality considerations also enter the equation. Specialized surgical teams can fail to gain sufficient experience or lose their effectiveness if they do not have the volume of cases necessary to keep their skills at a professional level.

Too many hospitals have financial borrowing and payback problems, especially when two older, relatively obsolete facilities are on different sides of the same street. Private donors and government agencies are asking a tough question with increasing frequency in recent years: Should these hospitals undertake major changes that would lead to overbuilding and duplication? Lending agencies are looking for larger volume operations and want greater assurances of full use of the hospital and an adequate cash flow to pay back a loan or a mortgage.

Population shifts, demographic trends, and cost trends—these are powerful stimuli coming from the environment. But hospitals do respond. The managers who make them run are sensitive organisms; they feel the stimuli. They shape and form their institutions and give them a human substance. Most managers are led by a desire for growth, control of operations, survival and power. Other managers are moved by religious and missionary beliefs; still others by profit.

Hospitals are not only service institutions, but also highly competitive organizations that want to stay in business; they desire many of the changes sought by government and have found many ways to cooperate and share. They are developing strategies to deal with stimuli coming from the environment.

GOVERNMENT INFLUENCES

The Congress has moved in a consistent pattern in the last ten years or so to solve these problems. More people are covered under federal and federal-state health care programs, and special programs for illnesses like chronic kidney disease. For many reasons, however, an estimated 30 million Americans are still without coverage.

As Congress has moved to expand coverage, it has also assumed a measurement orientation aimed at improving use of facilities and the quality of care. Utilization review has always been required under Medicare. Congress mandated nationwide peer review to begin by July 1, 1976 through the Professional Standards Review Organization program in an attempt to ensure *quality of care* while holding costs down.

Many hospitals are still trying to recover from the impact of the Economic Stabilization Program (ESP) when charges were frozen at predetermined levels, but costs were not. The four phases and one freeze of the ESP remain as a vivid reminder of the power in the hands of the federal executive and legislative branches. Congress and the administration have begun to slow down in their rush toward national health insurance. But they have stepped up efforts to regulate the cost and quality of health care.

At the state level, power is evident also. Massachussetts, New York, Connecticut and Maryland now have mandatory rate-setting laws in effect. Other states have voluntary rate-setting programs, and the pros and cons of rate-setting are being debated across the nation.

Over the years, Congress has moved in other ways to meet the social need for medical and health care services. One of its most consistent orientations has been to create coordinated, regional systems of care.

Congress enacted the Hospital Survey and Construction Act in 1954, creating the Hill-Burton Program. This act is a sweeping policy statement. It says that Congress would meet a need and help improve access to medical care by helping finance construction of thousands of new and modernized hospital beds. The intent of the act is to create overall state health care plans by placing the final authority where beds are to be built in the hands of a state health agency. Many small hospitals unfortunately were built without a clearly established need and without much thought given to relationship of the parts to the whole. There is also a caveat in the original act that became an issue in 1970. Each Hill-Burton hospital is to provide a reasonable volume of free or below cost care to those who cannot pay. This legal question is an issue as a result of legal actions in another part of the power bloc—the consumers of care working through public interest attorneys.

The mid-1960s brought Medicare and Medicaid. These programs pumped new dollars into an old system and increased problems of organization. The middle 1960s were also a time for the Congress to try and push the health care delivery system into regional orientations through two other new laws: The so-called heart disease, cancer, and stroke amendments to the Public Health Act, better known as Regional Medical Programs (RMP), an attempt to bring the benefits of research and technology to the people; and the Comprehensive Health Planning Act (CHP), a law designed to sift out the need for facilities and sevices and prevent overbuilding and duplication.

The architects and workmen who made up the RMPs appeared to be frustrated at every turn. RMP floundered and was never carried out fully. CHP program authorized state and regional ("A" and "B") planning agencies, but it suffered a similar fate. The specifics of these two laws are vague, but the intent is clear: regionalization, cooperation, and integration of facilities and resources into systems to serve defined areas of population.

Hill-Burton, RMP, and CHP, are giving way now to Public Law 93-641, the National Health Planning and Resources Development Act of 1974. This act urges all providers of care to work together as a system. Congress specified ten national health priorities and said that they were proper "to be used in the formulation of national health planning goals and in the development and operation of Federal, State, and area health planning and resource development programs."[6] These ten priorities are:

(1) The provisions of primary care services for medically underserved populations, especially those which are located in rural or economically depressed areas.

(2) The development of multi-institutional systems for coordination or consolidation of institutional health services (including obstetric, pediatric, emergency medical, intensive and coronary care, and radiation therapy services).

(3) The development of medical group practices (especially those whose services are appropriately coordinated or integrated with institutional health services), health maintainance organizations, and other organized systems for the provision of health care.

(4) The training and increased utilization of physician extenders.

(5) The development of multi-institutional arrangements for the sharing of support services necessary to all health service institutions.

(6) The promotion of activities to achieve needed improvements in the quality of health services, including needs identified by the review activities of Professional Standards Review Organizations.

(7) The development of health service institutions of the capacity to provide various levels of care (including intensive care, acute general care, and extended care) on a geographically integrated basis.

(8) The promotion of activities for the prevention of disease, including study of nutritional and environmental factors affecting health and provision of preventive health care services.

(9) The adoption of uniform cost accounting, simplified reimbursement, and utilization reporting systems and improved management procedures for health service institutions.

(10) The development of effective methods of educating the general public concerning proper personal (including preventive) health care and methods for effective use of available health services.

Priorities 2, 3, 5, 7, and 9 clearly mandate and set up national policy that is again pushing health care delivery system into systems configurations. The Health Systems Agency is the key arm of government created by the act. Two hundred and two of these agencies are to be named through federal regulations in 1976.

A few months after P.L. 93-641 was signed by President Ford, the director of HEW's Bureau of Health Planning and Resources Development, the agency responsible for carrying out the law, said: "We are now very definitely intervening in the private practice of medicine and in the organization and operation of health care institutions . . . and the primary reason is dollars. As inflation has eaten up all of the benefits of Medicare, there's been an overwhelming need to say that government can no longer play the passive role of simply paying the bills."[8]

Herman M. Somers, professor of politics and public affairs at Princeton University, said critics of Congress and government "tend to overlook or understate the extraordinary volume and variety of past and present governmental efforts. . . ." People complain about a lack of national health policy, he said; but "they are really saying that they are displeased with the policies, or, more frequently, they complain that the various policies lack coherence, that they are frequently contradictory, often fragmentary, tentative and halting." The same is true in every area of public concern, whether it be foreign, economic, labor, or welfare policy.

"In a country of continental dimensions," Somers said, "large issues cut across a multitude of diverse and conflicting interests, and the stakes are often high. We are sometimes told government is not responsive. Yet the problems people point at usually are direct consequences of the fact that governmental machinery, both legislative and administrative, dances to many tunes because it *is* responsive. It is, as it must be, responsive to diverse constituencies pursuing different goals. It marches to discordant beats of varied drummers, each of whom has a large enough drum to be heard and respected—each of whom has some power base among the multitude of power centers in our society, rarely powerful enough to get its own way but influential enough to be able to stop the opposition from getting theirs."[9]

CONSUMERS AND PRIVATE INSURORS

A second community of interest, allied with federal and state government, is represented by consumers and the organizations they support through fees and premiums paid to Blue Cross, Blue Shield, and insurance companies.

The consumer arm of this power bloc is hard to define, but the usual reference is to local, state and national organizations that in one way or another want to bring about change in the medical care system. The organizations vary from the so-called medical left, and their slogan that *Health Care is a Right,* to the Grey Panthers and the National Association of Patients on Hemodialysis. Their complaints generally, can be summarized as a desire for more humanistic, compassionate and economical medical care. Other consumers are concerned more with the outcome of their individual treatment. When the outcome is bad, they are beginning to sue more often and ask for more compensation.

Some consumer demands have been put in the health care system. The federal government has stated as official policy that health care is a right. Chronic kidney disease is now covered by Medicare. Many hospitals have adopted a patient's bill of rights. Courts are routinely awarding large malpractice settlements—$100,000 is not unusual, and the $1 million or more award is no longer rare.

Blue Cross, Blue Shield, and the other health insurors are working closer with management and unions in industries where consumers work because of the cost of care. The 74 Blue Cross plans, for example, must have now a majority of consumers on their boards of advisors in the service area. Consumer advisory boards are also found in large businesses or industry plans. Not long ago the director of employee benefits for General Motors Corporation was asked to name his largest annual expense associated with the manufacturing of cars and trucks. "The Blue Cross and Blue Shield plans are by far our largest single supplier,"[10] he said—not steel, tires, or parts but health care coverage for union employees.

Blue Cross Association (BCA) and the National Association of Blue Shield Plans are making attempts to sell the public (and the federal and state governments) on their accountability, community orientation and cost consciousness through national advertising campaigns. Medicare and Medicaid, and Blue Cross need to convince consumers and the first power bloc (government) that they are doing a good job as the primary fiscal intermediaries. The community orientation of the BCA does appear clear.

BCA President Walter J. McNerney certainly thinks that way. In an interview, McNerney said he saw:

> the need for more aggressive institutional management in hospitals. The problem, as I see it, is that the whole field is getting more complex. It is demanding of the administrator a large amount of outside activity as well as inside activity—relating the hospital to the community it serves . . . creating liaisons with increasing numbers of groups.
>
> The community no longer wants to have its hand held. It wants to be an effective participant. Technology is growing so fast that there is a greater diversity of services available. The gap between the user and the provider tends to widen under those circumstances. The administrator's job, of course, is to close to gap.[13]

Health is no longer being defined in restricted terms, McNerney feels, for it includes environmental, industrial, and personal components. The old administrator who was concerned only with having enough doctors and beds "now finds himself in a demand economy where productivity is essential. The whole question of what pays off is of over-riding importance."

Cost containment and the judicious use of community resources rest squarely with hospital managers and boards of trustees, because "it is a set of convictions and policies and a management context that make the difference. I am talking about the guts and balls the board of trustees has to address the payoff on investment, vis-a-vis alternative ways of doing the job and making the decision stick. . . . against a provider field that is dominated very heavily on the professional side."

Asked whether there were any signs that top health care managers were beginning to address these issues, McNerney said, "Few are sophisticated enough to admit that the hospital is a hazardous place and may be counterproductive to health in addition to being uneconomical. But a few administrators are beginning to worry about some of these things."

When McNerney refers to community, he is "talking about a responsible board, a group of gutty men and women who are well-oriented by a strong administrator and who are facing up to a series of options with the pros and cons and payoffs in front of them so they can make gut decisions. Now, this is difficult ... difficult. And I am not pretending it isn't ... either to find boards like that ... to create boards ... or to find administrative manpower of that force." But the time and money involved are worth it, for "without a strong user community orientation in institutions, all of the economies of scale could go right down the drain."

PHYSICIANS AND HOSPITALS ORGANIZE

A third community of interest is trying to balance its need, philosophy, professional orientation and desire to survive against the first two coalitions. This third group is made up of physicians and hospitals. They are coming together in some new ways: many doctors are now on hospital governing boards, as they should be; and the trend toward salaried practice is stepping up, creating what one administrator calls "the common meeting ground between hospital management and medical practitioners."[12]

The American Hospital Association's (AHA) *Policy Statement on Provision of Health Services* is the first comprehensive document from a professional trade association calling for the evolution and reorganization of health services into systems configurations. This idea has been put in the proposed National Health Care Services Reorganization and Financing Act—HR 1, a bill introduced in the 94th Congress by Rep. Al Ullman of Oregon.

A systems orientation is inherent in the AHA-Ullman proposal to set up a series of Health Care Corporations (HCC) around the nation. AHA defines "Health Care Corporation" as an organization that "would synthesize management, physicians, personnel, and facilities into a corporate structure with the capacity and responsibility to deliver comprehensive health care in the community, either directly through its own facilities and services or by contract with other health care providers."[13]

The association proposed that a sufficient number of HCCs be set up to give care for everyone in the United States: "Each HCC would be a new corporate organization. It could be established in a variety of ways, depending on community need, resources, and precedent. Its sponsorship could be local, or it might be broadly based."[14]

In his floor speech introducing HR 1, Rep. Ullman, the pragmatic chairman of the powerful House Committee on Ways and Means, called the HCC "an exciting new concept of responsible localism ... The health care corporation which would be the coordinating unit of the system at the local level would provide a geographically based system for synthesizing and coordinating local health resources. These corporations would be built upon the existing delivery system, but with mandatory reorganization and reorientation to meet local needs, under the supervision of newly mandated State health commissions."[15] The architects of Public Law 93-641 adopted many similar ideas.

There are many forces pulling and tugging at the health care delivery system, a term that "refers chiefly to the methods of organizing and financing all the resources that are involved in the processes of providing personal health services for the people who require them."[16]

The various communities of interest are demanding economy and improvements in accountability, accessibility and quality of care. In the process, the various forces want power also. These are the central issues facing the system.

Some people believe that there is too much power in Washington, D.C. and the state capitols. Money is power and as long as governments control one of the major blocs of money available to pay doctors and hospitals, they will continue to have power. The central government issue is the cost of care; and the central issue facing hospitals is survival.

NOTES

1. C. W. Weinberger, "A View of the Federal Government" (An address before the Commonwealth Club of San Francisco, July 21, 1975).

2. Ibid.

3. *Hospital Statistics,* 1975 edition, published by the American Hospital Association, Chicago.

4. *The World Almanac and Book of Facts,* 1976 ed., p. 201.

5. *Hospital Statistics,* op. cit.

6. U.S. Congress, Senate, Committee on Labor and Public Welfare, *Report No. 93-1285,* 93rd Cong., 2d sess., 1974, p. 77.

7. Ibid.

8. See Gregg W. Downey, "Healthcare Planning Gets Muscles," *Modern Healthcare* (March 1975), p. 32.

9. H. M. Somers, "Health and Public Policy" (the Robert D. Eilers Memorial Lecture, Leonard Davis Institute of Health Economics, University of Pennsylvania, February 26, 1975).

10. This statement is frequently made by health experts at national and local meetings.

11. Interview with Walter McNerney, Chicago, Illinois, August 2, 1975. All subsequent quotations were taken from this interview unless otherwise noted.

12. "Experts See New Balance of Health Care Forces," *Modern Hospital,* (April 1970), pp. 39, 40, 40a-40d.

13. "Policy Statement on Provision of Health Services," *American Hospital Association* (August 24, 1971), p. 4.

14. Ibid.

15. Al Ullman, "The National Health Care Services Reorganization and Financing Act—H.R. 1," *Congressional Record,* 94th Cong., 1st sess., 1975.

16. "Everyone Has A System—Except Those Who Need One," *Modern Hospital* (August 1972), p. 7.

Chapter 2
Strategies for Change

Federal and state governments want hospitals to hold down costs and in the end improve the quality and availability of services to more people. Consumers and the Blue Cross plans have similar goals. Trustees, administrators, and physicians are looking for ways to gain economies of scale, finance new and improved services, and accumulate enough power that will allow them to survive and go on with their mission of serving the sick. Each community of interest has developed its own strategy.

There is one major strategy that meets the needs of all the competing forces: the development of integrated hospital systems of care.

Hospital systems can range from informal discussions aimed at coordinating efforts of two or more institutions—to formal relationships taking in ownership, operations and control of all levels of health services in an area. The services can be classified as preventive, primary, secondary, tertiary, restorative and custodial.

Hospital systems can be integrated horizontally across geographical areas or integrated vertically within a geographical area or a combination of the two.

The thesis of this book is that hospital systems can achieve economies and qualities of scale and at the same time improve quality of care, comprehensiveness and continuity between levels of care.

There are many hospital systems in the making that are adopting this strategy to meet public demands and at the same time, reaching their own goals consistent with resources available to them.

Any institution, forced to change rapidly, like a hospital, must find a balancing point between its resources and interests and the environmental demands. A hospital either finds that balance or it doesn't survive.

Many doctor-owned hospitals have gone out of business, mainly in small towns, because their owners did not want to cope with government regulation and changing population demands.

Many Catholic-sponsored hospitals have either closed their doors, merged with other institutions, transferred ownership to a community group or sold to a profit-making organization. Congregations have made these decisions because they could no longer carry the financial burden of running a hospital, particularly with a shortage of nuns to provide management and religious guidance.

Nonprofit community hospitals in decaying cities are struggling along too, watching their neighborhoods change and their indigent patient loads skyrocket as they try to operate under what they consider to be inequitable reimbursement systems. Religious-sponsored community hospitals are experiencing these same difficulties.

Once relatively healthy suburban and rural hospitals are in trouble too because they are being forced to compete with newer proprietary and not-for-profit hospitals built in their service areas. The final blow in a struggle to survive often comes as the result of a new road or interstate highway that changes flow of traffic, making one hospital easier to get to than another.

Every hospital needs a strategy to survive. The trends of recent years can be a way to sift out the health care delivery system, forcing weak institutions out of business but making sure stronger institutions survive. Who will survive could become the province of the Health Systems Agencies created by Public Law 93-641.[1]

EVOLVING A STRATEGY

How does a strategy evolve? An institution must look closely at its environment, changing health needs of the population, available community resources, its strengths and aspirations, the medical practitioners involved and demands being made by consumers, agencies and organizations that buy care.

On the basis of this evaluation, the hospital organization has to come up with long-range goals. The linking of goals and objectives to policies and programs forms strategy—the method a manager uses to translate his objectives and plans into realities.

An important part of strategy is the management organization that must either be developed or modified for a hospital to reach its long-term goals. The organization must have people with the skills and experience to make sure that good decisions are made. The organization must also have enough internal and external power to influence decision making by physicians, regulatory and planning agencies, reimbursement agencies and community leaders.

University medical centers, for example, usually say their goals are teaching, research and service. They set apart university teaching hospitals from most other hospitals in two ways: (1) their involvement in under-graduate education of medical students, and (2) their basic and clinical research programs. University hospitals must cope with expensive federal and state demands for research and teaching while their competitors, neighboring community hospitals, concentrate on less-expensive primary and secondary care.

Medical school hospitals, to survive as centers of excellence, must have grassroot support in a region or state with long-term financial support and a sufficient supply of patient referrals to fill their teaching beds. Environmental demands, particularly the demand to do something about the doctor-gap, are forcing university medical centers into new strategies that are known as community service, community medicine, extramural programs and Area Health Education Centers.

Community hospitals have adopted some of the same strategies to meet the needs of patients in their service areas. At the same time, they have established new ventures—ambulatory services and satellite hospitals, for example—to control utilization and costs, to keep access to their doctors and to keep up with urban sprawl and shifts in population.

Rural hospitals have developed similar strategies to survive; some close beds and scale down service programs in outpatient clinics. Others form joint ventures with nursing homes and long-term care facilities by converting beds. Still others are seeking outside help through shared service arrangements, contract management agreements and affiliations with chains and systems of hospitals or urban-based medical centers.

Most hospitals, however, still run in an autonomous way. When these hospitals control a large number of beds and are fiscally strong, they probably don't need to adopt a new strategy. But many autonomous hospitals are having a hard time keeping up and coping with demands of their environment.

The years ahead will be marked by a managerial and operational revolution leading to rapid development of systems of hospitals under single management organizations, unless the current economic, regulatory, and political environment changes radically.

Under this new strategy, vigorous, existing hospitals will probably expand their sphere of influence by bringing into their system (or creating new systems) those hospitals that fit some combination of this profile: (1) chronic low occupancy, (2) deficit operations, (3) rural or inner-city location, (4) changing patient clientele with increasing medical needs but a reduced ability to pay for services, (5) geographical area having trouble attracting skilled and trained administrators and physicians, (6) new suburbs and new towns without a well-developed community group to pursue health care needs aggressively and furnish the start-up capital, (7) hospitals of small bed size and (8) hospitals with older, deteriorating physical plants.²

This profile applies to hospitals considering merger and also to a set of circumstances before a board of trustees discussing pros and cons of contract management. Many of these same characteristics are leading boards and administrators to the decision to build a satellite facility to make sure the financial survival of a base hospital.

The fact that a hospital needs help doesn't mean that someone will rush in and save the day. Existing multiple-unit systems will want to know: What is the potential for turning the operation around? What is the potential for modifying the mission (and strategy) of the institution so that a break-even point or a profit can be reached in a reasonable amount of time? Organizations that are apt to answer the needs of faltering, struggling hospitals are those that have the necessary management talent for growth and the support of their trustees and medical staff. They also will have ways to get money and know the rate of return they need on invested capital. The system will also want to be sure that the local institution will yield sufficient autonomy to let the new management develop an effective operation to meet local needs.

This assessment may seem crass, blunt and oriented to the dollar and not to the humanitarian aims of hospitals; but the missionary zeal of a hospital is of no value if it cannot survive. There must be new ideas of the type that led Henry Ford to the assembly line concept. There must be leaders around like Alfred Sloan, who in the early 1920s, felt the competition from Ford's superior economies of scale and "conceived the idea of bringing together half a dozen independent companies each in a different price and marketing area—a single company which would share countless services while creating a new, strong, competitive organization which would serve the public well. From his idea, General Motors was born."³

These innovators "helped remove 'caveat emptor' from the regular vocabulary, [and] ... also did for industry and commerce ... what public reaction is demanding we do today in hospitals.... They faced unique business pressures.... We face similar pressures and in a sense some of our answers may come from the methods these men pioneered."⁴

MULTIPLE SYSTEMS CAN MEET
CONFLICTING DEMANDS

The pressures haven't changed too much in the last ten years though they appear more intense. The late Ray E. Brown, a giant in his own time who made prophetic statements with ease, said in 1965: "As with all enterprises in a free society, and especially those performing an essentially social function, the hospital has tried to listen to all sides, and sideliners, and to observe as many of the divergent demands as possible. It has turned and squirmed organizationally in an effort to accommodate to the diversity of calls confronting it. In a large way the hospital has succeeded more than any other enterprise or agency in contemporary society in satisfying conflicting demands made upon it."

Brown said that "multiple hospital units under single management represent a response to some of the conflicting demands confronting the modern hospital." For him administrators should be cautious in seeking simple solutions to complex problems. Multiple-unit systems are not a panacea, but should be considered to see where they fit into the balance of things. Multiple systems are attempting to meet contradictory demands, but he suggested how multiple-unit systems might help meet these criticisms:

1. To the community's demand for "optimum size and optimal use of expensive personnel equipment," Brown replied, "Multiple units permit a systemization of facilities on a graduated care basis that might permit a reduction in duplication of resources and underutilization of services."

2. To the problem of local pride and community identification conflicting with economies of scale, Brown said "the multiple-unit arrangement can provide a local entity with which the neighborhood can identify while at the same time providing a means of shared volume and central administrative expertise."

3. To the natural drive of administrators to want their hospitals to grow, which is often in conflict with the need for community balance, systems offer "some built-in, community-wide planning features."

4. Small-sized hospitals which can't always attract talented administrators would find that "the creation of large administrative units might permit greater challenges, status, and salaries and thus increase the attraction of hospital administration."

5. The ability to provide quality patient care is often diluted by fragmentation of available physician manpower into small, independent units. "The multiple-unit organizational arrangement could help serve to maintain a more comprehensive and cohesive medical staff organization. By bringing the medical work of the component units into a relationship with the total medical staff organization, it could provide a greater visibility of the work of the individual physicians practicing in the separate units. It might also serve to define the sorts of medical procedures to be undertaken in the individual hospital units."[5]

Brown, who made his comments as he introduced Duke University's First National Forum on Hospital and Health Affairs, found other speakers disagreed strongly with his views. They wanted autonomous community hospitals. They argued for concentrating future efforts to meet the needs of the present users of their services and not on further expansion and development of community hospitals into systems configurations.

But more than ten years later, U. S. health care providers are changing rapidly into systems configuration. This organizational response is primarily a result of the stimulus given by federal and state regulation. Hospitals can survive by adopting new strategies, particularly the multiple-unit management system.

This book proposes that hospital systems under single management offer certain advantages over autonomous hospitals. These primary advantages are (1) economy, (2) quality, (3) accessibility and (4) power. Hospital systems also offer specific advantages in terms of community accountability, responsiveness to consumers and comprehensive care programs.

While the degree of central management control varies by system, the U. S. health care scene of today is very different from the (often-supposed) single-unit hospital operating without regard to the rest of the world. There are a variety of approaches being taken to regionalize and integrate hospitals into systems. A variety of purposes and motivations generated this movement and it is gaining momentum. The systems that are discussed in the following chapters represent new strategies for meeting community needs. They represent spontaneous innovations; and they represent voluntary choices made in a pluralistic society.

NOTES

1. See Gregg W. Downey, "Healthcare Planning Gets Muscles," *Modern Healthcare* (March 1975), p. 32.

2. M. Brown, "Contract Management: Latest Developments in the Trend Toward Regionalization of Hospital and Health Services," *Hospital & Health Services Administration* (Winter 1976), pp. 52-53.

3. P. Groner, (An untitled address before the Tennessee Hospital Association), October 2, 1975, Memphis, Tennessee.

4. Ibid.

5. R. E. Brown, "Forces Influencing Development," *The First Duke University Forum on Health and Hospital Affairs* (May 1965), pp. 3-5.

Chapter 3
Cooperation and Sharing

The rapid evolution of autonomous hospitals into systems is occurring in an environment long characterized by cooperation and sharing and competition for physicians, patients and financial support.

Health care literature is filled with reports of shared services, contract services, mergers, affiliations and contract management. These terms suggest that two or more entities have come together to produce goods, services, and engage in planning, as well as new trends toward integration of health services under various organizational and structural forms.[1]

SHARED SERVICES

The W. K. Kellogg Foundation, for example, has exerted considerable influence among hospitals to promote shared services. Robert A. DeVries, Program Director of the foundation, defines shared services as "those clinical or administrative functions that are common to two or more institutions, that are used jointly or cooperatively by them in some way for the purpose of improving service and/or effecting economies of scale, and that hold all participating parties at risk in the sharing venture."[2]

One of the most extensive national surveys of shared services was made in 1971 by Adrienne A. Astolfi and Leo B. Matti. According to their report: "Of the 5,727 short-term community hospitals contacted, 82.5 percent completed the survey questionnaire and of these, 66.6 percent reported that they share from 1 to 73 services with an average of 6.2 services shared per hospital. The five services most frequently shared by reporting hospitals are blood bank, purchasing of medical and surgical supplies, data processing, disaster plans, and professional staff in laboratories. . . ." They found that most sharing was in purchasing—group buying of medical and surgical supplies, linens, drugs, housekeeping and laboratory supplies.

Considerable interest was also shown in increased use of group purchasing as a way to effect economies. Responding hospitals were interested in shared administrative services and joint programs in continuing education and inservice education. Astolfi and Matti concluded: "Clearly, both the extent of present involvement in sharing programs and the degree of interest (29,890 instances of interest in sharing reported) strongly suggest sharing's potential as a major method of delivery of health care services. Sharing indeed may serve as the foundation for the many recent concepts which have emerged regarding health care delivery through formal cooperative arrangements."[3]

CONTRACT SERVICES

Many hospitals have taken, however, a different approach to sharing and cost containment. They have opted for contract services—negotiation of arrangements with outside agencies to manage a specific function or service, such as data processing, electronic equipment, food service, laundry and linen, plant operations, and other services in the housekeeping and support category.

Kenneth T. Wessner, president of Servicemaster Hospital Corporation, said that benefits from contract services are:

> Greater control in the areas of personnel and finance; Experience that grows out of research, study, and firsthand acquaintance with a wide spectrum of proven methods and techniques; Flexibility to meet changing demands as hospitals grow in size and complexity; Continuity of day-to-day management; A supportive team to handle the details of work scheduling so as to eliminate critical disruptions due to illness, vacations, and emergency situations; Versatility to handle routine departmental needs and to meet emergencies as they arise; Resources to support the administrator in the areas of cost control, technology, personnel, and materials management; A philosophy of service on the part of the department head and his staff that should help to eliminate such comments as 'that's not my job,' 'we're short of help,' and 'if we had better people.'[4]

A study of the extent of contract services on the departmental level in 259 hospitals in five geographically diverse areas was made by Bernard L. Brown, Jr. He charted trends in contracting for 15 different services, including 9 clinical services, and found smaller hospitals (1 to 99 beds) contracted for the most services, followed by hospitals in the 100-199 and 200-299 bed categories. More than 40 percent of the smallest hospitals had outside contracts for pathology, radiology and laundry services.[5]

Computers and the electronic data processing equipment represent one of the newest areas of contract service. Some hospitals have gone to facility management agreements; many others, particularly small facilities which usually don't own any equipment, have turned to computer service centers for help. These hospitals buy the software system, send information—generally business office, financial, budgeting, and payroll information—to the service center for processing, where it is returned by courier as printouts, or received directly via Dataphone (telephone) hookup.

MERGER

Another current trend is merger—when two or more institutions join together as a single entity. One source charted this phenomena and found twelve mergers between United States hospitals from 1947 through 1961.[6] American Hospital Association data show another 135 mergers occurring in the nine-year period of 1962 through 1970.[7]

Most sources warn that these data are very likely incomplete, usually adding that many more mergers have probably taken place. It is believed, however, that many mergers have been concentrated in New York, New Jersey, and Pennsylvania. And there have been extensive studies of merger activity in Pennsylvania and New England.

James R. Neely, president of the Hospital Association of Pennsylvania (HAP) calls merger "the ultimate act of sharing costs and services." In October 1971, the HAP Board of Trustees approved a nine-point program for the association and included a statement to encourage hospitals to develop systems. The HAP goal was to "develop a program to create systems (health care corporations, health maintenance organizations, mergers, consortiums) of health care institutions throughout the state." The HAP said it would "provide encouragement, consultation, and assistance to institutions to achieve institutional consolidation," and would "encourage legal and economic sanctions to stimulate the development of systems."[8]

As part of this effort, John R. Clark, a project officer with HAP, was commissioned to study interinstitutional cooperation in the state. He found, by reviewing the available literature and interviewing administrators, planning agency officials and health planners, that there were 18 mergers (and one "demerger") among Pennsylvania hospitals from 1946 to 1969.

The usual reasons given to justify a merger, he said, include desires to improve educational programs, eliminate duplication, broaden the range of available services, increase community support, and improve planning; but the real reasons for the merger, according to him are operational and political.   Hospitals lack money for modernization and replacement of facilities; they can't purchase the equipment they need, and they need money to operate their facilities. From 1920 to 1940, a number of specialty hospitals merged with general hospitals "because changing medical technology was creating the need for common equipment. However, economic forces are *primarily* responsible for the more recent merger trend which is occurring in an environment of increasing cost controls, higher standards for facilities and services, pressures to improve the utilization of personnel and services, and public concern for higher quality and more accessible services."[9]

The organizational aspects of mergers between hospitals in the New England states from 1960 to 1970 were extensively studied by Sally E. Knapp and Robert R. Lovejoy. Although unable to determine precisely the number of mergers in the area during the decade, they did provide valuable information on ten selected mergers and eight case studies in which hospitals decided to merge or not to merge. They concluded that "there appears to be an increasing likelihood that in the future external demands from state and regional authorities, coupled with national redirection of health policy, may furnish the most compelling rationale for hospital mergers."[10]

AFFILIATIONS

Affiliations represent another trend toward systems development. Richard Wittrup defined this trend "as an arrangement under which two or more institutions are engaged in a single program, with each responsible for separate parts. . . . The most common examples are found in education where students rotate from one institution to another, receiving some element of instruction in each. Other examples include formal arrangements between hospitals and nursing homes, between hospitals and neighborhood health centers, and between hospitals which refer patients to each other."[11]

Certainly the affiliation phenomena is widespread. There are 447 teaching hospitals in the United States[12], most of which are affiliated with one or more of the 114 medical schools. And of the 175 VA hospitals in the United States, about 95 percent of these are affiliated with a medical school. Wittrup believes these relationships tend to be more political than financial and that an element of dependency builds up between affiliated institutions. It is not difficult to see why: Medical schools need patient referrals and teaching patients; affiliated hospitals need house staff. "The dependency factor also causes affiliations to bind hospitals together more closely than do shared services," he says, "because a hospital using a shared laundry usually can get its linens washed elsewhere, but a teaching hospital usually has difficulty arranging another medical school affiliation. While each party to an affiliation retains its corporate autonomy, it can exercise its independence only at the expense of sacrificing program." And he adds: "Hospitals commonly attach great importance to educational programs, particularly in medicine. For that reason, a medical school and its affiliated hospitals often are bound together, and that relationship can serve as the basis for a variety of other cooperative endeavors."[13]

CONTRACT MANAGEMENT

Still another trend toward systems development can be seen in the contract management of a hospital by an outside corporation. This rapidly growing phenomenon has important implications for systems development. In one report, over 150 management contracts in hospitals of 40 beds to more than 200 beds had been studied. The organizations furnishing the management expertise included investor-owned chains, not-for-profit multiple-unit hospital systems, and a shared services organization.[14]

Under contract management, either the owners or a board of trustees contract with an outside organization that assumes responsibility for the general, day-to-day management of the institution. The managed hospital retains total legal responsibility and ownership of the facility, its assets and liabilities.

The individual brought in as administrator reports directly to the board of trustees, which must approve the appointment. The administrator serves as the chief executive officer. He prepares agendas for the board, usually in consultation with his contractor organization. The administrator and members of the contracting organization attend board meetings and participate fully. The administrator carries out policy, implements the budget, and works with medical staffs and community groups.

A top notch administrator is the key to a management contract. This individual must know hospital operations and have an extensive knowledge of reimbursement formulas, cash flow, and manpower cost control systems. But the administrator does not work in a vacuum. His contractor organization also brings specialized backup services to the contracting facility in key areas of management. A recent study shows that some managing companies can offer advisory services in 35 areas of need—ranging from patient admitting practices and labor relations to systems analysis and physician recruitment. Where the contractor organization is a medical school teaching center, the available backup medical, professional and management services may number over 100.[15]

Precontract feasibility studies indicate the services most needed by the managed hospital. Attempts are made to avoid overwhelming a hospital with all services simultaneously. Not all contracting organizations offer all services. Some but not all services would be provided without extra compensation above a basic agreement.

Contracts generally run for three years or longer. They provide that the hospital pay the contracting organization five to seven percent of either gross charges or gross revenues. Some not-for-profit contract management organizations charge only for direct costs incurred. The hospital may also pay the salary of the administrator. In a typical situation, say a 100-bed hospital, the gross revenue might be $2.7 million. The contracting company would receive $189,000 and a typical administrator's salary of $30,000 a year. All such expenses are legitimate expenses of the hospital and thus eligible for reimbursement by insurance agencies and government purchasers of care. In some cases, the hospital must also pay other administrative expenses and costs.

Investor-owned chains of hospitals, community hospitals, and church-owned facilities see many of the same advantages in selling management contracts. They increase revenue with little capital investment, spread overhead costs, gain new specialized personnel, serve new communities, cement important relationships with neighboring hospitals and possibly avoid the entry of new compettion into their service areas.

Preliminary research shows that there are at least a dozen environmental forces that push a hospital toward contract management. Hospitals of small bed size, chronic low occupancy rate problems, deficit operations and old physical plants are prime candidates. In other instances, a hospital's clientele has increasing needs for medical care but a diminishing ability to pay for services. Some of the forces relate to geography: Inner city and rural areas, for example, can't always attract skilled and trained administrators and physicians. Still other forces relate to philosophy: Some trustees want their hospital run "like their own business." Other trustees no longer want to cope with increasing complexity without assured technical backup in every area of management. Finally, physicians as well as trustees seem more confident of an administrator who has a team of specialists to consult.[16]

Contract management seems easier than other options such as merger. It can be negotiated quickly with the only potential for immediate change in personnel limited to the administrator. Boards, physicians, and employees retain their positions. A management contract can be terminated to place the institution back in full control. There are also psychological reasons why a contract makes sense: Hospital personnel appear to develop few of the fears associated with mergers. Physicians express less opposition. Board members retain their autonomy and control without the threats to their existence implicit in other arrangements.

Possible disadvantages to contract management are: Backup advisors may be spread too thinly to give proper attention to the variety of institutions being managed. Standardized reporting systems may decrease the flexibility normally available to any individual unit even though they are often an improvement on existing information systems. Corporate personnel may lack sensitivity to local needs. The institution may find itself with a board which loses its capacity for probing investigation and an administrator whose loyalties are to a system outside the local institution. Potential conflicts may be resolved in favor of the contracting unit to the potential detriment of the hospital without full knowledge of the board.

Contract management provides, however, an easy method for boards of small hospitals to gain quickly an experienced administrator. This administrator (who might not take the job at all if he were isolated from needed management backup) has working access to specialists who can handle the complicated legal, regulatory, technological and financial problems facing all hospitals.

An early example of cooperation and sharing can be seen in the formation and growth of hospital associations and councils in cities, counties, states and regions. These are voluntary membership organizations that have been formed to deal with common problems. Associations represent forms of interinstitutional and intrainstitutional cooperation. They were originally established to raise standards, share educational programs, develop charitable resources and represent the collective interest of hospitals with federal and state governmental agencies and law-making bodies. Association staffs began to grow with the passage of the Hill-Burton Act in 1945. They have continued to expand in response to government regulation and the complexity of problems and issues that their constituents must deal with.

Shared services, mergers, contract service, contract management and associations all represent system trends. Not all of these trends lead to the development of hospital systems, but they represent steps in that direction.

The previous two chapters have assessed the current environment and forces trying to bring about change and some of the strategies for change. The trends examined in this chapter represent attempts by providers to form more integrated approaches to the delivery of health and medical care services. And the studies discussed in the next chapter show that this integration is occurring rapidly all across the United States.

NOTES

1. M. Brown, "Current Trends in Cooperative Ventures," *Hospitals* (June 1, 1974), pp. 40-44.

2. "Kellogg's Role in Fostering Shared Services" *Hospitals* (February 1, 1973), pp. 86-87.

3. A. A. Astolfi and L. B. Matti, "Survey Profiles Shared Services," *Hospitals* (September 16, 1972), pp. 61-65.

4. K. T. Wessner, "How to Purchase Contract Services," *Hospitals* (September 1, 1972), pp. 104, 108, 112.

5. B. L. Brown, Jr., "Contract Services: Outsiders on the Hospital Team," *Hospital Topics* (August 1965), pp 62-64, 71.

6. "A Coordinated System for Institutionally Based Health Care Services," Hospital Educational and Research Foundation of Pennsylvania, report of one-year study by John R. Clark, August 1974.

7. Ibid.

8. Ibid.

9. Ibid.

10. S. E. Knapp and R. E. Lovejoy, *Hospital Mergers in New England: Organizational Perspectives* (Durham, New Hampshire: System Educators, Inc., 1972), p. 76.

11. R. Wittrup, "The Consortium Approach" in *A Decade of Implementation: The Multiple Hospital Management Concept Revisited, A Report of the 1975 National Forum on Hospital and Health Affairs,* Duke University, pp. 49-58.

12. 1975-76 AAMC Directory of Medical Education, pp. 305-326.

13. R. Wittrup, op. cit.

14. M. Brown and H. L. Lewis, "Ideas for Action," *Harvard Business Review* (May-June 1976), pp. 8, 13.

15. Ibid.

16. M. Brown and W. H. Money, "The Promise of Multihospital Management," *Hospital Progress* (August 1975), pp. 36-42.

Chapter 4
Autonomous Hospitals versus Systems

A variety of hospital systems operated by a single integrated management structure already exists in the United States. All signs point to expansion and growth of hospital systems capable of balancing a need for strong central control with the needs and desires of local communities. At the same time, systems growth will mark the continuing decline of the freestanding institution as the prototype American hospital.

GOALS, CLASSIFICATIONS AND DISTINCTIONS

Sophisticated, yet practical goals have characterized the development of hospital systems. Some managers are looking for economy of scale that will also make them more attractive to lenders. Other managers have adopted the multiple-system approach as a means for growth and survival. Still others, who want to serve multiple markets, for example, short-term and long-term care, have found systems integration to be the best way to achieve their specialized objectives. Finally, others have adopted a generalized strategic position with the goal to combine medical education, community service, applied research, profit-making, survival and growth.

Hospital systems can be classified in many ways: governmental and nongovernmental, for-profit and not-for-profit, or geographically—local or city, county, regional, multistate. Some systems are confined to either urban, suburban or rural areas; but nationwide multiple systems are also in the making. Groups of health care providers are beginning to think, and look like the huge industries that serve them on an interstate basis and giant health care conglomerates are emerging.

At the same time, some distinctions between hospitals are becoming diffuse. For-profit hospitals and not-for-profit institutions have to have some return on investment in order to progress. Attempts are being made to

27

remove governmental hospitals from political control and either place them in the hands of the consumers they are supposed to serve or have them managed by a third party for the community.   The objective is to sever at least partially the control of government agencies ill-equipped to manage properly such complex, specialized operations.   The source of financial support, the most obvious distinction betweeen hospitals, is also rapidly disappearing.   More than 40 percent of all care is paid for through government programs.   As long as a hospital is either accredited or certified and delivers good care, governments don't care whether the facility's orientation is for-profit or non-profit.

The major distinctions that remain between hospitals are: (1) bed size, (2) teaching or nonteaching, (3) types of services offered and (4) whether the facility is part of a hospital system.

STUDIES OF MULTIPLE UNIT SYSTEMS

A discussion of "The Multiple Unit Hospital" in 1965 defined this phenomenon as one whereby "a general hospital operates as a second unit at a point geographically removed from its parent institution." The Hospital Planning Association of Allegheny County, Pennsylvania, studied the second-unit hospital trend in the early 1960s and found these common character-istics: Each second unit facility was sharing with its parent institutions: "1) a single governing board, 2) a single administration, 3)a single medical staff organization, 4) acute general bed care and 5) a distance of more than one mile separating the units."[1]

According to one source, the first hospital known to operate a second-unit facility was the Youngstown (Ohio) Hospital Association that established its Northside Unit in 1929.   The second multiple-unit development supposedly didn't come until thirteen years later when the Detroit Grace Hospital opened its Northwest Unit in 1942.[2]

Until recent years, there has been no accurate accounting of the number of hospital systems in the United States.   It is clear, however, that there is no longer any validity in considering that the United States population is being served by 7,123 individual hospitals.   The veterans and branches of the military services have their systems.   Mentally ill patients are cared for in state systems.   Indigent and poor patients in cities and counties are sent to local and county government hospitals that are sometimes part of large systems.

The development of systems was studied by Barry A. Cooper, who in 1973 wrote: "Presently, there are at least 222 systems operating across the country—forty-five of which were included in the survey.   These forty-five systems, which averaged a highly skewed 543 beds per system, operated a total of 126 health care facilities consisting of an average of 2.8 facilities per system. Each system consisted of 2.4 hospital units averaging 226 beds per unit. Hospital size ran from a low of 16 to a high of 799 beds, with an average distance of 7.3 miles separating the branches from the most central or parent facilities."[3]

Even more systems were found existing by Michael F. Doody: "Today approximately 15 percent of the nation's hospitals are members of multi-hospital system arrangements. . . . In 1973, 350 such systems were identified, and it was speculated that their development will increase so that within the next 10 years most hospitals will be members of integrated systems of providers."[4]

More recent research has been completed by the Health Services Research Center of Northwestern University, and the American Hospital Association's affiliate, the Hospital Research and Educational Trust in Chicago. This study, published here for the first time, provides the best current accounting of the hospital system phenomenon in the United States.

The study, begun in late 1974 and early 1975 as part of the AHA's annual survey of hospitals, had a detailed, two-page questionnaire with six major sections: reporting period; classification; facilities and services, unit beds, and visits; beds and utilization; financial data, and personnel on payroll as of a specific date. Under Section B of the 1974 questionnaire, institutions were asked to indicate whether they are part of a multihospital system. Lists of multiple-hospital systems collected by the AHA supplied leads to different types of institutions with varying rural-urban characteristics, geographic dispersion, educational affiliations and organizational and management philosophies. Given the paucity of data on existing systems, no statistical sampling techniques were used in selecting the actual systems studied.

Interviews were conducted by telephone, on site, and during national meetings. Published documents and other sources of information were also used. An attempt was made to look at older systems, newer systems, and competitive systems in various areas of the United States.

Following this census intensive follow-up efforts were made through telephone calls, letters, questionnaires, personal visits and interviews with administrators and managers of hospital systems. Questions such as these were asked during the spring and summer of 1975: Are you part of a system? How many units of care and how many beds are involved? Where are those units and beds? Who is your chief executive officer? Do you own all of your facilities? Do you lease facilities? Do you contract manage facilities? Do you know of any other systems?

The AHA usually has a 90 percent or better return on its annual census of hospitals. The survey is vitally important to the AHA, hospitals, and researchers. The information is tabulated by computer and published in two volumes: *AHA Guide to the Health Care Field* and *Hospital Statistics*.

These valuable reference sources have been used extensively in this book. Unless more current information was available from primary sources, information from the AHA's 1975 editions of the *Guide* and *Hospital Statistics* has been used throughout this book.

The AHA *Guide Issue* lists health care institutions by state, county and city. Statistics are given for each hospital—such as type of control, short-stay or long-stay, beds, average census, occupancy rate, expenses and total full-time employees. *Hospital Statistics* provides this information according to the nine U.S. Census Divisions and the U.S. Associated Areas and hospital statistical information according to standard metropolitan statistical areas. Both reference works are invaluable sources of information about the number of physicians, house staff, service programs, educational programs, and many other pertinent statistics.

Data from the hospital system study were compiled according to the nine census divisions. All registered, nonfederal hospitals in the United States were included in the study. The results of that study are presented in the map and table titled "Number of Nonfederal Hospitals that are Members of Systems: by U. S. Census Divisions" (See Figure 4:1). This information is repeated and discussed in more detail in Chapters 5 through 12. Chapter 13 is devoted to Catholic-sponsored systems.

The study showed that 1,834 nonfederal hospitals of all types are part of systems; most of the hospitals are in the 100 to 199 bed category. The largest number of hospital units in systems are in Alaska, California, Hawaii, Oregon and Washington. The smallest number of systems hospitals are located in Connecticut, Maine, Massachusetts, New Hampshire, Rhode Island and Vermont. About 126 of the hospitals in multiple-unit systems are managed through contract arrangements. Most (41) of these hospitals are in the 50 to 99 bed size. And most (36) of the managed hospitals are located in Iowa, Kansas, Minnesota, Missouri, Nebraska, North Dakota and South Dakota.

The study shows that there are about 370 systems now operating in the United States. This number does not include the federal government systems, such as those operated by the Veterans Administration and military services. It does include some of the state-operated mental hospitals.

The community hospital systems (see Table 4:1) range from many systems of only two hospitals operated under a single management to 91 hospitals located in 14 states operated under a central management. Of the total 926,000 community hospital beds available in 1975, 293,000 or 32 per cent of those beds can be placed significantly enough in the hospital system category. It is fully recognized that many survey respondents are in hospital systems where the ownership or sponsoring body has very little central operating

Figure 4:1

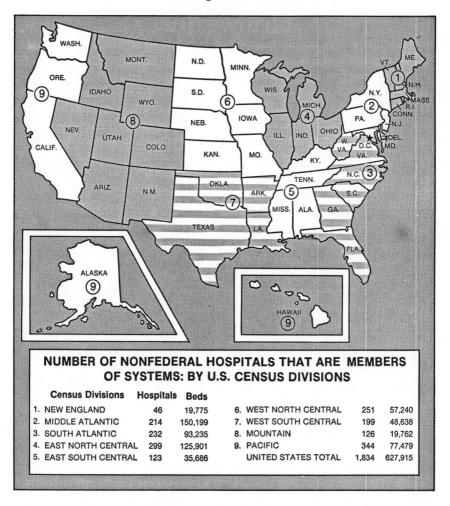

NUMBER OF NONFEDERAL HOSPITALS THAT ARE MEMBERS
OF SYSTEMS: BY U.S. CENSUS DIVISIONS

Census Divisions	Hospitals	Beds			
1. NEW ENGLAND	46	19,775	6. WEST NORTH CENTRAL	251	57,240
2. MIDDLE ATLANTIC	214	150,199	7. WEST SOUTH CENTRAL	199	48,638
3. SOUTH ATLANTIC	232	93,235	8. MOUNTAIN	126	19,762
4. EAST NORTH CENTRAL	299	125,901	9. PACIFIC	344	77,479
5. EAST SOUTH CENTRAL	123	35,686	UNITED STATES TOTAL	1,834	627,915

control over the decision making of the individual units. However, as we shall show, the ownership tie is being used as a base for building a strong central management group in many organizations.

Some of the associations and consortia not reported as systems represent a form of organization which frequently leads to merger, contract management and other stronger ties.

While the degree of central management control varies by system, the United States health care scene is different from the often supposed single-unit hospital operating without regard to the rest of the world. As we hope to

Table 4:1   Community Hospitals and Beds in Hospital Systems
by Type of Ownership

Ownership Category	Total Hospitals	HS	Percent	Total Beds*	HS*	Percent*
Nongovernmental, not-for-profit........	3,355	940	28	649,000	210,000	32
Investor-owned for-profit....................	755	309	40	70,000	37,000	51
State and local government..............	1,745	156	8	207,000	46,000	22
Totals.....................	5,875	1,405	24	926,000	293,000	32

HS—Hospital Systems
* Rounded Numbers
Source: These data were collected as part of the American Hospital Association's 1975 survey of the health care field, but not published. The data were confirmed by the authors through telephone calls and interviews.

show, a variety of approaches are being taken to regionalize and integrate hospitals, which has been generated by many different purposes and motivations, and this movement is gaining momentum. Hospital systems discussed in following chapters represent alternative strategies for responding to community need as well as spontaneous innovation and voluntary choices made in a pluralistic society.

In the following chapters, twenty-seven systems are discussed in detail. Other systems are mentioned in summary form. The organizations discussed in detail include five public hospital systems, two for-profit chain systems, and twenty not-for-profit systems that are either religious-oriented or nondenominational.

NOTES

1. "The Multiple-Unit Hospital" *Currents in Hospital Administration,* Ross Laboratories (November-December 1965).

2. Ibid.

3. B. A. Cooper, "A Study of the Organization and Operation of Multiple-Unit Hospital Systems in the United States" (Unpublished report, February 1973).

4. M. F. Doody, "Status of Multihospital Systems" *Hospitals* (June 1, 1974), pp. 61-63.

Chapter 5
New England and the Middle Atlantic States

The nationwide study of multiple hospital systems showed only 46 nonfederal hospital members and 19,775 beds located within organized systems in Connecticut, Maine, Massachusetts, New Hampshire, Rhode Island and Vermont. There may be several reasons for this low count: (1) all of the existing systems may not have been reported, (2) system·activity may be related to large geographical areas and distances, and the New England states are generally compact entities and small in area, (3) there is very little for-profit chain activity in this region, and (4) hospitals in the six states tend to be older and more established, perhaps even set in their ways with a go-it-alone style of management. There is, however, a lot of presystem activity in the New England states, such as the organization of special associations and consortiums.

In comparison, the highly populated Middle Atlantic states of New Jersey, New York and Pennsylvania were identified as having 214 nonfederal hospitals and 150,199 beds included within multiple-unit systems. These states also show a high level of presystem activity. For-profit chains have been expanding into these states. One of the largest chains, American Medicorp, has its corporate headquarters at Bala Cynwyd, Pennsylvania, and owns four hospitals within the area, although most of its facilities are located in California and Florida. The Middle Atlantic states also contain many hospitals that are part of Catholic-sponsored systems.

MASSACHUSETTS' HOSPITAL SYSTEMS

West of the Boston area, 13 institutions now make up the West Suburban Hospital Association (WSHA). The hospitals range in bed size from 113 to 330, a membership complement of 2,800 acute care beds. Representatives of the trustees, medical staffs and administrations of the hospitals voted in 1973 to formalize the association through incorporation and a set of bylaws.

33

According to Albert S. Deane, Jr., administrator and executive vice-president of Framingham Union Hospital, one of the WSHA members, the general goals of the association are: "The utilization and coordination of the efforts of the sponsors to provide and arrange for the resources and diagnosis of the treatment of illness and the continuity of care; the efficient use of the resources, equipment, and facilities of the sponsors; minimizing the cost of medical and health care; improving the quality of the educational programs and patient care, and coordinating hospital planning and hospital activities."[1]

These purposes clearly represent systems trends. And they can be directly related to the rationale the Congress used in stating the need for Public Law 93-641. WSHA is using cooperation as its philosophy and the region as its sphere of interest. In 1974, the association had several programs underway in inservice and continuing education. It was looking toward meeting common needs through shared service projects for emergency equipment and supplies, a master price list of equipment, an equipment loan program and a regional cancer therapy unit. The association was taking other steps that would bring it closer and closer to becoming an integrated, coordinated system by consolidating financial and statistical information. Another objective was one of developing "stronger liaison with the state and regional health agencies to examine a means toward attracting and sharing the services of physicians in the scarce medical subspecialties. . . ."[2]

Another group of hospitals in Massachusetts signed formal incorporation papers in July 1974, to form South Middlesex Hospital Association with Alan C. Nichols hired as fulltime executive director in January 1975. Nichols said both negative and positive reasons led to the association. The hospitals, sensing the encroachment of government into their affairs through a rigid state certification of need law and the federal planning law, "needed to assess the impact of these laws and they needed to set up an organization to deal with the new Health Systems Agency. The positive aspect of the association came about through the persuasive arguments of Walter P. Allen, executive director of Mount Auburn Hospital, Cambridge, Mass. He convinced the hospitals that they should work together."[3]

Harvard University's medical institutions and affiliated teaching hospitals in the Boston area formed in 1972 a Medical Area Service Corporation (MASCO) in an effort to economize through shared services. "Services are provided to the member institutions under formal contract. Not all institutions purchase all the services. Several years ago, hospitals in Boston organized a joint laundry. It also is separately incorporated and provides service under contract," explained an administrator of one of the hospitals. MASCO's goal "was to create an entity which would operate like a business with its services shielded as much as possible from the internal politics of the hospitals being served."[4]

The Affiliated Hospitals Center in Boston began several years ago as a consortium of three well-known institutions: the Boston Hospital for Women, the Peter Bent Brigham Hospital and the Robert B. Brigham Hospital. In 1974 these institutions merged to become one corporate structure.[5] These hospitals have 648 beds and are major teaching hospitals of the Harvard Medical School. They will very likely add new members, with a specialty hospital a primary candidate in the years ahead as they develop sophisticated and high-cost subspecialty programs.

CONNECTICUT'S CAPITAL AREA HEALTH CONSORTIUM

One of the most interesting trends in the New England area is the Capital Area Health Consortium (CAHC) organized in the Greater Hartford, Connecticut, area. On a historic day in May 1974, the representatives of eight hospitals stepped forward and signed a compact to share services, programs, staffs and the host of problems now facing all hospitals

When the corporation came into being, the eight institutions had about 150 board members, 1,800 physicians, 10,000 full and part-time support personnel, 3,300 beds, a capital investment of $270 million, and service areas for an estimated 1.5 million persons (see Figure 5:1). A ninth institution, the 183-bed Veterans Administration Hospital at Newington, was expected to join the consortium in late 1975 or early 1976.

The hospitals have agreed "to coordinate and further the health care delivery, medical, educational, research, administrative and other activities of its members. . . ." These objectives are further spelled out in five statements: (1) the highest possible quality of medical services at the lowest practicable cost to all persons; (2) the most advanced coordinated programs possible in the areas of preventive care and research; (3) the coordination of members' services to eliminate to the greatest possible degree both unnecessary duplication and incomplete coverage in the providing of services and facilities; (4) the greatest possible integration of educational programs in medicine, dentistry, nursing and allied health; and (5) the education of the public as to the health care needs of the community.

"The power of the consortium is contained in a section of its bylaws that covers rights and obligations. Each hospital has three members on a board of directors—one administrator, one hospital board member and one member of the medical staff. The dean of the school of medicine at the University of Connecticut is also a member. There is a dollar limit ($25,000) on the cost of a new capital improvement that can be made without approval of the

Figure 5:1

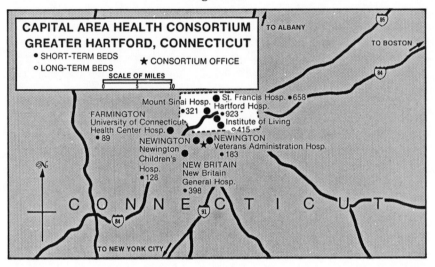

CAPITAL AREA HEALTH CONSORTIUM
GREATER HARTFORD, CONNECTICUT
● SHORT-TERM BEDS   ★ CONSORTIUM OFFICE
○ LONG-TERM BEDS
SCALE OF MILES
0   5   10

TO ALBANY
TO BOSTON

Mount Sinai Hosp.   ● St. Francis Hosp. ●658
●321   ● Hartford Hosp.
FARMINGTON   ●923
University of Connecticut   ● Institute of Living
Health Center Hosp. ●   ○415
● 89
NEWINGTON ●★● NEWINGTON
Newington ●   Veterans Administration Hosp.
Children's   ● 183
Hosp.   NEW BRITAIN
● 128   New Britain
            General Hosp.
            ● 398

C O N N E C T I C U T

TO NEW YORK CITY

trustees. Service and clinical care programs were frozen at their existing levels and consortium members must have approval from the board before they begin new programs."

CAHC also created obligations in budgets and financial statements, sharing of services and facilities, common standards of care, and a pledge to cooperate with one another. A specific power given to the board was one "to monitor the quality of patient care provided by its members, to prescribe standards of patient care, with specific reference to preventive care and inpatient and outpatient care and, alone or in cooperation with others, to implement programs designed to attain and maintain the highest standards possible among its members in all areas of patient care."

The formation of the consortium was a substantial victory for T. Stewart Hamilton, M.D., president and general director of Hartford Hospital and first president of the consortium. He recalled that administrators in the city had been meeting periodically for about twenty years to discuss common issues and problems. At one time a council was formed, but it was abandoned after the issues and the membership became so diffuse that they couldn't be resolved within the structure of the administrators' organization. In late 1972 several events occurred that made the time ripe to move toward organizing a consortium.

The regional "B" agency and the Connecticut Hospital Planning Commission urged Hartford area hospitals to made a strenuous effort to cooperate. Studies of open-heart surgery facilities in the city and high energy radiotherapy facilities in the state had shown duplication and competition for patients and had also raised serious questions about the quality of medical care in underused facilities. Hartford had several hospitals but no trauma or burn units. The city is headquarters for a number of major insurance companies. Many of them are in the health care underwriting business and have urged the hospitals to work more closely together.

Several months passed before all the problems could be worked out. The primary issue to resolve was how the consortium would affect private practice. A specialist in ENT who was trying to keep the peace talked about the opposition among his physician colleagues: "There is sort of an attitude, what are you going to do *to* us, and not *for* us. Full-time people are concerned about the consolidation of services. It might mean the elimination of some positions. There's also a feeling that the medical school [University of Connecticut] will gobble us up and that we'd jump to a different tune."

There were also concerns about who would have the responsibility to keep the beds full. Several months before this issue was resolved, Dr. Hamilton said: "The biggest stumbling block at the moment is to persuade the medical staffs of the value of this and the fact that it won't be a threat."[6] Patients cross service areas in order to receive care, he said, and doctors will have to do the same in order to deliver care. Ideally, patients will go into the proper unit for care.

The medical staff issue was resolved by giving each doctor a primary appointment in his original hospital and a secondary appointment at all other consortium hospitals.[7] Like the hospitals, the doctors have taken the option of togetherness. The consortium provided something of a buffer zone between them and governmental regulatory agencies. And physicians have one-third of the consortium votes. Individual hospitals are responsible for credentialing and screening. All of the hospitals regard credentialing in the primary hospital to be of equal competence to their own system. New appointments are circulated to the various hospitals and doctors are then eligible for consortium-affiliated status appointments. The affiliated doctor observes the rules and regulations of the hospital in which he practices. And the staffing procedure has been made a part of the bylaws of each hospital's medical staff.

Dr. Hamilton predicted that the consortium could provide new opportunities—a common medical record, for example, and a common voice that could speak in a strong tone to a new Connecticut State Hospital Commission that is a rate-setting body.

And in 1975 the first executive director of CAHC, John M. Danielson, told *Business Week:* "I think we are the cutting edge of something very important." The early programs of the consortium involved inventorying resources, establishing various educational programs and joint sharing projects. Danielson said the CAHC would place considerable emphasis on preventive medicine: "You can save nickels and dimes by combining laundries, but you save hundreds of thousands of dollars by keeping people out of that high-cost hospital system."[8]

NEW YORK'S HOSPITAL SYSTEMS

Many consortiums begin as low-key efforts to create unity on a regional scale. For example, four hospitals in northeastern New York established in 1972, the Iroquois Hospital Consortium. They said their purpose was to "foster and encourage cooperation and consultation among hospitals to improve the quality of hospital service provided for patients." The Iroquois consortium was formed by the presidents of 763-bed Albany Medical Center Hospital, 233-bed Memorial Hospital and 420-bed St. Peter's Hospital, also in Albany, and the 323-bed Samaritan Hospital in nearby Troy. The initial objectives were to: "(1) sponsor cooperative programs, including one for joint central services; (2) develop new techniques in hospitals procedures, administration, and service that would lead to more effective and efficient patient care; and (3) explore and develop new concepts in health care aimed at insuring maximum quality of care for patients."[9]

NEW YORK CITY HEALTH AND HOSPITALS CORPORATION

Organized system activity in New York State is marked by one significant example: the New York City Health and Hospitals Corporation (NYCHHC). This public benefit corporation was established by an act of the state assembly. And on July 1, 1970, the city's municipal hospitals were, in theory, taken out of politics to be run as a public trust.[10] But things haven't worked out that way.

This system is the largest of its type in the United States. In 1974, there were 12,924 beds in 20 facilities. The 16 hospitals had 10,279 beds and 4 long-term care institutions had 2,645 beds. Their combined budgets came to around $462 million. The overall occupancy rate was 77 percent. There were 45,000 employees and about 6,000 interns and residents. Kings County Hospital, with 1,745 beds, is the nation's largest public hospital.

An estimated 2 million persons, mostly impoverished blacks and Puerto Ricans, rely on the public hospitals for practically all of their care. There are about 4.9 million inpatient admissions and outpatient visits each year. In addition to hospitals, the corporation has a growing network of outpatient facilities and runs a fleet of almost 150 ambulances that make about 90 percent of all the calls in the five boroughs.

After five years in operation, the corporation's problems remained much the same as before. In the late 1960s, Joseph V. Terenzio, then commissioner of hospitals and now president of United Hospital Fund, pushed for the law creating the corporation. In 1975, he said NYCHHC "hasn't worked out the way it was intended. The city basically retains leverage over it, especially in financing . But the idea remains sound. It should be restructured to be more independent."[12]

A sixteen-member board of directors makes policy. But five members of the board are appointed by the mayor and five others hold seats on the board by virtue of appointments as chiefs of health-related agencies. The city council appoints the other five members and the sixteenth member is the president of the corporation. Half of the operating budget comes from city tax revenues.

The first president of the corporation was Joseph English, M.D., former physician for the Peace Corps and now chairman of psychiatry at St. Vincent's Hospital & Medical Center in New York. The second and current president is John L. S. Holloman, Jr., M.D., an internist and liberal black physician who had practiced in Harlem and been an early critic of the NYCHHC concept. Early in 1975, Holloman said: "My opinion has gradually come around to the positive. I believe the corporation has great potential. But I don't expect its potential to be realized for some time.[13] By mid-1975, New York City was nearly broke. The mayor ordered cutbacks in personnel and Dr. Holloman refused. Late in the year, the mayor cut all department budgets and the municipal hospitals began reducing services.[14]

The future of this system appeared bleak and confused as the year ended. Adding to the uncertainties was the potential impact of Public Law 93-641 on NYCHHC. Three organizations were competing to become the official Health Systems Agency (HSA) designated by the Department of Health, Education & Welfare. The HSA would be powerful, as Lowell E. Bellin, M.D., the city's health commissioner pointed out: "This is no longer review and comment. This is review, comment, and decision."[15]

As a multiple-unit system, the NYCHHC had not really had a chance to prove itself. Dr. Holloman had visions of a network of family health care centers, increasing ambulatory care services, and possibly even starting a nontuition "public" school of medicine. Economies of scale, central management, and other systems concepts were cast aside by the double problems of political interference and fiscal crisis. And yet, no city needed an organized system of medical and health care any more than the city of New York.

PENNSYLVANIA'S HOSPITAL SYSTEMS

Central Pennsylvania contains one of the newest organizations of the consortium type, a group of six hospitals called the Susquehanna Valley Health Care Consortium (SVHCC). Formally organized in 1974, the

SVHCC covers a five-county mountainous and rural area traversed by two branches of the Susquehanna River. Virtually all of the communities in this economically depressed area were damaged in 1972 by the flooding caused by Hurricane Agnes.

The six institutions are: 163-bed Berwick Hospital; 154-bed Bloomsburg Hospital; 136-bed Evangelical Community Hospital, Lewisburg; the 109-bed Shamokin State General Hospital; the 109-bed Sunbury Community Hospital, and the 428-bed Geisinger Medical Center, Danville. These hospitals have collectively 1,100 beds and admit in excess of 40,000 patients a year. They provide more than 400,000 outpatient visits, including nearly 100,000 episodes of care in six emergency rooms. They have a combined professional and support staff of over 3,000. Total expenses in 1974 were $36 million.

This consortium is organized around Geisinger Medical Center, which contains a large group practice as the primary care hospital and teaching center. The consortium is controlled by a board of directors made up of three representatives from each hospital. Acording to its bylaws, the consortium wanted "to insure to its communities, patients and health care personnel":

A. The availability and delivery of the highest quality of health care services at the most reasonable cost to all persons requiring them.

B. The most advanced, coordinated programs in preventive care.

C. The coordination of services to minimize to the greatest extent possible both unnecessary duplication and voids in services and facilities.

D. The greatest possible integration of educational programs in medicine, nursing, and other health industry disciplines.

E. A means of taking a unified position when dealing with health care issues of mutual concern."[16]

Western Pennsylvania contains two organizational examples of trends that fall roughly into the consortium category. These organizations began with shared services orientations, but they have become effective voices to promote the regionalization of care. And they could develop into multiple hospital systems under single management.

UNIVERSITY HEALTH CENTER OF PITTSBURGH

University Health Center of Pittsburgh (UHCP) was granted a state charter in 1965. It is a corporate management superstructure, something like the Detroit Medical Center Corporation see (Chapter 7), that has pulled together academically-oriented institutions into a voluntary, cooperative arrangement. The nine organizational entities are located in the Oakland district of the city.[17]

They are the 235-bed Children's Hospital of Pittsburgh, the 172-bed Eye and Ear Hospital of Pittsburgh, 357-bed Magee-Womens Hospital, 480-bed

Montefiore Hospital, 561-bed Presbyterian-University Hospital, the Ambulatory Care Program (Falk Clinic and the Matilda H. Theiss Health Center) and the University of Pittsburgh through its six Schools of the Health Professions and 150-bed Western Psychiatric Institute and Clinic. Affiliate members of the center are the Central Blood Bank of Pittsburgh, the Pittsburgh Child Guidance Center, and the 949-bed Veterans Administration Hospital.

Walter J. Rome, while executive director of Children's Hospital, said the new corporation provided an answer to the question: "How do you structure and organize a group of independent institutions so they can work together, develop shared services, and, at the same time, preserve the essential independence of each institution?"

The Center's bylaws state that the members want to grow and develop into "an efficient, well-rounded, and effective community and regional health resource."[18] By 1968, when Rome made his report, the center was involved in several shared service projects. Uniform policies were developed in some areas of medical and allied health education. And the center had become a central voice in community health planning.

UHCP, however, had only begun to tap its potential. In July 1974, the University of Pittsburgh named Nathan J. Stark, J.D., as Vice-Chancellor for the Health Professions and President of UHCP. Stark had had extensive experience in health and medical affairs and is well-known nationally.

By December 1974, Stark outlined his "protocol for effective governance" that pointed UHCP to the future as a regional resource for western Pennsylvania and the nation. In what he called an "internal coherence thrust," Stark proposed a larger corporate organization and the creation of top management jobs in professional affairs, finance, development and fund raising, physical plant development, administration, industrial relations and the development of corporate structure.

Stark pointed out that the state assembly had studied the need for an additional medical school in Northwestern Pennsylvania: "The Commonwealth study urged the University of Pittsburgh to meet the needs of this region for improved health education, research and care as a corporate responsibility." Stark's protocol said: "The U.H.C.P. must open lines of communication between community hospitals and agencies in Western Pennsylvania so that we can learn the perceived needs of these institutions. We must know our collective educational strengths so that we can participate as a cohesive unit in supplying these programs to our neighbors."

And in looking at "the needs of external constituencies," Stark began to orient the UHCP toward multiple system development. He said one external goal was, "To integrate the U.H.C.P., including both the schools and the hospitals, with other appropriate institutions and agencies as components of a regional system providing health education and delivering health care to the people of Western Pennsylvania. . . ."[19]

NORTHWEST ALLEGHENY HOSPITALS CORPORATION

Just two years after the incorporation of University Health Center of Pittsburgh, nine other hospitals in the area formed Northwest Allegheny Hospitals Corporation (NAHC). A ninth hospital joined the organization in 1974.

The Pittsburgh-area NAHC members are: 158-bed Ohio Valley General Hospital, McKees Rocks; 237-bed Sewickley Valley Hospital; 215-bed Suburban General Hospital; 278-bed St. John's General Hospital; 123-bed Divine Providence Hospital; 641-bed Allegheny General Hospital; 272-bed North Hills Passavant Hospital; the 60-bed D. T. Watson Home for Crippled Children, Leetsdale, and the 68-bed Harmarville Rehabilitation Center.

According to its bylaws, the NAHC was formed "to bring better health to the people . . . through coordinating and implementing action by the health organizations that are members of the Corporation."[20] The bylaws protect the individual financial autonomy of the hospitals while also providing that NAHC shall be apolitical. Specific objectives of the consortium sound similar to the priorities stated in the federal planning law. Under its bylaws, NAHC said it shall:

> (a) be an agency for inter-communication, planning and cooperation among the member organizations, especially in areas concerning health services, facilities, manpower, research and education;
> (b) be the corporate mechanism for planning health services coordinations among member organizations, including but not limited to ascertaining and continuously reviewing the current health needs and resources; projecting future needs; and develop and work toward an areawide health delivery system that balances needs and resources of the area in the most economical manner;
> (c) investigate and develop innovative systems of health care delivery and improvements in the system of health care delivery;
> (d) explore and develop shared or joint services in order to obtain maximum use of resources, expand scope and quality of services, reduce duplicate facilities and services, improve efficiency and contain operating costs;
> (e) become involved in the comprehensive long-range planning processes of member organizations;
> (f) consider, and if approved, endorse (i) comprehensive long-

range plans and (ii) specific expansion and redevelopment plans
of member organizations; and

(g) be an advocate before appropriate private and public review
agencies of expansion and redevelopment plans of member organizations endorsed under (f) above.[21]

During its formative years, NAHC moved slowly into such areas as
studying the need for a joint laundry (later developed for six members),
developing in-service education programs for nurses and the coordination of a
common home care program for all members. In the early 1970s the
corporation tackled tougher problems. It coordinated the closing of two, low-
use obstetrical units. It also was instrumental in developing a regional
pediatric care program, strengthening referral patterns between the eight
hospitals, and coordinating the development of an alcoholic-drug rehabilitation center. NAHC also began to coordinate a continuing education program
for physicians, an emergency medical communications system, a management
development program, a vendors' guide and a joint data processing project.

The corporation's major accomplishment in 1974, according to a report by
F. J. Terrance Baker, chairman of the board, and Terrence N. Manke,
coordinator, was the adoption of a health care policy statement. This
statement says: "The delivery of better health care requires optimal efficiency of operation and cost effectiveness in the services now provided, the
development of new, innovative delivery systems where appropriate, and
further exploration and implementation of shared/joint services." Manke said
national organizations have called the guidelines "the first effort... in
voluntary, local level creation of guides for the overall development of multi-
health care systems. The guidelines are specific ... dealing with ambulatory
and bed capacity needs areawide for certain target years in medical/surgical,
obstetrics, pediatrics, and mental health. This provides an opportunity to
relate 'what is' and 'what might be' to 'what's needed'."[22]

NOTES

1. A. S. Deane, Jr., "Consortium Achieves Mutual Goals," *Hospitals* (July 1, 1974), pp. 95, 96.
2. Ibid.
3. Telephone interview with Alan C. Nichols, September 29, 1975.
4. R. D. Wittrup, "The Consortium Approach" in *A Decade of Implementation: The Multiple Hospital Management Concept Revisited, A Report of the 1975 National Forum on Hospital and Health Affairs,* Duke University, pp. 49-58.
5. Ibid.
6. H. L. Lewis, "A Togetherness Spirit in Connecticut" *Modern Healthcare* (July 1974), pp. 25-29.

7. From a telephone interview with John M. Danielson, October 28, 1975.

8. "Performing Major Surgery on Hospital Costs," *Business Week* (May 19, 1975), p. 149.

9. "1st Annual Report," Iroquois Hospital Consortium, 1972.

10. H. L. Lewis, "'Buffer' Corporation Offers New Hope to New York City Hospitals," *Modern Hospital* (February 1970), p. 84.

11. L. Frederick, "The Toughest Hospital Job," *Modern Healthcare* (February 1975), p. 35.

12. Ibid.

13. Ibid.

14. New York City Health and Hospitals Corporation press release, November 13, 1975.

15. "The City Has a Deadline for a New Health Services Agency but It Must Define It First," *New York Times* (January 14, 1976), p. 23.

16. "Planning and Implementing Integrated Primary Health Care Services Through the Susquehanna Valley Health Care Consortium" Undated and unsigned document.

17. "The University Health Center of Pittsburgh" Undated and unsigned document.

18. W. J. Rome, "A Design for Shared Services," *Hospitals* (May 16, 1968), pp. 51-54.

19. N. J. Stark, "Organizational Goals of the University Health Center of Pittsburgh: A Protocol for Effective Governance" (Unpublished, December 1974).

20. Northwest Allegheny Hospitals Corporation, 1974-1975 Annual Report.

21. "Health Care Guidelines," Northwest Allegheny Hospitals Corporation, June 1974.

22. Ibid.

Chapter 6
South Atlantic States and Federal Systems

The special research program conducted by the Health Services Research Center of Northwestern University and the Hospital Research and Education Trust, an affiliate of the American Hospital Association, shows that the South Atlantic census area is active with systems development. At least 232 nonfederal hospitals and 93,235 beds in the region can be counted within multiple-unit organizations. The region comprises Delaware, Florida, Georgia, Maryland, North Carolina, South Carolina, Virginia, West Virginia, and for statistical purposes, the District of Columbia is included within this census grouping.

FEDERAL SYSTEMS

The District is headquarters for some of the largest governmental systems—those set up under the control and power of the Department of Defense, the Department of Health, Education and Welfare, and the Veterans Administration. For example, the four branches of the military services run these domestic systems: 37 Army hospitals; 27 Navy hospitals, and 68 Air Force hospitals. The Marine Corps is served by Navy hospitals. The Defense department's three systems also include 54 hospitals overseas and a domestic-foreign total of 458 medical clinics and 794 dental clinics. Overall in fiscal year 1974-1975, there were 27,754 operating beds in the three service systems with a daily load of 19,860—an occupancy rate of 72 percent. There are now about 10 million Defense Department beneficiaries who can use military hospitals, including 2.1 million persons on active duty. When military personnel and their dependents are more than forty miles from a government hospital, they are eligible to use civilian hospitals, such as through the CHAMPUS program.[1]

The Department of Health, Education and Welfare has eight Public Health Service Hospitals, located in eight states. These special purpose facilities are responsible for the care of American Indians, natives of Alaska, and others such as members of the U.S. Coast Guard.

VA HOSPITAL SYSTEM

But the biggest federal hospital system in terms of beds and patient load is that of the Veterans Administration. The VA has 175 hospitals located in the 48 continental states and Puerto Rico. These facilities are located within 27 medical districts. The medical care division of the VA employs about 213,000 persons. In 1975 VA hospitals had over 1 million admissions. The average census in 1975 was about 79,000 patients per day. VA hospitals had general operating expenses of approximately $4.38 million. VA general hospitals had about 162,000 full-time, part-time, and intermittent employees. The employee to patient ratio goals are 2 to 1 in general medicine and 1 to 1 in general psychiatry.[2]

The top manager of the VA system is John D. Chase, M.D., Chief Medical Director of the Department of Medicine and Surgery with headquarters in Washington, D.C. In 1975, Dr. Chase outlined a regionalized management structure that represents a new direction for this huge system.

The new service emphasis is one of outpatient care and long-term care. Writing in *Military Medicine* in October 1975, Dr. Chase said six new outpatient clinics had been established and seven additional ones were opening, and the VA would probably reach its authorized capacity of 10,000 nursing home beds in the next few years. The VA was building one totally new hospital, a 204-bed facility at White River Junction, Vermont, but it was also constructing replacement hospitals (2,810 beds) at Loma Linda, California; Bronx, New York; Phoenix, Arizona; Los Angeles and San Francisco, California.

The vast sweep of legislation passed by Congress in recent years, such as the Professional Standards Review Organization (PSRO) program, and Public Law 93-641, contain caveats that exempt VA hospitals. But the VA has instituted its own peer review system, which is done by a VA Health Services Review Organization that "parallels the P.S.R.O. activity in private hospitals." VA hospitals also "will be surveyed every two years by a team composed of Central Office and Medical District VA staff, assisted by the medical school or county medical society representatives—an external or peer review."[3]

Dr. Chase, mentioning the specialized services being added to several hospitals, said "such resources are added to a VA hospital only if it has been determined by the medical district involved to be a rational and justifiable need. The VA Sharing Program fosters full and effective utilization of the resources of both VA and community health care facilities. This program continues to grow, and substantial benefits are accruing to both the local community and to the VA. In fiscal year 1974, there were 82 VA hospitals participating in 152 sharing agreements totaling $6.75 million. In long-range planning, VA is considering ways to facilitate its sharing agreements on a more flexible basis...."

Dr. Chase also said that "the VA is committed to regionalizing its nationwide system of health care facilities, while at the same time avoiding needless and costly duplication of specialized equipment and manpower in both VA and community facilities. Examination and implementation of all phases of this program have been assigned as the full-time responsibility of a staff member of the office of the chief medical director."[4]

Earlier in 1975, Dr. Chase told a federal hospitals executive meeting in Chicago that the central problems facing the health care delivery system —cost, accessibility, and utilization—require providers to "function *together* along a pathway of planned action to deliver care with a minimum of false effort and a maximum of effectiveness. Further, that there be positive incentives for maintenance of quality and this be done with retention of individual identity. We in the VA have deliberately organized our institutions to facilitate these objectives and have termed the effort 'regionalization.' We believe this organizational structure offers the best prospect for solution of the stated problem. Further, that it permits positive interaction with non-VA providers, and is adaptable to changing conditions within the private and public sector; to wit, the National Health Planning and Resources Development Act of 1974."[5]

Dr. Chase said the regionalization approach would be built on the basis of consortia of "geographically dispersed institutions of differing capabilities." He said the VA plan was based on "cross-utilization" of resources and that the VA would have a "mission in the context of the community as a whole." He added that "we see both VA and non-VA institutions cooperating in the provision of patient care. So, too, we wish to see each VA health care facility participating in the comprehensive care planning of its immediate community." He gave an example of the VA's new orientation: "The guidelines we have drawn up for the acquisition of computerized axial tomographic instruments illustrates our policy. We are placing this equipment only in VA hospitals serving districts in which such facilities are either totally inadequate, or nonexistent, and therefore can be made available as a community resource."[6]

There have been proposals over the years that the VA hospitals should be closed or turned over to the medical schools; over 95 percent of VA hospitals are affiliated with medical schools. But Dr. Chase's comments clearly state the VA position that its hospitals plan to stay around as integrated segments of community-based systems, and that the VA wants a voice within the Health Systems Agencies.

Meanwhile, the VA is extending its political and economic influence into medical education in some new ways. In 1975, the VA facilities were involved in training of about 73,000 students in some 40 different health care fields—ranging from doctors of medicine to nurses and technicians. Public Law 92-541, the Medical School Assistance and Health Manpower Training Act of 1972 authorizes the VA to give grants to medical schools. That same law allowed the VA to develop Regional Medical Education Centers.[7] Through these programs, the Chicago Medical School made plans to move out of the inner city area to the campus of the 1,915-bed Downey VA Hospital north of Chicago in Lake County and is now using the VA hospital as one of two major teaching facilities.[8] The 180-bed VA Hospital in Huntington, West Virginia, will be used as a teaching facility by the developing Marshall University school of medicine.[9] And the VA has been instrumental in developing its "own" medical schools in other parts of the United States by using the money and power available under Public Law 92-541.

AREA HEALTH EDUCATION CENTERS

Other Washington-based dollars have led to new medical school and community hospital efforts called Area Health Education Centers (AHEC).[10] AHECs could rapidly transform some parts of the health care delivery system into regional system configurations. AHECs link together the human and material resources of medical schools with those of community hospitals some distance away.

In 1970 a special report by the Carnegie Commission on Higher Education recommended and urged the nation's medical schools to attack the need for more health manpower by increasing enrollments, shortening curriculums and putting more emphasis on primary care. The report said that every metropolitan area of 350,000 or more persons should have a university health sciences center, which should lead the way in graduate and continuing education for professionals and paraprofessionals by establishing satellite AHECs in lesser populated and medically underserved areas of the United States. The report suggested that 126 AHECs be established, using one or more community hospitals as the nucleus for education. Students also should receive experience in neighborhood clinics and other health care facilities as well as teaching hospitals. If all 126 AHECs were developed, the expertise of a major medical center could be made available to 95 percent of the nation's population.

The Congress responded with the Health Manpower Training Act of 1971 that authorized the AHEC experiment. In October 1972, the HEW made five-year contract commitments totaling $64 million to eleven medical schools in eleven states to establish one or more AHECs.

The next month, Edmund D. Pellegrino, M.D., a well-known medical educator, pointed out the rationale of AHECs. Indicating that university teaching hospitals only treat 10 to 15 percent of the problems of illness, he said, "They do not, cannot and should not provide much in secondary care, primary first-contact care, long-term care, or health maintenance. Yet these latter comprise the largest bulk of the health needs of society, for which we must specifically train more—and perhaps the bulk of—new health professionals." Another reason that AHECs make sense, he said, is economy: "If clinical campuses [community hospitals of sufficient size and patient mix] can be coupled with a series of basic science campuses, the educational capacity of most university health science centers can be enlarged materially without loss of quality education."[11]

Practically any sizable metropolitan area can become a center for health care education. The resources are usually there: doctors and nurses, hospitals, nursing homes, clinics, colleges and universities and—most important—interested people willing to do those things necessary to insure that good care is available and provided.

Under HEW guidelines, a single community hospital or consortium of hospitals can become a clinical campus, although HEW emphasizes that the AHEC is a concept and not a building. As the prime contractor, a health sciences center has the responsibility to carry out and control: (1) clinical instruction for undergraduate, medical or osteopathic students; (2) residency training programs, with emphasis on primary care and family practice; (3) continuing education for physicians, dentists and other practitioners; (4) clinical instruction for other undergraduate professional students in fields such as nursing, dentistry and allied health; and (5) assistance to education institutions and health care facilities within the region in developing training and preprofessional programs.

The AHECs systems orientation is easy to see when projects are considered in detail. West Virginia provides a good example. An oddly-shaped state with diverse geography, West Virginia has an area of 24,181 square miles, northern and eastern panhandles, and a total population of 1.7 million. It ranks thirty-ninth in doctor to patient ratio and is especially low in some specialty ratios, such as psychiatry. The state medical school is located in the northern part of the state at Morgantown. The population center is 180 miles to the south at Charleston, the state capital and a prosperous business center.

In 1971, recognizing these facts and political demands that some more innovative way be found to keep doctors in the state, Charles E. Andrews, M.D., provost for health sciences at West Virginia University, proposed that a series of clinical campuses be developed at Charleston and in other urban areas. The AHEC contract provided the necessary "seed" money to establish a clinical campus at Charleston, focused around the new Charleston Area Medical Center, the result of a merger between three hospitals. The center provided 902 teaching beds in three physical facilities.[12]

The health care needs in the Charleston area were clear. The average age of doctors in the area was increasing, and the proportion of foreign medical graduates on the staffs of hospitals and in private practice was increasing too. Young graduates from the state medical school were going elsewhere for internship and residency programs; they tended to setup practice where they received postgraduate training.

The Charleston AHEC opened for business in 1972 in the context of a Charleston Division of the West Virginia University Medical Center, and a prime subcontractor, the Charleston Area Medical Center. By the fall of 1974, residency programs had been established in family practice and psychiatry, in addition to those already existing in medicine, surgery and other fields. Doctors were soon beginning to stay in the area and open practices.

What has the AHEC meant to southern West Virginia? The area's health resources are being inventoried. Goals have been set in terms of the need for training more professionals and paraprofessionals. Four small colleges and another university in the state have been brought into the training of health manpower. Consumer health education programs are getting off the ground. In these ways, the AHEC has pulled community and state resources together as a system to deliver care to a defined population in West Virginia.

There are ten other AHEC programs under way that are creating a matrix for systems development.[13] The University of California's San Francisco and Los Angeles campuses are cooperating in a program for a six-county area in the San Joaquin Valley. The University of Illinois is trying to develop regional health care education systems in Chicago, Peoria, Champaign-Urbana and Rockford. Tufts University in Boston is trying to increase the doctor supply in Maine through a cooperative program with the Maine Medical Center at Portland. The University of Minnesota established an AHEC in a health care-poor area around Saint Cloud and later expanded its efforts statewide. The University of Missouri at Kansas City has an AHEC program in the western part of the state. The health care needs of Navajos in a 25,000 square mile area around Arizona, New Mexico and Utah is the objective of an AHEC sponsored by the University of New Mexico. Programs by the University of North Dakota, University of North Carolina and University of South Carolina are concentrating on links to community hospitals in order to train medical students and increase available medical manpower, particularly physicians. And the University of Texas at Galveston has carved out a 16-county area in the extreme southern part of the state for manpower planning and allied health education.

As an anomaly within the South Atlantic census area, Washington is the control point for federal multiple-hospital systems located all over the United States and in many foreign countries. The power of the administration and agencies within HEW is also being used to influence systems development, although the approach might not be a direct one.

SOUTH ATLANTIC STATES

Washington, however, is not the universe. There are many community-based multiple systems located within the borders of the eight states—West Virginia and the seven contiguous states that sweep from Delaware down the Atlantic Coast and up the Gulf Coast to Florida's western panhandle. These systems include the Wilmington (Delaware) Medical Center; the Charlotte-Mecklenburg Hospital Authority, Charlotte, North Carolina; the Carolinas Hospital and Health Services, Charlotte, North Carolina; the Greenville (South Carolina) Hospital System and the North Broward County Hospital District, Fort Lauderdale, Florida. Another anomaly within this census region is the Hospital Research and Development Institute, Pensacola, Florida, a management think tank that could develop into a technical advisor to hospital systems.

WILMINGTON MEDICAL CENTER

The Wilmington Medical Center (WMC) is in a unique position. It is not only an urban and suburban multiple-hospital system but also a statewide hospital system, the major medical and health care resource for Delaware. This situation can bring promise and problems.

A centrally-organized system like WMC should certainly be able to affect economies, ensure accessibility and accountability and wield enough power to survive and prosper. But there are always growth pains present in any new organization, which intensify when hard choices have to be made, such as moving the main hospital and finding a way to finance indigent patient care.

WMC became a corporate entity on November 1, 1965[14] and the first full corporate merger between three voluntary, nonsectarian, acute care general hospitals in the United States. These long-established institutions are now divisions of the medical center and include the Delaware Hospital, the Wilmington Memorial Hospital and its rehabilitation facility, the Eugene duPont Memorial Hospital and the Wilmington General Hospital.

Wilmington, established in 1739 as the first city in the first state, remains closely tied to the vast chemical complexes established in the area by the duPont family, whose corporation is headquartered there, along with Hercules Powder Co., and related industries and research facilities.

A committee studying the possibility of merger in the early 1960s "learned that the opportunity in Wilmington was unique because of the small geographical area involved, its proximity to medical schools in Philadelphia, and the obvious similarities of the three hospitals: their mutual problems, their triplicated attempts to be all things to the same community, their shared medical staffs, and the close ties binding many members of the three governing boards."

The merger question was also approached with candor, for "the committee had come to recognize that any proposal grounded in the expectation of major savings in costs was unrealistic—simply because the cost of medical advances was sure to rise, and the cost of training and retaining the very more highly skilled employees required was sure to rise as well—but that the merger could hold down costs through avoiding unnecessary duplication and through consolidation of services wherever possible."[15]

Although the capital of this small state is Dover, the center of activity is metropolitan Wilmington. No part of the state is much more than three hours' driving time from the city. Wilmington is similar to a lot of other cities. The inner-city population is around 80,000 but the New Castle County population is an estimated 400,000 and the metropolitan area contains about 510,000 persons. In the decade since WMC was formed, the population has continued to move out of the city to the south and west into suburbs and communities such as Newark, home of the University of Delaware. Between the 1960 and 1970 censuses, for example, Wilmington lost 15,000 persons and Newark gained 10,000.

WMC supplies 85 percent of the acute care beds in the city and New Castle county. There are only eight general hospitals in the state with 2,234 beds; four of the hospitals and 1,069 beds are controlled by WMC. WMC is the major resource for emergency, outpatient and rehabilatative treatment for the surrounding area and parts of three other states—Virginia, Maryland and Pennsylvania.

In 1974, the 1,069 WMC beds provided for 38,599 admissions. The average daily census was 935 and the average occupancy rate was 88.3 percent. Expenses were $47.1 million, including a payroll of $27.1 million for 3,431 full-time employees. There are more than 400 members of the combined medical and dental staffs.

Before the medical center was formed, each of the four hospitals competed with each other. That competition has been fairly well dampened, but there are other short-stay hospitals in the metropolitan area; the 60-bed Alfred I duPont Institute; the 100-bed Riverside Hospital, and the 185-bed St. Francis

Hospital. There is also a large, 351-bed Veterans Administration Center and a 92-bed long-term care facility, Emily P. Bissell Hospital for chronic diseases.

There is no medical school in Delaware. But through an affiliation arrangement between the medical center, the University of Delaware and the Jefferson Medical College of Thomas Jefferson University in Philadelphia 20 premedical students are admitted to Jefferson each year; they receive their two years of clinical education at WMC.

Three years after the merger, Norman L. Cannon, M.D., president of the center's medical and dental staff, and the first physician to formally suggest the merger, said: "It seems almost axiomatic that as Wilmington goes, so goes the medical care for the rest of the state. In fact, the problems of rural health care are almost identical to those of depressed urban areas. Both have become isolated from the national health care system, don't know how to enter it, and are somewhat resentful of outside restrictions. To overcome this obstacle, Wilmington is developing a concept of satellite neighborhood health centers, which will reach into areas where there is no practicing doctor, no dentist, nor pharmacy. The object: To generate intake facilities indigenous to the community, but varied in staff and function as the situation warrants. Such centers will be tied to Wilmington's program by a health transportation system."[16]

Dr. Cannon also pointed out that the very future of the location of the tertiary care center was in doubt, however, because of the need to consolidate physical facilities downtown and provide an inpatient facility in the suburbs.

WMC has a 67-member board of trustees, including many trustees from the three premerger hospitals, and a 13-member board directors.[17] The center's chief executive officer is James G. Harding, a former administrator of Cleveland Clinic, who came to WMC as president in 1971.

Unlike many other multiple-unit systems and some urban medical centers, WMC is not involved in so-called "outreach" efforts to any large extent because of its geographical compactness. Shared purchasing is handled by the state hospital association. The outpost-like clinics that Dr. Cannon proposed in 1968 have not been built, although there are some neighborhood clinics in the city.

WMC has concentrated on its immediate environment through a $3.5 million construction program for an ambulatory emergency facility at the Delaware division in the heart of the city. The new walk-in facility is to open in late 1976. In fiscal year 1973-1974, WMC had a whopping 209,791 outpatient visits and 79,652 emergency visits. WMC has been functioning as the indigent care facility for the state. This has put a severe strain on existing resources and has prompted a continuous debate with the state about its responsibility to cover reimbursement for charity care. This financial drain combined with discounts to Blue Cross led WMC into deficit positions in three of its first four years. And the problem had not abated by the 1974-1975 reporting period when the center had a loss from operations of $2.2 million. The center was able to balance its books, however, because of income from endowments and gifts.[18]

In recent years, the managers of WMC have had to make some hard choices. Many multiple-unit systems have developed in a unit of service configuration like a doughnut with the acute care tertiary care center occupying the hole of the doughnut and satellite or branch facilities located on the periphery. WMC hospitals are all within the hole of the doughnut, but this configuration will change in the next few years.

After long and detailed discussions, proposals and counterproposals by various community organizations and controversy about the economic impact on the city, WMC announced in late 1975 that it will build a new 800-bed acute care facility on a 200-acre site near Interstate 95 south of the city. The Wilmington division will be upgraded and essentially replaced with a new 325-bed primary care and emergency care facility to serve the inner city. Total cost of the two projects was estimated to be $72 million. The Memorial and Delaware divisions will be converted either to other purposes, such as long-term care, or torn down.[19]

There was considerable debate among community groups and in the local newspapers about this decision and the potential economic impact on the center city. Before the decision, Dr. Cannon told a reporter: "Today, the city is barely more than 70,000 and the county is well up into the 300,000s. And these people are not finding it very appetizing to come into the city for health care; they've made their lives in the suburbs. So the pressures are now for a hospital located in the suburbs."[20]

After the decision had been made, Joseph A. Dallas, chairman of the board of trustees, wrote in the local newspaper: "While we are proud of the quality of care being given in these facilities, this result is being obtained only by inefficient use of personnel, a practice which cannot continue indefinitely because of soaring hospital costs." Adding that WMC provides primary care for all of the county and is a referral hospital for a large region, he noted: "The center of the population we serve has shifted to the southwest and is forecast to shift further in this direction. The I-95 site is near the center of our primary area and therefore optimizes convenience for all patients."[21]

NORTH AND SOUTH CAROLINA'S HOSPITAL SYSTEMS

Of all states within the Middle Atlantic census division, North Carolina and South Carolina stand out as primary examples of hospital system activity. It was on the Duke University campus in 1965 that the late Ray E. Brown suggested that hospital systems should be examined to "see how they fit into the balance of things."[22] Although it was not clear whether Brown was referring to the balance of political power or that related to other health care delivery system approaches, he got his point across: it was time to experiment more widely with an integrated systems approach and time to cooperate, share and see if central management was more efficient than solo management. In Charlotte, where the idea had come to life in 1943, a different type of Charlotte-based experiment was beginning in 1969. And in Greenville, South Carolina, a model multiple-unit system was already in the making (See Figure 6:2).

CHARLOTTE-MECKLENBURG HOSPITAL AUTHORITY

The Charlotte-Mecklenburg Hospital Authority (CMHA), established in 1943 under a special charter issued by the secretary of state. The multiple-unit system includes four hospitals with a total 1,330 beds in the short and long-term care classifications. A long-range development plan adopted in 1975 could mean that the system will evolve into one of the most comprehensive county-wide organizations in the United States.

The Authority grew out of an atmosphere of restiveness. In the late 1930s, community leaders in the city-county area decided that they needed a coordinated hospital system. They wanted to establish a vehicle that would authorize and empower them to respond to health care needs while also insulating their organization from local and state politics. The North Carolina Hospital Authorities Law, written by Charlotte attorney Fred B. Helms and passed by the state legislature in 1943, provided for the buffer organization they wanted.

This law gives CMHA limited taxation powers and the right of eminent domain. It charges the Authority to be sensitive to the medical and hospital needs of the community, and to establish programs for technical and medical education. The Authority may build, own, operate, buy, lease and rent any facility as long as it meets its statutory charge. The Authority may issue revenue bonds for the purposes of financing new construction and adding new facilities and services. Community bond referenda, local votes of confidence, public subscriptions and private philanthrophy have been the major routes that CMHA has taken to obtain money for capital improvements and growth.

CMHA is a systems concept, for the Authority may (and does) operate more than one institution for the purposes of health care delivery. R. Zach Thomas, Jr., executive director of the Authority since 1961, said the comprehensive health planning "B" agency in the area has coordinated the health care needs of the citizens well: "I don't know that a health facility planning decision has ever been made that has resulted in serious duplication."[23] There are three nonauthority hospitals in the area: the privately owned 62-bed Charlotte Eye, Ear and Throat Hospital; 349-bed Mercy Hospital, and 507-bed Presbyterian Hospital.

For its first seven years, the Authority owned and operated only the Charlotte Memorial Hospital. This institution now has 889 beds and its name has been changed to Charlotte Memorial Hospital and Medical Center. Charlotte Memorial is the Authority's flagship facility, the county's tertiary care center and a major medical education resource for the state. All of the Authority's acute care beds are concentrated in this hospital, whose beds comprise about 40 percent of the county total.

The Authority's influence grew in the 1960s as government officials began to see the wisdom of an integrated system. At the turn of the decade, the Authority agreed to a city request to assume responsibility for the oldest (circa 1872) all-black hospital in North America, the Good Samaritan Hospital, an act which demonstrated the flexible characteristic of the Authority concept. Thomas explained: "It was a horrible place to house any patient with an illness . . . the only place in Charlotte, however, that a black could get medical attention. Incidentally, it was the only place where a black physician could practice, even in my time, and I say that with much embarrassment."

So the Authority became a progressive mechanism for integration in more ways than one. The worn-out structure that was Good Samaritan received a new coat of paint, and the acute care section was closed. Acute care patients were transferred to Charlotte Memorial. Black physicians were allowed to apply for membership on Memorial's medical staff that now became fully integrated. The city provided $1 million for a new 108-bed long-term care facility that was built near the original Good Samaritan, the name of which was changed to Charlotte Community Hospital and reopened in 1962 as a long-term care facility.

Also added to the Authority system in the 1960s was an old county tuberculosis sanitorium—a series of wooden, barracks-type buildings, complete with sleeping porches, built during World War I. Thomas recalls that county officials came to the authority and said: "Will you take this off our hands?" The Authority agreed and the old buildings were promptly razed. Citizens of the county approved a $7-million bond issue to replace the original complex with a 73-bed long-term care unit which was named Huntersville Hospital. Another 200-bed unit, The Oaks, was added to this long-term care facility in 1974. Because of legal technicalities, the Authority operates this modern 273-bed long-term care hospital under a twenty-five year, renewable lease.

A fourth facility was added to the system in 1961—Carolina Spastics Hospital which was converted during the late 1940s to the care of poliomyelitis patients in response to a severe polio epidemic at that time—when the hospital's trustees asked to become a member institution. Through a public bond referendum this facility was completely rebuilt and modernized and renamed Charlotte Rehabilitation Hospital. It now contains 89 beds, including a new 32-bed spinal cord injury center which opened in 1975. The center is considered to be one of the finest facilities of its type in the South.

The four-unit system would appear to have come into existence with relative ease. But building any system is not easy, as Thomas explained: "There was a certain amount of trauma ... a certain amount of diehard attitude on the part of the governing boards at Good Samaritan Hospital and Carolina Spastics Hospital. They did not want to totally lose their identity by marrying into this family. So, we tried about 10 different approaches to consolidated governance and representation."

North Carolina hospital authority law specifies that the total governing authority rests with the twenty four commissioners who make up the CMHA. A representation approach that worked was to absorb a majority of the members of each of the three prior governing boards into an enlarged hospital authority. The Authority then created separate boards of managers for each of the hospitals by subdividing the new consolidated authority into four managing "committees," augmented by additional "noncommissioner" appointees where indicated or desired. The noncommissioner board members vote in their own hospital meetings, although they have no official vote within the Authority.

"So we retained, on the surface, the identification of the hospital and its board in just about the same profile as that hospital had before it came into the authority," Thomas explained. Each hospital board was asked to draw up its own by-laws and outline its own medical staff organization, which it must submit to the overall Authority for ratification.

Overall power of the Authority is vested in an eight-member executive committee made up of the chairman, vice-chairman, secretary, treasurer of CMHA and the four chairmen of the four hospitals' boards of managers. Thomas provides day-to-day management continuity by his frequent contacts with administrators of the four hospitals. He attends all of the hospital board meetings, although the administrator prepares the agenda and conducts the meeting. Authority-wide problems percolate up from the individual boards to Thomas and the executive committee. The committee's word is law, particularly in any matters involving income and expense, as relates to decisions which have to do with corporate business.

CMHA works on the basis of what Thomas calls "economically, a low rate of metabolism." The central staff operation cost $102,000 in 1974. Each hospital pays twenty cents per day per occupied bed to finance the operations of the Authority's small executive staff—Thomas, a part-time controller, and one secretary. The four hospital units had combined 1974 expenses of $36 million, including $19 million for payroll, and 2,780 employees.

Unlike most multiple-unit systems, CMHA takes a low key approach to centralized functions. Thomas says this philosophy "has a uniqueness which is a strength, yet it has a looseness which can work to a disadvantage unless programs are properly coordinated at each institution." There are shared services in dietary and purchasing, but there is no central personnel office, because of differences in compensation levels and skills required among employees in four diverse facilities.

The central office does handle the critically important job of managing the Authority's cash flow and financial reserves and is careful to keep idle funds invested at maximum earnings in keeping with the schedule of utilization of such funds for their ultimate purposes.

Thomas sees other systems' advantages. The four hospitals may freely transfer patients to another CMHA institution without going through the costly process of readmission, for it is considered to be "a valid transfer, just like moving a patient from one room to another room on the same floor." This cooperative procedure saves physician time for it eliminates the patient discharge summary and the patient's money for it eliminates duplicate medical workups and admission laboratory tests.

As a $36-million-a-year corporation, the Charlotte-Mecklenburg Hospital Authority is a considerable economic force in a growing region. The standard metropolitan statistical area, of which Charlotte is the hub, showed a population growth from 316,781 in the 1960 census to 409,370 in 1970. It is the largest urban area in the state. Traditionally known for such industries as textiles and tobacco, which remain strong, the region has also developed a thriving commerce in industrial chemicals and has over 150 electronic data processing installations. The city is also home for four higher education facilities, including a branch of the University of North Carolina system. And Charlotte Memorial Hospital and Medical Center is one site for the state's network of six Area Health Education Centers.

There is a bullish outlook for growth in the area. The hospital authority has sensed the existing and coming health care needs through a planning document that argues for decentralization and integration of facilities. CMHA has divided the county into five sectors related to the transportation catchment areas created by the criss-crossing of Interstate 77 (north-south) and Interstate 85 (east-west).

An overall argument in the plan is that all hospitals in the city-county metropolitan region should rely and build upon the tertiary care status of Charlotte Memorial. The statement strongly suggests that new facilities must follow a feeder-line concept—patients going from one level of care in one institution to another level in a second. As Thomas said: "The most direct service rendered to patients in the community is the separation of levels of care. Doctors don't always cooperate with this philosophy because of their tendency to consolidate practices. You can come closer to mandating stratified clinical care under a system . . . than you can if you didn't have a system.

"Perhaps that element of its [the Authority's] profile which justifies its existence more so than any others is the flexibility of patient service at each of its four hospitals. . . . Given a reasonable amount of governmental cooperation, beds may be assigned to reflect an appropriate response to community health needs. The more finely and accurately we can tune the stratification of clinical needs in our community, the more efficiently we are then permitted to employ the beds. When this 'capacity to respond' is placed under one governing authority it is obvious that objectives can be much more easily attained."

The five sector plan also emphasizes the need to integrate acute care facilities with an emergency care transportation system of life-supportequipped ambulances. Each sector would be considered a medical service area; each would include a medical service center. The planning document recommends that by 1980 CMHA should acquire four new building sites of thirty to fifty acres each. These sites would be used for the Authority's expansion into a number of outpatient facilities and services—emergency vehicle stations, health information centers, public health annexes, physicians' office facilities and outpatient ambulatory care clinics. The only totally new inpatient facility proposed would be a 200 to 600-bed hospital located near the University of North Carolina at Charlotte in an area of the county where planners estimate a large population growth will occur over the next two decades.

CAROLINAS HOSPITAL AND HEALTH SERVICES

Carolinas Hospital and Health Services (CHHS) with main offices in Charlotte, North Carolina (see Figure 6:1), is listed in the American Hospital Association's 1975 guide book as a shared service organization. CHHS provides group purchasing for dozens of hospitals in North Carolina and South Carolina. CHHS also makes available management engineering, biomedical equipment maintenance, electronic data processing and financial services.[24]

And in October 1974, CHHS took a great leap forward by signing a contract agreeing to provide day-to-day management for 21-bed Our Community Hospital in Scotland Neck, North Carolina. CHHS thus became more than a service organization; it had evolved into a hospital system, an organization similar to the management contracting arm of either a nonprofit or for-profit hospital system. CHHS's closest comparable model is the Great Plains Lutheran Hospitals, Phillipsburg, Kansas, an organization that manages twenty-one hospitals on a lease basis (see Chapter 9).

The contract with Our Community Hospital was a small venture that caught on rapidly. When CHHS decided to offer facilities management services, it had projected to be managing six small Carolinas hospitals within three years. But seven months after the program was offered, CHHS had five contracts. Since then, the organization has expanded its central office capabilities and hopes to be managing sixteen hospitals by October 1978.

Ben W. Latimer, executive director of CHHS, says the organization "makes geography no barrier to economy of scale.... The organizational model that CHHS demonstrates is especially applicable to states in which size, density, and health care patterns have precluded the existence of enough mid-size hospitals to support shared services economically."

Latimer explained the early history this way: "The North Carolina and South Carolina hospital associations were instrumental in CHHS's organization in 1969 and the association-corporation relationship remains strong and somewhat unusual among shared programs. Through independence of direct association control or ownership, CHHS does serve *in effect* as the associations' operational arm for some services developed or wanted by them for hospital members.... However, CHHS is not limited to direct association initiative in service development and may operate as an expansion-minded company would in assessing user needs and organizing services to meet them."[25]

CHHS has 70 employees, including professional, technical and clerical personnel. Most of these employees are headquartered in Charlotte but the corporation also has regional center offices in Raleigh and Lumberton, N.C., and Columbia and Greenville, S.C. The estimated 1976 operations budget was $2.2 million.

The corporation receives its direction from a seventeen-member board of trustees made up of four representatives from each of the two state hospital associations (executive director of the association and three working administrators) and a cross-section of seven other persons in different professions. The subscribers and users of services are represented on management advisory committees for each of the following five service divisions.

Carolinas Affiliated Purchasing Program, a division that buys for more than 100 hospitals and offers, according to the corporation, "savings and price protection through volume supply purchases, greater reliability in quality and delivery, and professional development opportunities for their professional staffs."

Carolinas Hospital Improvement Program was the initial division formed in 1969 to provide management engineering shared services. Latimer

Figure 6:1

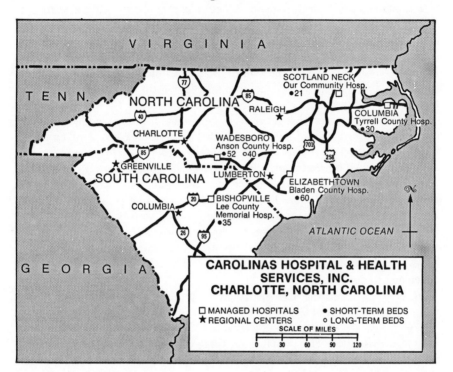

explained that "the division in 1976 will provide regular and special services to more than 75 hospitals on an expense budget balanced by hospital fees, which compare very favorably with those of similar shared programs and private enterprises."[26]

The clinical engineering division is called Carolinas Hospital Engineering Support Services and was expected to serve 55 hospitals in 1976, the fourth year of its operation,

Of these programs, often referred to as CAPP, CHIP and CHESS, Latimer said their "development has corresponded to that of similar shared programs in other states for management engineering, clinical engineering, and group purchasing. As foreseen by the foundations which funded the pioneers as demonstrations, these programs now constitute informal national networks through which cooperation and communication are growing in each field."[27]

The data processing division began operations in early 1975 by using the Burroughs Corporation's Charlotte data center. A year later this division was offering administrative and fiscal management data packages to three hospitals. Future plans call for developing a complete electronic data processing package for hospitals including advanced patient care modules.

The management services division began operations in late 1974 and in early 1976 had contracts with these five hospitals: the 21-bed Our Community Hospital, Scotland Neck, North Carolina; the 35-bed Lee County Memorial Hospital, Bishopville, South Carolina; the 30-bed Tyrrell County Hospital, Columbia, N.C.; the 60-bed Bladen County Hospital, Elizabethtown, N.C., and the 92-bed (including 40 long-term beds) Anson County Hospital, Wadesboro, N.C.

Latimer emphasizes that this division is not-for-profit and community oriented: "By renewable agreement with the hospital's board of trustees, CHHS assumes responsibility for the hospital's active day-to-day management and provides staff for that management. Ownership of facilities is retained by the community. The hospital's board of trustees, acting in the community's behalf, retains legal responsibility for assets, liabilities, policy-making and budget functions. A CHHS agreement detracts in no way from the board's traditional perogatives. In effect, the hospital board is choosing to hire an executive *department* instead of one person as administrator." Latimer believes that facilities management is "the 'definitive' shared service fully developed to potential."[28]

In 1974, four of the five managed hospitals (Tyrrell County is not included) had a total of 208 beds, 5,052 admissions, an average daily census of 164 patients, an average occupancy of 71.3 percent and 396 employees. Financial statistics were available on three of the hospitals—Our Community, Bladen County and Anson County. These hospitals have 173 beds and showed total expenses of $3.1 million, including payroll of $1.2 million for 171 employees.

The management services fee is based on a percentage of gross patient revenue, although CHHS retains the option of setting a flat rate for smaller hospitals. Latimer said: "The fee includes the salary of the in-hospital director, and it is considerably lower than the fees charged by most investor-owned contract management organizations."[29] Most for-profit companies charge 7 to 10 percent of gross revenue; CHHS charges 2 to 4, and this fee includes the salary of the administrator.

The outlook for CHHS is good. This organization although only six years old is well-known in the Carolinas. The working relationships with over 100 hospitals in the two-state area offers an excellent base for growth.

There are 203 community hospitals in the Carolinas, including 157 hospitals with under 200 beds. And 96 of the 157 hospitals have fewer than 100 beds and would seem to be primary targets for facilities management contracts. Although for-profit chains are very active in the Carolinas, CHHS has a natural advantage in being set up by the state hospital associations with the help of The Duke Endowment. The Endowment, the W.K. Kellogg

Foundation, and the Kate B. Reynolds Health Care Trust are supporting its activities. All of these organizations give CHHS credibility in the communities where its programs must be sold.

Latimer sums up the potential this way: "C.H.H.S. as a model is based on the American enterprise principle of risk-taking and the corresponding concept that the innovative, expansion-minded, well-managed organization will survive and grow." Jack Milburn, director of the management services division and the line supervisor of the in-hospital directors, believes that the "shared multi-hospital management programs can serve as the voluntary sector's alternative to the new regionalization and health care delivery forms forecast as governmental requirements for the future. Shared multi-hospital management plans demonstrate that voluntary efforts can be effective. If multi-institutional arrangements should be further dictated by government, the voluntary plans can serve as proven, workable lead-in vehicles."[30]

GREENVILLE HOSPITAL SYSTEM

The Greenville Hospital System (GHS), Greenville, South Carolina, is a model multiple-hospital system that has attracted national and international attention. This system is a vertically and horizontally integrated organization of nine facilities and 1,107 beds located in the western part of the state. (See Figure 6:2).

The top managers of GHS are systems advocates, who have written and spoken widely about the need for systems. GHS is the prototype urban-rural model of the public authority type. Economy, accessibility and accountability, quality of care and power describe GHS.

Robert E. Toomey became general director of the GHS in 1953, and, significantly enough he was a member of the American Hospital Association's Perloff Committee that recommended the Health Care Corporation concept, almost an exact copy of the Greenville Hospital System.[31] A philosopher in the health policy field, he firmly believes that systems managers should help make national policy, and was an early pioneer of federally supported medical education in community hospitals. He helped establish one of the nation's first allied health-technical schools.

Toomey has pushed the concept of primary care. The so-called Greenville Plan was adopted in 1971 by the South Carolina Appalachian Health Policy and Planning Council.[32] The idea was to develop primary care centers to serve defined populations in the county using the Health Care Corporation concept. This project was allowed and funded through Section 202 of the Appalachian Regional Development Act. Through this program and other grants, family practice has become a way of life and a way of service to residents in Greenville County. And through those experiences, Toomey has

Figure 6:2

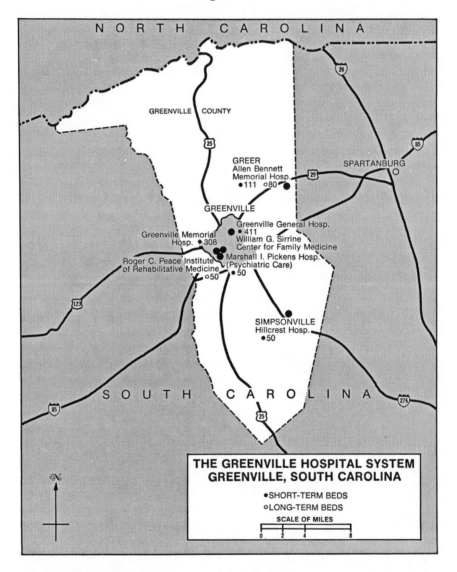

THE GREENVILLE HOSPITAL SYSTEM
GREENVILLE, SOUTH CAROLINA

gained a breadth of experience in dealing with power structures—doctors, trustees, communities, planning agencies, state and local governments.

Through the years, Toomey has developed a systems philosophy. For him, "Hospitals, it should be emphasized, are social instruments for the attainment of better health for all the citizens. Basically, all health care institutions are expressions of concern for the health and welfare of each and every family in the community."

Social, medical, economic and political reasons led to the original separation of patients into a variety of nonintegrated institutions, which "left only the acutely ill and—as if in a kind of penance for its exile of the long-term ill—the community rallied to the support of these patients. Nothing was too good for them, and the development of autonomous general hospitals became a matter of national pride."

And he proposed that "hospital managements are now sufficiently advanced and sophisticated to assume responsibility for the establishment of institutions that care for all the sick. The association of all health care institutions within the current hospital milieu will enable medicine and science to seek cures for all forms of illness, to the ultimate benefit of all families and individuals." This, then, was the philosophical basis for his fundamental argument: that only an integrated system of care could really meet the needs of people. He concluded: "The social thrust of the future will be for total and comprehensive health care services under single management. In the future, hospital authorities will no longer operate individual, autonomous hospitals devoted to one aspect of the total need. They will operate hospital systems in which the organizational structure will be different, the management function will be different, and the skills needed will be different, but all will be related to the total needs of the community."[33]

This total needs concept, and his push for integrated hospital systems, has not always left Toomey a safe haven. He has occasionally been attacked by newspapers and conservative physicians for his opinions and positions on health care issues. But with a certain charm and charisma, he has developed physician and manager friends too. They know he wants the Greenville system to be a leading organization of its type in the United States. Toomey and his associates have built a system that has strong citizen input and solid backing from local government.

Over the years, Toomey also has developed a superior management team, including such individuals as Jack A. Skarupa who has been executive director since October 1971. Like Toomey, Skarupa is active at the higher levels of the American Hospital Association policy structure and has written widely about the Greenville system.

This system attracted nationwide press attention in 1972 through an article in *Medical Economics* headlined, "General hospitals are going the way of G.P.s," which noted that, "The system is based on the premise that doctors habitually deal with a range of illness extending far beyond acute disease. 'They're often frustrated,' says its director, Robert E. Toomey, 'when it comes to geriatric patients, or those in need of long-term physical or psychiatric rehabilitation, because there's no place to put them except outside the circle, out of the physician's purview. Our system is a pragmatic attempt to bring these patients back into the circle, and to enable our doctors to offer the right facility to the right patient at the right time.' "[34]

The complete circle created at Greenville is vertically integrated with a strong central management. There are three divisions, each managed by an administrator. The general division has day-to-day responsibility for the 430-bed Greenville General Hospital located in the center of the city. This division also has management control over the William G. Sirrine Center for Family Medicine, the site of a family practice residency program. A suburban division has responsibility for four facilities: The 110-bed Allen Bennett Memorial Hospital at Greer; the 80-bed Roger Huntington Nursing Center, a long-term facility also located at Greer; the 50-bed Hillcrest Hospital at Simpsonville, and the 29-bed North Greenville Hospital.

The newest and potentially largest operating unit is called the center division because it is located near the geographical center of the county in an area called Grove Road. Most of the major development, including a new tertiary care center, is located here. The facilities are: the 308-bed Greenville Memorial Hospital that will be expanded to 700 beds by 1980; the 50-bed Roger C. Peace Institute of Rehabilitative Medicine, and the 50-bed Marshall I. Pickens Hospital that concentrates on psychiatric care.[35]

There are also three non-GHS hospitals in the county: the 60-bed Shriners Hospital for Crippled Children; the 195-bed Saint Francis Community Hospital, and the 79-bed W. J. Barge Memorial Hospital.

There are two system support facilities located at the Grove Road campus: the Frank H. Earle Management Services Center where personnel, fiscal programs, patient accounting, billing and data processing are centralized, and a supply and distribution center. The GHS organization is relatively clear-cut. Toomey reports directly to the trustees and is responsible for development and external relations (specifically planning), the treasurer's office and community services. Skarupa reports to Toomey and is responsible for the three hospital divisions and institutional support services. Although the medical staff organization is institutional in nature, the medical staff as a whole is noninstitutional. Doctors work within clinical departments but they can cross institutional lines to treat a patient in any GHS facility.

Over all, the nine institutions with 927 acute beds, 100 specialty beds, and 80 long-term beds constitute a comprehensive system tied together by roads and highways, for no facility is more than thirty minutes driving time from the administrative offices at Grove Road. In 1974 the eight GHS facilities then open for care had 39,709 admissions and provided 292,683 adult days of care. The average daily census in the five acute care facilities was 882 patients and the average occupancy rate was 69.1 percent. Total expenses for all the facilities were $27.9 million, including payroll of about $18 million for

2,717 employees. There were 338 physicians and 79 dentists providing care within the hospitals and 67 interns and residents.

Greenville is a major site for the University of South Carolina's Area Health Education Program. The system's current gross assets are $63 million.

Act number 432 of the 1947 South Carolina General Assembly established the authority for a hospital system serving the county. As early as 1895, when there were two cases of typhoid fever in a city of about 9,000 persons, private citizens led a movement for a hospital. The agitation continued for over a decade and a citizens' group responded in 1909 with money for a two-room emergency hospital similar to a clinic. That facility was phased out and replaced in 1912 with 85-bed Greenville City Hospital. The city assumed responsibility for the facility in 1918 and by 1935 the hospital had been expanded to 275 beds and renamed Greenville General.

In 1947, Greenville County was experiencing a surge of population growth. Another private citizens' group proposed that the city hospital be operated for the benefit of all residents of the county. Act 432 was passed that year "providing for the establishment of an independent, self-perpetuating board of trustees to govern and operate the hospital as a community, non-profit, voluntary institution on behalf of all citizens of Greenville County."[36]

The one hospital officially became a system in 1952 because citizens of Greer, a community about 12 miles northeast of the center city, had petitioned for a hospital. The 27-bed Allen Bennett Memorial Hospital was opened and that development marked the beginning of continuous system expansion to catch up with a rapidly growing population.

Greenville County, a prosperous area with a diversified economic base, is a burgeoning manufacturing area for textiles, machinery and chemicals. General Electric makes generators there and Michelin, a French company, opened its first United States tire plant there. South Carolina's population in 1970 was 2.59 million. The Greenville-Spartanburg standard metropolitan statistical area had an estimated population of 299,502 in 1970 which exploded to 473,226 persons by 1975. Between the 1960 and 1970 national censuses, however, the city of Greenville lost about 5,000 persons.

Interstate 85 runs all the way from Richmond, Virginia, to Charlotte and through the Greenville-Spartanburg area on to Atlanta. All along this major artery, there is a high level of industrial activity, particularly in the Greenville region and throughout the Piedmont Crescent. This growth has also helped spawn the development of two other South Carolina systems. One has grown up around the 525-bed Spartanburg General Hospital (S. C.). Another has developed around the 486-bed Anderson Memorial Hospital at Aderson, South Carolina.

The official name of GHS was adopted in 1966 through an act of the state legislature. The city board became the system board. There are seven trustees of the GHS, who are charged to make overall policy. The system is a creature of city, county, and state, Toomey explained. The city deeded its property and hospital to an independent board set up by state law and created for that purpose. The county matched the value of the city property with cash. The seven original members of the board were commissioned by the governor—three members who reside in the city, three who are outside the city but residents of the county, and one at-large member. The commissioners serve six-year terms and new members are approved by the city and the county governing units.

In 1966, county voters approved a referendum for a constitutional amendment allowing the system to incur a debt not exceeding 25 percent of the assessed property valuation in the county. The general assembly and governor agreed in 1969 thus setting off a major expansion to keep up with population shifts, population growth and the need for modernization and consolidation.

Over the years, the GHS has used funds from a variety of sources—federal, state, gifts and grants—to finance capital projects. About 40 percent of its money has come from sources outside the county. The other 60 percent of its capital needs have been supplied by a $22 million bond issue made in 1968 and 1969, and $30 million in bonds authorized for the current development program.[37]

A consolidated statement of revenues and expenses for a twelve-month period ending in September 1975, showed the GHS with total operating revenues of $35.9 million, including $56,772 earned as interest on investments. The net total income from all sources after expenses was $575,021. In the previous year, the system had an excess of revenue over expenses of $324,214.

Major studies of the health care needs of the county have been developed and examined by managers and medical staff committees. The major conclusion reached was to consolidate the programs and services of the old downtown hospital at the new site on Grove Road. A two-phase development plan was conceived; phase one was completed in 1972 when the first Grove Road facilities were all opened. Phase two will continue into 1980 and include closing the old downtown hospital as an acute care complex, which will be converted to other uses, probably long-term or ambulatory care.

In July 1976, the GHS was to offer some $7 million in tax exempt bonds for sale as the initial financing phase of the new bond issue. This money will allow an expansion of Greenville Memorial to 700 beds. A mental health center also will be built at the Grove Road site, a 147-acre campus that should provide plenty of room to expand in future years.

The Grove Road site will take on the atmosphere of a total medical complex when the phase two development is completed. There will be additional ambulatory care and emergency care facilities, a trauma center, in-and-out surgical center, walk-in clinic, and a cancer treatment center. Other facilities to be built there include: physicians' office facilities; an Area Health Education Center building; housing for interns and residents; housing for other staff, students and employees; an office building for voluntary and official health agencies and residences for the aged.

GHS's development plan makes a strong case for only one major acute care hospital within a system and within the limits of geography, for "maintaining the continued simultaneous operation of two major acute care facilities, each of 300 beds or more, requires many duplications of manpower, equipment, supplies and services and is considerably more expensive per unit of service rendered than if the total activities are carried out in one 700-bed acute care Greenville Hospital Center," according to a consolidation and development report. The report also notes that "transfer of patients between two hospital locations [a distance of three miles] for diagnostic and therapeutic procedures is tiring, annoying and sometimes uncomfortable for patients."[38] The separation of acute facilities also costs physicians' time.

With such a broad expanse of service and programs, however, GHS has retrenched in one area. After graduating 1,654 women from a diploma school of nursing established in 1912, the nursing education program was phased out in 1974 for "economic and academic reasons."[39] The system assisted in the development of alternative nursing programs in area universities and schools.

The system has forged links to its communities through four, fifteen-member Community Advisory Councils named in 1974. These councils represent the county's four service areas—Greer, north Greenville, Greenville, and the south area. Councils meet monthly, are briefed on system plans and urged to "advise hospital leadership concerning needs and problems in their own areas which require attention. The Councils have participated in naming a new hospital, assisting in the creating of an auxiliary for the new hospital [at Greer], a survey of health care needs, development of a 'no smoking' policy in each hospital, and recruiting physicians."[40]

Toomey believes GHS, like many other hospital systems, has many advantages over autonomous hospitals because of the ability to vertically integrate services: "We have ambulatory care, long-term care, a school for emotionally-disturbed children, inpatient psychiatry, outpatient psychiatry—I can't tell you what it will cost any more than anyone else can that is doing the same thing. The cost factor is subjective.

"Economy? It's hard to prove a difference. . .terribly difficult to find proof."[41] Toomey said he'd often suggested that Ph.D. candidates go at the economy question through modeling. Meanwhile, the economy questions persist. "We have a monitor in the coronary care unit that has a simulator to measure the monitor. The simulator takes a normal heartbeat and measures it against the monitor. So, what's known? It is hard to measure my total operation against anything."

For Toomey, "there *are* economies in systems that can't be measured, and services provided individually or within a group cost more. There are community services and medical education services because of the way we operate. I can take my entire medical education program, and charity care, and divide it up among all units of the system. I have an opportunity to distribute costs throughout the entire county. That makes it equitable."

The ability to pool depreciation and resources is another advantage. As Toomey said, "When we need eight or ten beds some place we can use the money where it is needed rather than just in the hospitals that generate the most depreciation. This is something planners have hollered for. We've been able to do this. It's great."

What about power? "There's no doubt that we have power. But the person with power doesn't use it. We have economic, social and education power—and a certain degree of political power. We never flaunt it at anybody. It stays in the background; people know it's there. How do you use it? You don't. You don't tell them. We have 3,000 employees and a $45 million operating budget. We have had an impact in a number of areas—and even in the nation."

FLORIDA'S NORTH BROWARD HOSPITAL DISTRICT

The North Broward Hospital District (NBHD), Fort Lauderdale, Florida, is one of the oldest hospital systems of the public authority type. Established in 1951 as a geographical district by the Florida legislature, NBHD serves the northern two-thirds of the county north of Miami with three acute care hospitals: the 613-bed Broward General Medical Center; the 259-bed North Broward Hospital at Pompano Beach, and the 130-bed Imperial Point Hospital, newest facility built by the authority. These facilities had in 1974 36,965 admissions and an average daily census of 770 patients. The average occupancy rate was 72.2 percent. Total expenses were $30.7 million, including $17.4 million in payroll costs for 2,224 full-time employees.[42]

The Fort Lauderdale region served by the authority has changed radically since the 1920s when area citizens were in desperate need of hospital facilities. In 1920, the population of the village of Fort Lauderdale was only a little over 2,000. A great hurricane in 1926 had pointed up the need for sanitary conditions and medical facilities in the area. Several hospitals were established during the 1920s but they were all short lived ventures. Meanwhile, the population was growing.

The district traces its history to 1938. By that time citizen interest had led to the establishment of 45-bed Broward General Hospital. By 1948, the hospital had grown to 142 beds and additional citizen pressure led to the legislative enabling act in 1951 creating the hospital district. Broward County has not stopped growing; the 1970 census shows a population of 620,100. Mainly tourism, but also boating industry, electronics and surgical instrument manufacturing have spurred the area's economic growth.

And as the Broward North Hospital District has raced along keeping up with population growth by building new hospitals, fifteen other facilities have been built in the county, including several for-profit hospitals. "At one time, the authority had one-half of the hospital beds in the county," said Bernie B. Welch, district director and administrator of Broward General Medical Center. "Now," Welch added, "every hospital chain in the county has a facility here—they got in before certification of need."[43]

The state law created a special geographical hospital district that has an area of 800 square miles. There are about 40 other hospital districts in the state. The law provided for seven authority directors who serve four-year terms and are appointed by the governor. Said Welch:

> They receive no compensation for their positions. The Board enjoys complete control of the District including selection of its management team, policy setting, working with the medical staff to establish standards of patient care, and limited authority to levy ad valorem taxes. . . . In the . . . district we feel that our board . . . has used its taxing authority to a minimum degree but has utilized this authority in other ways which have strengthened the financial programs of the district. Tax funds are used for two purposes only. Primarily they assist in financing the cost of medically-indigent patients' hospital care not otherwise covered by local, state, or federal programs. Secondly, taxes are used for financing selected capital projects. While the maximum authorized millage . . . is 2.5 mills, during the past five years the average millage levied has been only 1.09 mills. Approximately 50 percent has been used for indigent care with the remainder for capital project requirements."[44]

Since 1951, the taxing authority has provided millions of dollars for indigent patient care and other millions for capital improvements, including a $10 million bond issue to build Imperial Point Hospital. The large issue was made possible by revenues generated within the system "without pledging any tax funds whatsoever. An important factor, however, is that when the New York money market evaluated the financial capabilities of our district, they were aware of the underlying taxing authority and impressed by the hospital system's financial performances independent of taxes. . . ."

Welch argues persuasively that "multihospitals within special hospital districts offer many distinct advantages, especially in the area of operational costs. The . . . district is able to operate its hospitals which are on a par with the best available, at lower rates and provide more services because of a combination of factors. Centralization of services such as purchasing, personnel, printing, accounting and accounts payable, hospital relations, certain laboratory equipment, and coordination of construction and renovations are major areas. These not only help our patients who pay lower rates but contribute to a better operation of our hospitals, making people and services available that would not be available in our smaller facilities."

There are many other advantages to the hospital district concept, Welch argues, including the fact that excess revenue is plowed back into services for patients and the community. Although once wary of the open press coverage required of a hospital district coverage, he said, "We expect our entire operation to be completely in the best interests of the people in our district, and we have nothing that we feel we need to keep from the public." At a time when people all over the United States are questioning the motives of hospitals, he feels "that the 'openness' of a district hospital cannot only help the public be better informed but help them gain full confidence in their own hospital."[45]

Each of the authority's hospitals is a full-service facility, including general medical, surgical, emergency and outpatient services. Broward General Medical Center, located on a sixteen-acre site, received its first patient in 1938. Its services include three intensive care units, thirty-eight beds in psychiatry, radiation therapy, kidney dialysis and an emergency room staffed by ten physicians. North Broward Hospital, located on a forty-acre site in Pompano Beach, admitted its first patient in 1961. This hospital specializes in medicine, surgery and pediatrics. There are three intensive care units and an emergency room staffed by five doctors. A medical office building will be built at this site. The newest facility, Imperial Point Hospital, a medical-surgical hospital built on a twenty-two-acre site, began receiving patients in 1972 and also has a physician-staffed emergency room. A doctors' office building will be built at this site too.

Many of the services are sophisticated—including advanced equipment in diagnostic and therapeutic radiology. One hospital is equipped with a heliport. Each hospital has its own medical staff organization and there are some 800 physicians who are members of the medical staffs, including 481 active members.

The district management staff works under very detailed policies and procedures. For example, the administrator may approve an expenditure of up to $1,000. Purchases of $1,000 to $2,500 require the authority of the hospital department head, administrator, and Welch. Expense items of $2,500 or over require all those approvals plus the board of commissioners'.

A chart of management organization shows Welch reporting directly to the commissioners. He has these eight departments reporting to him: controller, construction coordinator, clinics, medical education, personnel, publications, public relations, and purchasing. These groups are called "district departments" and they perform the central service and control functions inherent in most hospital systems.

HOSPITAL RESEARCH AND DEVELOPMENT INSTITUTE

The Hospital Research and Development Institute (HRDI) with main offices in Pensacola, Florida, is discussed, because it is not a hospital system, but a unique and unusual organization dominated by the administrators of some of the best-known hospitals and hospital systems in the United States. HRDI is a technical assistance organization for twenty-two administrator members, and in many cases, their hospitals. HRDI became much more than an elite club in December 1975 when several of its members formed Hospital Shared Services with offices in Schaumburg, Illinois.[46]

The formation and early history of HRDI is discussed in a *Modern Hospital* article, "Shooting the gap with The Group," in which its evolution is divided into four stages.

Stage one began when several prestigious hospital administrators got together in the mid-1950s at American Hospital Association meetings to discuss common business problems. They became known simply as "The Group." The acknowledged "father" of HRDI is Donald C. Carner, executive vice-president of Memorial Hospital Medical Center, Long Beach, California. The Group was in touch by telephone and by mail for a few years too—exchanging information about personnel, admissions, receivables and other problems of management.

Stage two began when a friend in industry asked a member of The Group for advice on the acquisition of another company in the health care field. The administrators advised against it. Not long thereafter in 1961, a request came to The Group from another company for evaluation of a disposable infant feeding system, and that's when HRDI was set up as a nonprofit Florida corporation to handle the job. From 1965 until 1973, HRDI confined itself to exchanging information and providing a number of services for industry, such as educational programs and evaluation studies of devices, techniques, systems and corporate acquisitions.

In 1967, HRDI's brochure said: "The 20 Institute hospitals represent a concentrated market which can be accurately described and studied with a minimum of time and expense and with the least possible effort on the part of the client. Should such studies indicate areas of interest, the Institute stands ready to aid in the development of design specifications. All too often products and services have been placed before consumers in the health field, but serious oversights have contributed to their downfall or have required major redesign and retooling—needless to say at heavy expense. The Institute does not imply that these problems will be eliminated when its advice is followed, but it can state with positive assurance that the possibility is greatly reduced."

HRDI administrator-members pointed out that combined they had 500 years of hospital experience, directed more than 20,000 employees, provided care for about 8,000 patients a day, and engaged in negotiations with 6,000 physicians. The 1967 magazine article said HRDI member hospitals had more than $200 million in assets and that the twenty administrators were authorizing expenditures of $100 million a year.[47] A more recent brochure listed twenty-two administrators who were in charge of $519 million in assets and had served as administrators or consultants on construction projects amounting to $616 million.[48] Although the author of the magazine article detected a note of hyperbole in HRDI's description of itself and its administrator members in the late 1960s, there is no doubt that the managers had come a long way. They were wielding a tremendous amount of power in their own institutions and in state and national hospital organizations.

Stage three of HRDI's history began in 1973 when The Group considered a national posture on management and cost containment.[49] In April 1974, during its mid-winter meeting, HRDI set up a national cooperative for shared purchasing and is also establishing a captive insurance company for liability coverage.

The Group did not consider a national system for purchasing supplies and medications, however, citing "strong political reasons" for individual hospitals to stay in local shared purchasing groups; often, HRDI hospitals represented the core facility in a purchasing organization. The Group did see a tremendous potential for savings by negotiating national contracts for expensive technological devices, for example, the EMI brain scanner. Economies were also predicted through nationwide compacts on capital financing (shaving one-half of a percentage point off the cost of money) and nationwide leases.

Carner said HRDI's "real strength is in management. That's what HRDI fellows are best in and what we're going to try to do is pool some of our strength in management." In the labor union problem area, he said, "We might wind up having an individual or firm that specializes in dealing with labor problems to help us stay out of trouble in that area."

Pat N. Groner, executive director of Baptist Hospital, Pensacola, has been a major force in the development of the Institute. He pointed out that HRDI does not have central control or central authority over its members: "In essence we are dealing with a United Nations. Everyone has veto power, everyone has special circumstances and they can or they cannot participate."

He was optimistic, however; for he saw HRDI possibly taking a quantum jump from a local system to a national enterprise. His model was the for-profit hospital system:

> They've demonstrated that this type of organization . . . has application to a hospital. They have demonstrated that through their size they can gain certain economies and advantages from their personnel. They can fix up situations so people can transfer from one area to another . . . all sorts of career path opportunities. There's just no end to a lot of the advantages ahead. One of the biggest advantages early on, of course, was in capital financing. But as long as the market is depressed as it is now [August 1975] this has become a disadvantage. Also, the tax-exempt financing that's now available in a majority of the states has put the investor-owned chain at a disadvantage.
>
> I think a lot of the heart in this whole [for-profit] service is missing. They avoid the free service. By and large they avoid the educational commitment. Now, I believe that if we [HRDI] should develop into a national hospital voluntary federation, we would have disadvantages—we could not achieve the control that they have. But we would have advantages that they could never have. I think we could achieve greater economies of scale. We have more productive plants in relation to equity. They have what—40 percent equity? Our hospitals probably average 80 to 90 percent equity." Groner also said HRDI hospitals had less debt service to carry and the advantage of tax breaks over investor-owned chains. "So it seems to me," he concluded, "that we do have the potential of really developing a concept that other hospitals can follow, a not-for-profit alternative to the investor-owned chain. A lot of communities all over the country would welcome that alternative."

The fourth stage in HRDI's development began in December 1975, when Hospital Shared Services was formed and Donald M. Kilourie was named president.[50] Earlier in 1975, an HRDI "action plan" had been completed by Scott S. Parker, now president of Intermountain Health Care, a hospital system in the mountain states.   That plan built on the management consulting study.   Kilourie spent several months digesting the ideas and visiting HRDI member administrators throughout the United States.   In early 1976 Hospital Shared Services was ready to spin off in several directions, according to the response from HRDI members.

One service to be offered was a hospital financial planning model to bring about some commonality in budgeting between members.   The model would be one developed by Medicus Systems Corporation.   The second service would be a comparative price index in purchasing to see whether local and regional purchasing alliances were actually saving all the money they could. Kilourie was also planning a survey and analysis of malpractice liability coverage buying patterns, and a number of programs in inter-hospital consulting.

Kilourie said Hospital Shared Services also might consider seminars on contract management—"even an offensive-defensive strategy of what to expect when Hospital Corporation of America comes to town." Overall, he said, the objective of the new group was to give HRDI members an opportunity "to pool talents and see if they can make something bigger happen."

NOTES

1. From a telephone interview with Gordon K. Dowery, LTC, MSC, USA, Deputy Director for Facilities and Material, Office of the Assistant Secretary of Defense, Washington, D.C., January 29, 1976.

2. The information on the VA System was received from Aladino A. Gavazzi, Director, Medical District Six, and the *Annual Report,* U.S. Govt. Printing Office, 1975.

3. J. D. Chase, "Veterans Administration," *Military Medicine* (October 1975), pp. 690-693.

4. Ibid.

5. J. D. Chase, "Regionalization: Management by Consortium," A presentation before the American Hospital Association annual meeting, August 19, 1975.

6. Ibid.

7. Public Law 92-541, "The Medical School Assistance and Health Manpower Training Act of 1972."

8. A. J. Snider, "Med School Moving Out of Chicago," *The Chicago Daily News,* April 15, 1974, p. 1,20.

9. Telephone interview with Aladino A. Gavazzi, March 18, 1976.

10. H. L. Lewis, "Hospitals as Classrooms," *Modern Healthcare* (October 1974), pp. 57-60,62.

11. Ibid.

12. H. L. Lewis, "The Mastic of a Merger: Education," *Modern Healthcare* (October 1974), pp. 62, 66, 67.

13. Lewis, "Hospitals as Classrooms," op. cit., note 10.

14. "A Brief History of the Wilmington Medical Center" (Wilmington, Del.: WMC Department

of Public Affairs, April 27, 1973).

15. Ibid.

16. N. L. Cannon, "Three Years After a Merger: An Appraisal and a Look Ahead." *Hospitals* (September 16, 1968), pp. 55-59.

17. Annual Report, Wilmington Medical Center, 1974.

18. Ibid.

19. Ibid.

20. Excerpts of the interview were published in a television and news supplement of *The Philadelphia Inquirer*, October 15, 1975.

21. J. A. Dallas, "How the Medical Center Decision Was Made," *Evening Journal*, October 21, 1975, p. 19.

22. R. E. Brown, "Forces Influencing Development," in *The First Duke University Forum on Health and Hospital Affairs* (May 1965), pp. 3-5.

23. Recorded interview held by authors August 18, 1975 with R. Z. Thomas, Jr., in Chicago. All subsequent quotations were taken from this interview unless otherwise noted.

24. Carolinas Hospital and Health Services, Inc., 1973 Annual Report.

25. B. W. Latimer, "Multi-State, Multi-Service Corporate Model: Carolinas Hospital and Health Services, Inc.," *Topics in Health Care Financing* (June 1976), p. 25-38.

26. Carolinas Hospital Annual Report, op. cit., note 24.

27. B. W. Latimer, op. cit., note 25.

28. Ibid.

29. Telephone interview with Ben W. Latimer, December 22, 1975.

30. B. W. Latimer, op. cit., note 25.

31. This concept is the heart of a national health insurance plan introduced in the Congress by the Hon. Al Ullman. U.S. Congress, Senate, Committee on Labor and Public Welfare, Report No. 93-1285, 93rd Cong., 2nd Sess., 1974, p. 77.

32. M. Brown, "The Impact of Changing Interorganizational Relations on the Policy Structure of a Hospital: An Historical Case Study of a Health Planning Organization and a Hospital System," Dr. P. H. dissertation, University of North Carolina, 1972.

33. R. E. Toomey, "Developing a Comprehensive Hospital Community," *Trustee* (July 1968), pp. 1-7.

34. C. L. Rosenberg, "General Hospitals are Going the Way of G.P.s," *Medical Economics* (September 11, 1972), pp. 104-115.

35. "Greenville Hospital System Phase II Consolidation and Development 1975-1980," a planning document.

36. Ibid.

37. From a telephone interview with Robert E. Toomey, February 12, 1976.

38. Planning document. See note 35.

39. 1974 Annual Report, Greenville Hospital System.

40. Ibid.

41. Toomey telephone interview. Succeeding quotations are taken from this interview, unless otherwise noted.

42. From a telephone interview with Bernie B. Welch, November 11, 1975.

43. Ibid.

44. B. B. Welch, "The Special Hospital District," *Hospital Administration,* (Spring 1973), pp. 21-26.

45. Ibid.

46. From a telephone interview with Donald M. Kilourie, Oak Brook, Illinois, February 2, 1976.

47. "Shooting the Gap with The Group," *Modern Hospital* (December 1967), pp. 81-83, 111.

48. Hospital Research and Development Institute, Inc., undated brochure.

49. Discussed in a recorded interview in Chicago on August 18, 1975 with three members: Pat N. Groner, Donald C. Carner and Stanley R. Nelson. Succeeding quotations are taken from this interview, unless otherwise noted.

50. Kilourie interview, op. cit., note 46. Succeeding quotations are taken from this interview.

Chapter 7
East North Central States

The five-state area that makes up the East North Central census division—Wisconsin, Michigan, Illinois, Indiana and Ohio—contains 299 nonfederal hospitals and 125,901 beds that can be counted within hospital systems. These data were obtained in late 1974 and early 1975 as part of the American Hospital Association's annual survey of hospitals.

Systems activity is quite prevalent in two cities within the census division: Chicago and Detroit. In this chapter, two Chicago-based organizations are discussed in some detail—the Rush University System for Health and the Evangelical Hospital Association. This chapter also includes an examination of three Metropolitan Detroit systems: the Henry Ford Hospital; the Peoples Community Hospital Authority, Wayne, Michigan; and the Detroit Medical Center Corporation. Another Detroit-based system, the Sisters of Mercy, Detroit Province, is discussed in Chapter 13.

CHICAGO'S HOSPITAL SYSTEMS

In December 1974, the Chicago Hospital Council published a map locating all of the hospitals in the six-county metropolitan area of Cook, Lake, DuPage, McHenry, Kane and Will Counties. The council's tally showed 143 hospitals of all types—general, specialty, psychiatric, rehabilitation, chronic and tuberculosis.[1]

In November 1975, the *Chicago Tribune* published a news report entitled "Doctors seeking greener suburb pastures, flee city" related to the council's accounting detailing Pierre de Vise's latest study of the flight of doctors from Chicago to the suburbs.

De Vise, an assistant professor of urban sciences at the University of Illinois-Chicago Circle Campus, noted that Chicago "was once the nation's medical mecca" and is still national headquarters for the American Medical, American Hospital, Blue Cross, and American Dental Associations. Yet it "is the only large metropolitan area to have fewer private physicians today than 15 years ago," de Vise said. "Incredibly, metropolitan Chicago's physician-population ratio is today one-fourth below that of the average for the nation's large metropolitan areas—.98 doctors per 1,000 people versus 1.31 per 1,000." ... A major share of the overall increase in physicians would have been in hospital interns and residents, but they typically spend only one-fourth of their time in patient care, he said.... In the six-county metropolitan area, the total number of physicians rose from 9,270 in 1950 to 13,060 in 1974, he said. But the entire gain was accounted for by suburban practitioners and by salaried physicians.... The doctor exodus has not only shortchanged the Chicago area in its share of the nation's physicians, but has also greatly aggravated the "maldistribution" of physicians in the area, de Vise said. Doctors like to work in wealthy and densely populated communities—both for accessibility to patients able to pay for their services and to hospitals in which to see patients, and for closeness to fashionable neighborhoods in which to make their own home.[2]

This newspaper report came at a time when hospitals and hospital systems in the five-county Chicago metro area were beginning to sift out in new ways, creating new relationships and new power structures. Chicago, the city where the term "clout" was coined,[3] is usually thought of in terms of Illinois and national politics and most often related to the city government's power, specifically Mayor Richard J. Daley and the upstate political machine. But "clout" and "power" are terms that can be used in references to health and medical care too, particularly when in early 1976 various Chicago groups were competing to become the official Health Systems Agency. They wanted power and clout.

The Chicago metro area is dotted with hospital systems and pseudo systems. There are 298 hospitals of all classifications in Illinois and they contain 84,858 beds. Seventy-eight of the hospitals are affiliated with one or more of the state's seven medical schools.[4]

The University of Illinois school of medicine, for example, has thirty-four affiliations at four branches throughout the state, including the so-called Metro Six hospitals linked to the Chicago Circle branch for teaching purposes and tied together through an Area Health Education Center program.

The Northwestern University-McGaw Medical Center was established several years ago to bring about integrated planning and program development between nine institutions that have joined together as a consortium. A major step made through this development has been the merger of Wesley Hospital and Passavant Hospital into the 983-bed Northwestern Memorial Hospital. The original hospitals are now called pavilions.

Northwestern-McGaw has developed many shared service programs, including sophisticated management services that are provided to three affiliates: Women's Hospital, the Rehabilitation Institute of Chicago and the Psychiatric Institute. Two of the center's affiliates are located some distance from the medical center area—the Children's Memorial Hospital and Evanston Hospital. Evanston Hospital will become a system in 1977 when it opens a satellite, the 140-bed Glenbrook Hospital in a growing suburban area west of Evanston.[5]

The Michael Reese Hospital and Medical Center on the city's south side is affiliated with the University of Chicago Pritzker School of Medicine, one of twelve affiliates connected with the University. The Loyola University of Chicago Stritch School of Medicine has seven affiliated hospitals.

One of the area's most unusual affiliations occurred in 1974 between University of the Health Sciences, The Chicago Medical School and two federal hospitals.[6] The Chicago Medical School, founded in 1912, had long used the 423-bed Mount Sinai Hospital Medical Center of Chicago as its primary teaching hospital. In 1974 sixty medical students received their two years of clinical training at Mount Sinai. Early in 1974 it was revealed that the medical school would move out of the city. And in July, the rumors were official. The Chicago Medical School said it would migrate to Downey and use the 1,915 bed VA Hospital there, a long-term care institution primarily for psychiatric patients, as one of two primary teaching hospitals. The other primary teaching hospital would be the 400-bed Naval Regional Medical Center at Great Lakes, the basic training site.

The Downey facility also contains 300 general care beds. The Great Lakes facility handles about 1,000 outpatient visits a day and acute medical and surgical problems of veterans, servicemen, officers and dependents. The plans called for the Downey facility to gradually shift over to general care and become known as the North Chicago VA hospital. The medical school said it would build a multimillion dollar basic sciences facility on an 87-acre site adjacent to the hospital.

Eight key medical school department chairmen resigned in protest over the move. But the school said it was reaffirming its commitment to the inner city by maintaining teaching affiliations with three hospitals, including Cook County Hospital.

Mount Sinai and its clinical staff had the option to move out of the city too, but decided to stay although its neighborhood, called Lawndale, has changed radically in the last decade or so. Once primarily populated by Jews, the area is now predominantly populated by blacks. In early 1976, the physical move of The Chicago Medical School had not taken place. Meanwhile, Mount Sinai has lined up in a close association with another developing hospital system in the Chicago area, The Rush University System for Health.[7] Rush is also closely related to a suburban-oriented system in the Chicago area, the Evangelical Hospital Association (see Figure 7:1).

Systems-building in the six-county area of Metropolitan Chicago is nowhere near complete. In early 1976 other powerful alliances, some only rumored and others imagined, were part of the polite banter heard in occasional conversations about hospital-medical school systems developing in the area. Only two things were clear: The metropolitan area contained eighty-nine hospitals that were not affiliated with any medical school, and the HSA would have a tough time sifting out beds and services and relating them to needs in areas of population expansion and regression.[8]

RUSH UNIVERSITY SYSTEM FOR HEALTH

Rush-Presbyterian-St. Luke's Medical Center in Chicago has embarked on an ambitious dream known as the Rush University System for Health. It could become a prototype regional health care delivery system for other areas of the United States. Conceived in 1968 and born in 1972, the so-called "Rush Network" has the characteristics of a service-business conglomerate. There are medical and health care programs, education programs, research projects, business ventures, and new approaches to health care management.

Rush numbers are big, offering strong arguments for financial and political clout. The system is a combination of two networks, one educational, the other medical and health care.

In explaining their two networks, Rush managers often refer to concepts of a "health university," a "university without walls," and a "medical center without walls." They argue for the need to integrate the educational and care components involved in medical and health care.[9]

The educational network involves Rush University and its three schools—Rush Medical College, Rush College of Nursing and Allied Health Sciences, and the Rush Graduate School—in close academic affiliations with eleven other institutions. These institutions include nine members of the Associated Colleges of the Midwest, the Illinois Institute of Technology, Chicago, and Fisk University in Nashville, Tennessee. The educational affiliates provide undergraduate liberal arts training for health sciences students who complete their education within Rush Network facilities and receive joint degrees.[10]

A health and medical care consortium includes eight hospitals and 2,743 beds fanning out from the Chicago area to a distance of 180 miles (see Figure

7:1). In early 1976, Rush listed one "associated" hospital, Mount Sinai, and the remaining network hospitals are affiliates, the largest of which is 803 –bed Christ Hospital in Oak Lawn, the tertiary care hospital for the Evangelical Hospital Association's system.[11]

The network concept can be traced to the "Campbell Report," completed in 1968 and authored by James A. Campbell, M.D. He is professor and chairman of the department of medicine at Presbyterian-St. Luke's Hospital in Chicago, and president of the Rush-Presbyterian-St. Luke's Medical Center.[12] Dr. Campbell's report established the need for professional and paraprofessional medical manpower in Illinois. He urged the medical schools to make new commitments toward filling the gap by increasing enrollments and entering into outreach affiliation efforts with community hospitals.

Dr. Campbell was born in 1917 at Mowegua, Illinois. He received a bachelors' from Knox College and his M.D. degree from Harvard University. "Our commitment is to meet the health care needs of one and a half million people in northern Illinois," Dr. Campbell said in the medical center's 1974 "report of stewardship." "This is the population base which each of the nation's academic health centers must accept if the entire country is to be served equitably and well."

"Our response must be functional," Dr. Campbell continued, "providing access on the basis of individual choices by private physicians and their patients. Some 4,000 hospital beds are required to meet this standard. They must be distributed through all strata of society from crowded inner city to sparsely populated rural areas. From this requirement we have developed our affiliations with cooperating hospitals, and the rationale for our own branch hospitals.

"Each year more than 100 doctors, most of them in primary care, are needed to replenish and improve the professional capacity to provide medical care for the one and a half million people for whom we feel responsible. Each of these physicians in turn requires the support of five other health professionals, nurses, and other specialists, if the full health care team is to be available."[13]

These are ambitious goals. They mark the Rush Health System as an innovator that has plunged into the middle of most all of the issues now facing doctors' and hospitals—cost of care, accessibility, accountability, doctor supply and distribution and the need for innovative management.

The basic groundwork for the system was laid in October 1969, when Presbyterian-St. Luke's Hospital and Health Center merged with the Rush Medical College. Presbyterian-St. Luke's was formed in 1956 by the merger of St. Luke's, founded in 1864, and Presbyterian Hospital, founded in 1883. The Health Center is an outgrowth of the Central Free Dispensary, founded in 1867 as the first facility of its type in the Midwest, an outpatient center that now registers about 100,000 visits a year.

Rush Medical College traces its history to 1837. It was chartered two days before the city of Chicago. Rush, the first M.D. –granting medical school in Illinois and graduated 10,976 physicians before ceasing operations in 1942. After a twenty-nine-year lapse, Rush Medical College reopened its doors in 1971.

The medical center managers sometimes refer to their organization as the "hub-energizer"[14] of the Rush Network. In the fiscal year that ended June 30, 1975, there were 858 beds in service, 28,808 admissions and 289,394 days of care. The average length of stay was 10.5 days. Average occupancy rate was 88.8 percent. There were almost 90,000 outpatient visits and more than 25,000 emergency room visits. Educational programs were provided for 284 medical students, 254 nursing and allied health sciences students, and 264 interns, residents and fellows. The medical school has a faculty and staff of 1,200,634 attending physicians, and total employees were 5,014. Operating expenses for the year were $88.3 million and the budget for 1975-1976 was $102 million. Total assets were $128 million.

The center provides almost every conceivable medical and surgical service. It is one of the most active cardiovascular centers in the nation—performing 750 procedures in a recent year. Rush has an endowment of around $22 million. Its basic and clinical research scientists attracted some $5.6 million in grants and contracts in fiscal 1974-1975, the majority of which came from the federal government. The health network has received support from such benefactors as the W.K. Kellogg Foundation, The Commonwealth Fund, The Robert Wood Johnson Foundation and the Kaiser Family Foundation.

The Rush Network commitment to be involved in a major way with providing services for 1.5 million Illinois residents also includes a commitment to needy areas and needy people in Chicago. Rush estimates that it is responsible for about 100,000 to 200,000 inner-city people.

A neighborhood health center once sponsored by the Office of Equal Opportunity has now become a private community organization called Mile Square Health Center, Inc. This facility serves a black ghetto area and has recently signed a major affiliation agreement with Rush. Rush provides professional staffing and Mile Square is a source of inpatient referrals as well as a facility where Rush can refer unregistered outpatients.

In July 1971, Rush established a health maintenance organization called ANCHOR, a modified acronym for "a new comprehensive health organization." In February 1976, ANCHOR was providing coverage for about 11,000 persons, about one-half medical center employees and the other one-half obtained through a Blue Cross marketing plan called Co-Care. The HMO has a group practice office facility in Park Forest South, a community where Rush had hoped to expand into primary care through its own branch hospital, and another office at Arlington Heights, also a growing suburban area. In early 1976, ANCHOR was approved by the U.S. Civil Service Commission to offer benefits to federal employees under the Federal Employees Health Benefit Plan.[15]

Another commitment to Chicago's health care needs is Rush's Johnson R. Bowman Health Park. It is on the Rush campus adjacent to the Chicago rapid transit system. This facility is for senior citizens. It includes apartments, inpatient and outpatient facilities. The project director considers it a prototype. Rhoda S. Pomerantz, M.D., said "the time has come for aged patients to be given the same probabilities for quality of care and life, no matter what the prognosis, that we propose to give to others in our population. The older person must not be considered a second-rate citizen."[16]

The huge Rush enterprise is managed by a seventy-one member board of trustees, headed by Edward McCormick Blair in 1976. There is a smaller executive board of trustees. But the day-to-day management is vested in a Medical Center Cabinet directed by Dr. Campbell. The top operations manager is Gail L. Warden, executive vice-president.

Dr. Campbell is a charismatic leader with a vision of comprehensive, accessible care made available through the systems concept. Through his leadership the state has made a major commitment to support graduate medical education and allied health programs in public and private institutions. His report carved out a strong role for Rush. And when money to support new educational programs became available, Rush moved in rapidly with proposals.

The system objectives of the Rush University System for Health are being developed in five ways: (1) expansion through new construction and acquisitions, (2) associate and affiliate contracts with network hospitals and more limited program arrangements with other hospitals, (3) shared service programs and management contract agreements, (4) extension and enrichment of undergraduate, graduate, and continuing education programs in nursing and medicine in affiliated hospitals, and (5) affiliations with prestigious small colleges that feed students to Rush University.

Some of this strategy has worked. Some has not. And some of the strategy has yet to be fully implemented and tested.

A fundamental purpose of the strategy is to ensure the survival and growth of the medical center in two ways: (1) by increasing patient referrals, and (2) by forging links to community hospitals, and other service organizations. These goals must be reached if the Rush objective of providing comprehensive services to 1.5 million persons is to be reached. Rush faces the same problems as any other inner city medical center. Patients and doctors continue to move to the suburbs. And as suburban hospitals grow in bed size and service expertise, fewer patients are being referred into the city to receive care.

In the early 1970s, Rush managers identified two suburban areas that seemed natural for branch facility expansion and the medical center was invited to come to the communities. A site in Schaumburg, Illinois, was to be the site of a 160-bed hospital. A new city area called Park Forest South was to be the site of a second 160-bed hospital. Each hospital was estimated to cost $16 million; Rush would put up three-fourths of the money, or $24 million, and the two communities would each provide $4 million through philanthropy.

The cost estimates were based on the national economic picture in 1973. In early 1975, when final decisions had to be made, the construction estimates had doubled and the plans fell through. The medical center executive board said that its decision to drop the projects was "based on analysis of the economy both nationally and locally, excessive escalation of construction and financing costs beyond acceptable debt levels, and assessment of the potential of the respective communities to be served to provide equity capital at double the original estimates."[17] The statement called on the medical center's management to find other solutions to health care needs in the area.

There were no economic roadblocks in the way of acquisitions, however. In late 1975, Rush leased the 180-bed Northeast Community Hospital, a facility located on Chicago's north side not far from the Evanston city limits.[18] Rush had been managing the hospital on a contract basis for several months. The facility was renamed Sheridan Road Pavilion of Presbyterian-St. Luke's. Under the agreement, four trustees from Rush are members of the board of the ownership group—the Charity Hospital Association. Sheridan Road Pavilion is completely integrated into the Rush management system and will serve as something of a test bed for developments in central management and shared services.

Earlier in 1975, at the request of the state of Illinois, the Rush Network extended its reach some 500 miles south by signing an agreement to manage the 115-bed PADCO Community Hospital in Cairo, Illinois.[19] This agreement was to remain in effect until a permanent management team could be recruited. Rush recruited the team and then began providing backup management services.

In addition to these efforts, Rush has brought together a network of affiliate and associate hospitals located north, south, and west of Chicago (see Figure 7:1). During the first three years of this program, Rush invested almost $500,000 in network hospitals' educational and cooperative health care programs. The agreement of association "articulates the terms of an affiliation relationship" between Rush and the network hospitals, beginning with these purposes:

Figure 7:1

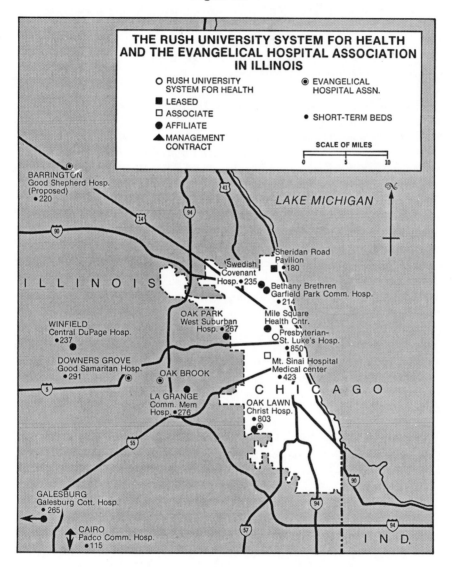

THE RUSH UNIVERSITY SYSTEM FOR HEALTH
AND THE EVANGELICAL HOSPITAL ASSOCIATION
IN ILLINOIS

○ RUSH UNIVERSITY SYSTEM FOR HEALTH
■ LEASED
□ ASSOCIATE
● AFFILIATE
▲ MANAGEMENT CONTRACT

◉ EVANGELICAL HOSPITAL ASSN.

● SHORT-TERM BEDS

SCALE OF MILES
0   5   10

For the purposes of fulfilling common goals of bringing the highest level of quality in medical care to their broad communities, providing high quality education in the health fields, enhancing research activities and achieving efficiency and economy in these and related activities, this cooperative effort is established.

Whereas, Rush ... seeks to provide a broad spectrum of health services to a population of a million and a half persons representing a broad socio-economic and geographical base through a system of relating institutions which unites the academic and care elements, which is manpower self-sufficient, is effective, efficient, and economic and, therefore, financially viable. ...

The agreements then go on to spell out the responsibilities and philosophy of the institution and finally state: "Whereas, (name of institution) and Rush ... desire to cooperate in the use of their respective facilities, faculty, and staff to accomplish these common goals and objectives, Whereas, to implement the foregoing, Rush ... and (name of institution) wish to enter into this agreement, this agreement is executed."

Corporate relationships are then defined. This begins with assurances that Rush and the affiliate hospital will continue to be autonomous corporations governed independently by their respective governing bodies. Joint corporate relationships are carried out through a Joint Policy Committee. These committees have ten members—five from each institution. "The function of this committee," according to the agreement, "shall be to review, hear, and decide upon policy issues which are brought to it by each separate governing body and which affects the well being of the programs and purposes elaborated in this agreement."

Finally, the agreements spell out operational relationships between Rush and the affiliate. "To implement policy to keep the corporate joint policy committee informed and to coordinate the conjoint functions," the agreement states, "a Joint Management Committee shall be established which will consist of four members: the executive vice-president and one other administrative representative from (name of hospital) and the executive vice-president and vice-president of medical affairs and dean of Rush Medical College from Rush-Presbyterian-St. Luke's. This committee shall meet monthly at call of the chairman which will be a rotating position and render an annual report to the Joint Policy Board regarding the status of their relationship and other matters."

In terms of patient care programs and planning, the agreements conclude with this statement:

The concept of inter-institutional programs for patient care is recognized as an effective mechanism for providing health care to a broad population. Both institutions are dedicated to the exploration of programs that will provide more efficient and effective methods of health care delivery at multiple levels. It is anticipated that this exploration will take place through the Joint Management Committee. Health care planning will be viewed in the wholistic sense giving consideration to such factors as demographic information, geographic distribution, manpower production and availability, existing institutional capacity, and need. It mutually recognizes that patient care is enhanced through education and research programs and, therefore, special attention will be given to the cooperative development and integration of these programs.[20]

An assessment in 1974 of the value of the affiliation agreements was mixed on the accomplishments to that time, although the future prospects were considered to be good. In early 1976, all of the affiliation contracts were still in force except one. The 103-bed DeKalb Public Hospital, located sixty miles west in the middle of prosperous corn country, was being converted to a long-term care facility. A successor facility, the new Kishwaukee Health Center, is being managed under a three-year contract by Hospital Corporation of America, Nashville, Tennessee.[21] When DeKalb Public became Kishwaukee Health Center, the affiliation was terminated. A Rush spokesman said: "We have given them [Kishwaukee] the opportunity to seek affiliation, and it appears that they will sometime in the near future."*

Rush's most successful effort in medical education occurred just a mile away in Chicago at Mount Sinai Hospital Medical Center. Rush wanted to widen its urban teaching base into a first class teaching hospital with an experienced faculty and staff. In 1975, Rush and Mount Sinai said in a statement announcing a cooperative course of action:

"In planning for a wider relationship, the two institutions recognize a common objective in encouraging the training of physicians in primary care and in meeting the health needs of urban life. The next stage of cooperation should provide for greater integration of graduate medical education programs, involvement of the Rush College of Nursing and the College of Allied Health Sciences and the Mount Sinai allied health programs, continuing education of physicians and faculties of the two institutions, and improvement of outpatient and inpatient programs and services in the inner city areas."[22]

Rush has moved rapidly to develop the system's management and business capabilities that will allow it to grow and expand. They employed Medicus Systems Corporation, an innovative operations research company that has done pioneering studies in nurse staffing, electronic data processing applications, and systems engineering.[23] Medicus is a part-time research and development arm for the network in addition to its role as operations

---

* In early 1976, HCA officials confirmed to the authors that Kishwaukee's board of directors had cancelled the management contract.

manager of two medical center departments. In many ways, Medicus has grown up with Rush.

Medicus' electronic data processing capabilities were considerably enhanced and broadened in late 1975 when the company acquired Spectra Medical Systems of Palo Alto, California.[24] Spectra is one of several U. S. computer companies that have developed so-called "total hospital information systems." This acquisition should help accelerate the development of Rush's systemwide medical information system.

Three years after the rapid system development program began, Warden said, the goals of the Rush University Network for Health remained as objectives and realistic goals. But who would initiate and coordinate the massive effort, and provide the drive? Warden proposed and the executive board agreed to create the Rush Health System Development Institute, a new organization to handle the massive task.

Institute managers were drawn from existing departments and asked to find out what would work, based on the experience of other sharing efforts around the United States, and what was cost effective and applicable to a broad socioeconomic base. Managers were also told to keep in mind and identify the external constraints and incentives that would influence the development of strategy for the Rush Health System. The constraints were classified as legal, economic, political and social. And they applied to other networks in the Chicago area and in Illinois, including the competition that might be perceived by network affiliated hospitals.

Managers were also asked to consider issues and opportunities in the patient services, nursing, medical education, ambulatory care and administrative services. "It is clear that we have come to agree upon the strategy that shared services be the major focus of the Institute," Warden said.[25] Institute managers developed voluminous and detailed business plans in: contract management; laundry services; EDP administrative services; management services, including affirmative action planning, labor relations and major equipment planning; administrative consulting services; business services; specialized laboratory services; and manpower development and training.

In the summer of 1975, Rush managers were frank about the competitive marketplace they were hoping to tap. If the network objectives were to be reached, they said, the "hub-energizer" (the medical center, including the university) would have to remain educationally and economically viable. Stated another way, Rush would have to weigh its various commitments—inner city, urban, suburban and rural—against each other and achieve a certain amount of balance.

Rush would like to develop an "associated" status with several other hospitals besides Mount Sinai. This would be a way to bring about closer working relationships than are available through affiliation. An obvious "associated" candidate was Christ Hospital.

There are assumptions that underlie the development of a system, Warden and an associate, Marie E. Sinioris, wrote in 1976: "The special role that medical schools and medical school-based hospitals can play in integrating the academic and care elements in the development of health systems must be recognized and capitalized upon. As health care institutions become increasingly aware of potential benefits that may accrue to these voluntary relationships, the full realization of the Rush prototype may be possible. The viability of the concept is directly related to each institution's willingness to exchange individual autonomy for system development."[26]

Ever since the system was conceived in 1968, and formalized on paper in 1972, Rush has lived and breathed the systems gospel. As he thought about Rush's innovative moves, an administrator of a teaching hospital in Chicago said: "I wish that I could get my board and the university to back a move like that for us. Rush will be so far out ahead of us if they pull off these network arrangements that we'll never really get back into the game."[27]

EVANGELICAL HOSPITAL ASSOCIATION

The suburban areas north, west and south of Chicago are booming with population growth. The Evangelical Hospital Association (EHA), sensing the need for hospitals in those areas years ago, decided to concentrate the development of its multiple hospital system in areas west and northwest of the city, "because they saw as suburban life becomes more centered in the local area in terms of jobs, recreation, and education, families are less likely to look to the city for medical services. The pressures of time and distance make local health care a desirable commodity."

Official statements also emphasize the role of EHA in meeting health care needs: "The quality of life many suburbanites seek in their local communities includes access to top caliber medical care. In many sections of metropolitan Chicago, this part of the good life is passing suburbanites by." The statement continues to say that EHA "has the experience, financial stability, and care credentials to deliver medical care in full-service, not satellite, hospitals. And it has the know-how to play a role in changing the health care picture by holding down the costs of medical care and by attracting top flight specialists and family doctors to suburban practices."[28] These are persuasive arguments and they clearly state the EHA strategy: survive and grow by moving with the population and providing primary care.

This focus partially distinguishes EHA from other systems in the Chicago area. EHA's closest counterpart is the 512–bed Evanston Hospital that is building a 140–bed satellite hospital in the growing suburban areas of Glenview and Northbrook west of its base hospital.

EHA's new focus is quite a departure from its orientation of a decade ago. The association, incorporated in 1906 as a nonprofit organization, opened its original Evangelical Hospital in 1911 on Chicago's South Side. By the late 1950s, the association, noticing a flight of doctors to the suburbs, responded by opening Christ Community Hospital in Oak Park as a satellite facility. This was a successful attempt to follow doctors and patients, for the satellite hospital prospered.

EHA moved out of the city altogether in 1972. Evangelical Hospital, sold to the fundamentalist Tabernacle Missionary Baptist Church for $150,000, is now the 150–bed Tabernacle Community Hospital and Health Center. "The EHA felt it couldn't keep operating the hospital with the quality of people and care we wanted to maintain, and the Missionary Baptists thought they could, so we sold it for a nominal price," said The Rev. Paul F. Umbeck, president of the EHA.[29]

The association has another distinguishing feature. It is an affiliate of the United Church of Christ. Although the church does not control the hospital system, there are strong ties.

Sixty-five United Church of Christ organizations in the Metropolitan Chicago and northern Illinois areas are members of EHA. And there are several church leaders on the seventeen-member board of directors. The religious orientation of the system comes through vividly in Umbeck's style. He is a powerful personality, a strong speaker, a huge imposing man. In a reference to the strong leadership within the EHA board, Umbeck wrote; "I have always felt and continue to feel that God brings to us those leaders we need at given times. We look forward to another year of 'Health Care in the Ministry of Christ.' "[30]

The purposes of EHA are educational and charitable, including the ownership of church-related hospitals and training for nurses, chaplains and medical doctors. The organization says it also will operate and maintain "other facilities as may be consistent with the Christian concern of this Association for the physical, mental and spiritual welfare of all persons."[31]

EHA has still another distinguishing feature: It is a multiple hospital system within a system because of a strong teaching affiliation with the Rush Medical School and the Rush University System for Health. The 809–bed Christ Hospital—the word "Community" was dropped in 1975—has six approved residency programs, including a new program in family practice, and in 1975 had a house staff of eighty-seven interns and residents.[32]

An educational orientation is present in other ways. The Evangelical School of Nursing, organized in 1911, is one of the few remaining diploma schools in the Chicago area, and has graduated over 1,100 students. There were 49 graduates in 1974. The school is affiliated with Elmhurst College for some instruction.

The number two manager in the EHA organization is Stephen F. Kasbeer, executive vice-president, who feels that "one of the aims of the EHA is a health care system as an alternative to single hospitals.... One of our objectives is lower costs. Common ownership with this systems approach is an attempt at economies of scale and qualities of scale."[33]

Umbeck, Kasbeer, other top managers, and a central support staff are located in an office complex at Oak Brook, Illinois, west of the Chicago Loop. Within the central staff, Umbeck has line responsibility for development, planning and properties, public relations, nursing service, and personnel. Kasbeer has line responsibility for finance, management information systems, personnel, purchasing, audiovisual programs and a new linen processing center. The association has six vice-presidents, including four persons who also hold the title of administrator, an associate administrator and three assistant administrators.

There are executive councils for each of the three hospitals and the Evangelical School of Nursing, and joint conference committees for each hospital. Overall association policy is made by the board of directors. But the day-to-day power is concentrated in a seven-member executive committee that includes Umbeck as a member.

In early 1976, EHA was involved in an $82.8 million development program aiming at a three-unit multiple hospital system by 1978. The idea is to have hospitals in a semicircle around Chicago. These facilities and the administrative center at Oak Brook will be tied together by telephone lines and the expressway system, making the units only thirty to sixty minutes driving time from each other (see Figure 7:1).

One unit of the system, Christ Hospital, has just undergone a major expansion—a new nine-story wing. This $22.8 million project made Christ Hospital the fourth largest voluntary hospital in Chicago and the fifth largest in Illinois. New facilities include cardiovascular and neurosurgery operating suites and a two-floor medical arts facility to allow the medical staff to incorporate hospital-based diagnostic services into their office practices.

In 1974, when Christ Hospital had 619 beds in service, there were 22,561 admissions, 3,039 births, an average daily census of 583, and an average occupancy rate of 94.4 percent. Total expenses were $23.7 million, including payroll costs of $13.5 million for 1,559 full-time employees. There were 208 physicians on the active medical staff.

Also constructed at Christ Hospital was a large parking garage and a modern, $2.3 million linen processing center that will serve all three hospitals. Other centralized services include group purchasing and an audiovisual center.

EHA officially became a system in early 1976 with the opening of a second hospital, the 291-bed Good Samaritan Hospital at Downers Grove, Illinois.

This $33.8 million facility will serve eleven communities and a population base estimated at 200,000 in central DuPage county.

In the early months of 1976, a third proposed hospital in the EHA system was still in doubt. This is the 220-bed Good Shepherd Hospital to be built near Barrington, Illinois. The estimated cost was $25 million. Six governmental agencies and consumer groups had been involved in discussion and debate about this hospital. Umbeck said there was no doubt about the medical need for the facility, since the closest hospitals are sixteen miles away, but the bed size was the main point of contention. There was a possibility that the size would be reduced by 50 beds, Umbeck said.[34]

DETROIT'S HOSPITAL SYSTEMS

Detroit, Michigan, is fairly typical of the urban industrial areas that sweep across the upper part of the United States. Minneapolis-Saint Paul, Milwaukee, Chicago, Detroit, Cleveland and Pittsburgh all have certain characteristics in common. Great centers of commerce, these areas remain plagued with a number of inner-city problems well identified, but certainly not solved. The litany is familiar: air, noise and water pollution; decaying, substandard housing; abandoned buildings; weakening tax bases; concentrations of older, sicker population groups and ethnic minorities, and explosive suburban growth.

Business and industry continue to move out of these areas. But very few health care institutions have closed their doors. In Minneapolis-Saint Paul (see Chapter 9), in Chicago and other areas, many hospitals and medical centers have made a commitment to help save the cities, eliminate urban blight, and help the people who remain in the cities and need medical care.

Detroit is the nation's fifth largest city with a 1972 population of 1.5 million and a three-county (Wayne, Oakland and Macomb) population of 4.25 million. The city stretches out over 139.6 square miles, several of which burned during the civil rights demonstrations of August 1967. In the ten years between 1960 and 1970, an estimated 156,000 persons moved out of Detroit.[35]

Capital of the U.S. automobile and truck industry, Detroit also has considerable diversification into other industries, such as machine tools, iron products, industrial chemicals, drugs, paints, wire products and office machinery.

There are 33 short-term, general hospitals in Detroit, 9,434 acute beds in the city and another 20,469 beds in the three-county area.

DETROIT QUADRANGLE CORPORATION

Most inner-city hospitals are watching their daily census and occupancy rates go down while their costs go up. Detroit's hospitals and medical centers have reacted to this problem in various ways. In the early 1970s four large hospitals in the metropolitan northwest formed an organization known as the Detroit Quadrangle Corporation. Their primary purpose is coordination of services and long-range planning. The institutions involved—558-bed Mount Carmel Mercy Hospital and Medical Center, 624-bed Sinai Hospital of Detroit, the Grace Hospital Northwest Unit (part of United Hospitals of Detroit), and 402-bed Providence Hospital—are located within a radius of three miles of each other. This organization grew out of a need to consolidate low census pediatric services. Discussions over this question began in 1968 between the chiefs of pediatrics at the four hospitals and two years later the units were consolidated. After another two years, obstetrical units were also consolidated.

Sister Gertrude Bastnagel, administrator of Providence Hospital, remarked:

> The administrators of each of the four hospitals have admitted that the most difficult change of all is to think quadrangle and to speak quadrangle. Each of us most certainly have our own hospitals, as it were, but when it comes to community needs, community resources—what we as a group can do to help cut hospital cost, to improve quality and to provide comprehensive health care services—we are committed to quadrangle thinking.
>
> In summary then, the quadrangle was formed to develop an organizational structure of hospitals and other institutions dedicated to the concept that purposeful planning can furnish the best type of health care on the most economical basis. Much remains to be done. At present however, the quadrangle provides a concentration of physicians, a core of nurses and paramedical staff, and centralized equipment and facilities that make available a far broader range of health care services than would be available if each hospital persisted in an attempt to provide by itself comprehensive medical services.[36]

Detroit Quadrangle Corporation is directed by a sixteen-member Board of Trustees made up of four representatives from each hospital. The five simple purposes of the organization commit its members to: coordination; determining community needs; providing health care services; development, construction, and operation of facilities, and cooperative relationships with other hospitals and health care organizations in the community. This organization is not a multiple unit system in itself, but it is oriented in that direction.

Two interesting observations can be made about Detroit Quadrangle Corporation. Mt. Carmel Mercy is a facility sponsored by the Sisters of Mercy of the Union and Providence Hospital by the Daughters of Charity of St. Vincent dePaul. Both of these hospitals are already tied to regional and national systems. Now they are being increasingly committed to local consortia efforts designed to vertically integrate services within a geographical region. These developments suggest that it is possible for strong national systems to develop while cooperative relationships exist at the local level.

Figure 7:2

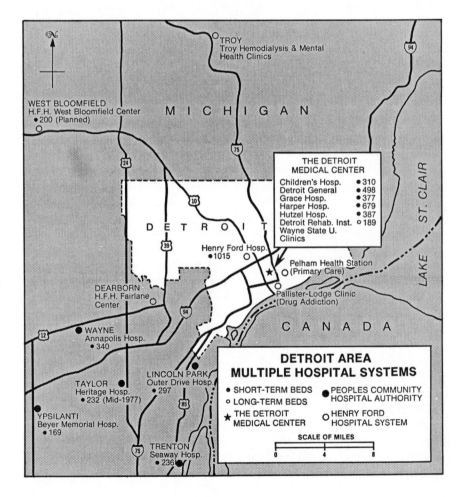

Two well-known hospital systems in the Detroit region are the prestigious Henry Ford Hospital and the pioneering Peoples Community Hospital Authority in Wayne. A third corporate entity, the Detroit Medical Center, is a developing system.

HENRY FORD HOSPITAL

The Henry Ford Hospital has long been a major health care resource for Detroit and Michigan. This prestigious institution is known throughout the United States and in many parts of the world for its excellent medical care. The AMA and private practitioners in the state, however, don't particularly care for one thing about Ford Hospital—all of the physicians there are full-time, paid members of the medical staff. The AMA has never favored a closed group practice and still doesn't. But like its founder Henry Ford, the hospital seems to be a step ahead of the times.

When Henry Ford established the institution in 1915, he went to Johns Hopkins Hospital and recruited the staff. As Stanley R. Nelson, executive vice-president, has said, "Henry Ford had a philosophy of self-sufficiency and he carried some of that right into the hospital."[37] And in many ways, the sixty-year-old medical complex is a combination National Institutes of Health, British National Health Service, and school of medicine.

There are 1,015 beds and eight major buildings on a 20-acre campus in downtown Detroit. This New Center area is in the shadows of the General Motors Corporation headquarters building and the Fisher Tower. The hospital is voluntary, not-for-profit. There are 230 staff physicians and 330 interns and residents who relate to one or more of fifteen clinical departments, each of which is headed by a chairman. There are seventy-eight clinical research programs under way and another thirty-one basic research projects in progress in the Edsel B. Ford Institute for Medical Research. The physicians staff thirty-three specialty clinics.

This huge professional staff is supported by another 4,500 employees. In 1974, there were 26,867 admissions. Expenses were $76.1 million, including $47.1 million for payroll. But the operating budget was about $120 million. Average occupancy rate was 86 percent in 1974. The total assets of the hospital are a whopping $200 million, including a $100 million one-time grant announced by the Ford Foundation in 1973 to provide one-third of the money needed for a massive building and renovation program.

Beyond sheer wealth and size, however, the Henry Ford Hospital is different in other ways. While other institutions are dropping out, this hospital has made a continuing commitment to its fifty-year-old diploma school of nursing. The hospital has had phenomenal growth in recent years into outpatient, outreach and ambulatory clinic programs. Its managers see their hospital as the nucleus for a multiple-unit health care delivery system for a growing metropolitan Detroit and the state. Henry Ford Hospital also wants to reach out to rural areas and develop comprehensive multiple-unit management systems. And all of these characteristics are present within a community hospital, not a giant medical center supported by either the state or federal government.

In summary, the hospital has made a continuing, lifelong commitment to the people of Detroit and the population crowding into the suburban areas of three contiguous counties—Wayne, Oakland, and Macomb. When the development program was announced, Benson Ford, chairman of the board, commented: "We believe in Detroit and are committed to its growth. We mean to contribute our fair share toward the revitalization of the city."[38]

The development plan will continue until 1983. Eight new structures are being added: a $10 million education and research building; an addition to the clinic building; a new outpatient entry; additional parking; housing for medical students, interns and residents; apartments and low residential units; a new service facility for laundry, storage and maintenance shops, and ambulatory housing for out-of-town patients and their families. Of the $300 million to be spent, $25 million will go for medical education, $27 million for research, $62.7 for construction and operation of the three suburban satellite centers, $74 million for remodeled and new housing, and $113.3 million for expansion and replacement of facilities and equipment.

The nineteen-member Board of Trustees operates through three major committees: finance, executive and planning. The board, once dominated by the Fords, now includes several community members, two members of the medical staff, and the two top managers. The executive office includes the two managers, Nelson, executive vice-president, and C. Thomas Smith, executive director. Major management positions reporting to Nelson and Smith are administrators for external programs, physical facilities, operations, institutional services, and staff and personnel services. There are also line positions in nursing, clinic administration and development. The administrator for operations, Dennis E. Sal, is in direct charge of the day-to-day operations of the main campus hospital. Four assistant administrators and the controller report to Sal.[39]

The Henry Ford Hospital Health Care system was outlined in a proposal made to the W. K. Kellogg Foundation in October 1974. The authors of the proposal argued: "The non-governmental, non-profit hospitals form a logical base for the development of a 'system' of institutions and services. Characteristically, they have (1) management talent, (2) financial resources, (3) medical leadership, and (4) community roots."[40] The authors added that such hospitals "are especially well-suited to demonstrate innovation and to seize the initiative in the development of a revised institutions network.

They have a history of leadership in serving the community. They tend to avoid some of the major limitations experienced by public hospitals, academic health science centers, and the proprietaries." Ford Hospital is not held back either by political constraints or the diffusion in lines of authority that can retard the innovation of public and university hospitals. And unlike for-profit hospitals, there is no profit motive and a firm commitment to education.

In the proposal, the hospital said its personnel had been answering an increasing number of requests in recent years for help from hospitals in Michigan and elsewhere: "The need for assistance seems to result from the shortage of skilled personnel and the increased pressures from various sources to improve effectiveness and efficiency of health care organizations. The extent of the need seems to vary from short-term help with a specific problem in a given area of an institution to overall management of an entire organization."

A multiple-unit hospital-based health care system could meet those needs with system objectives: "to strengthen the voluntary, non-governmental sector of the health services delivery system; to improve the coordination among various institutions and programs; to reduce unnecessary duplication and fragmentation of services; to improve the accessibility of health services; to increase the capability of delivering comprehensive health services, and to enhance the educational and research programs of Henry Ford Hospital."

Six program elements made up the hospital-based system. Ford Hospital asked (and was granted) $188,600 to support the program for three years. The objective was to make the systems management organization self-supporting by the beginning of the fourth year. If that didn't work out, the idea would be dropped.

The hospital proposed to continue the operation of the hospital and clinic, "including emergency and unscheduled walk in service." This objective was met with relative ease—for the hospital recorded thousands of emergency room and walk-in visits.

A second integral part of the health care system is the operation of three satellite clinics in suburban areas. The Troy Center, located about twenty miles from the hospital, opened in 1973. Specifically called the Troy Hemodialysis and Mental Health Clinics, this facility provides outpatient treatment for the victims of chronic kidney disease and individuals and families with psychiatric and social problems.

The Fairlane Center opened in 1975 on a sixteen-acre site in Dearborn, twelve miles from the hospital's main campus. This $6 million ambulatory care center provides 24-hour service and can handle up to 135,000 patient visits a year. Fairlane Center provides care in ambulatory surgery, internal medicine, pediatrics, OB/GYN, allergy, cardiology, ophthalmology, audiology, psychiatry, occupational medicine, dentistry, diseases of the ear, nose and throat, psychiatry, psychology and alcoholism therapy. The on-site staff is supplemented by doctors from the main hospital. A program in industrial medicine, including assistance and consultation to business and industrial companies in the area about various phases of occupational health, will be added to Fairlane Center in 1976.

Another suburban clinic, the West Bloomfield Center, also was opened in 1975. Even farther out in the suburbs—some twenty from the main campus—this $6 million ambulatory facility was built on 78 acres of land and includes 80,000 square feet of space. It is designed to be a primary care facility for the area's growing population. "Flexibility has been planned into the structure to allow for program change and future growth," a hospital brochure reported. Stated another way, the hospital's first satellite inpatient facility probably will be built in West Bloomfield. A similar range of comprehensive medical services, including dentistry and ambulatory surgery, is provided at West Bloomfield.

A third strategy under the Henry Ford Health Care System is the operation of four inner-city programs. The Woodrow Wilson Clinic provides comprehensive OB and newborn pediatric care to residents of a low-income community. The Pelham Health Station offers primary medical treatment and referral service to 28,000 low-income residents of another inner-city area. The Chass (Community Health and Social Services agency) clinic serves residents of a primarily Spanish-speaking area. And the hospital's Pallister-Lodge Clinic is operated for the treatment and rehabilitation of the victims of drug addiction. In still another outreach effort, the hospital has joined with Metropolitan Hospital, Highland Park General, and Kirwood Hospital in a shared preventive health education program for residents of the north central section of Detroit.

A survey was made in 1974 by an independent Boston company for the Ford Foundation on the hospital's impact on the community and it concluded: "The tide has turned in terms of the hospital's image in its immediate community ... the hospital has adopted a constructively activist role rather than a passive one in dealing with community groups and community problems."[41]

"One of the basic reasons we are doing some of these things," Nelson said, "is to increase accessibility to the hospital. We have lost patients because they either have no need to come here or it's not as easy to get into the hospital as before. An early symptom of better access is that the satellite clinic at Fairlane is reactivating a number of patients in that geographical area who are coming back to the base hospital for inpatient care."[42]

A fourth proposed objective was stated as "affiliation with additional hospitals, nursing homes, and ambulatory care centers."[43] Objective number five, the extension of management services to other institutions, would be done on the basis of management contracts, shared services on a prearranged basis, and consultations, according to the proposal to Kellogg. And the final objective under the systems concept was a program to extend the hospital's clinical and educational services within Michigan.

Specific guidelines were established in the management services area. The geographical limit is U.S. hospitals within a 250 to 300 mile radius of Detroit. Efforts are concentrating on marketing to Michigan hospitals. Only two to three management contracts will be taken on each year—up to a maximum of eight or ten.

A special Division of Institutional Services was set up to handle the consultation and contract management services. The job of administrator of this division was filled by Alan R. Case, who explains the program in an article for *Michigan Hospitals*.[44] In April 1975, he sent a formal letter outlining the program to prospective Michigan hospitals. Queries were invited. A detailed description of the institutional services available was enclosed with the mailing.

Contract management business, however, was another matter. Generally, Ford Hospital proposed that under this service it would make a joint appointment with the board of the hospital of a chief executive officer. Other appointments of Ford Hospital's executives would be made as needed. There would be written agreements stating Ford Hospital's support for the chief executive in the managed hospital. Another agreement would cover the extent of consultative services to be provided. Services were to be paid on an annual fee basis, billed and payable monthly.

Three hospitals expressed interest in the total management contract; two declined the Ford offer, and one prospect was turned down by Ford. The first hospital is a proprietary facility located fifty-five miles from Detroit that was available for purchase. This hospital was primarily seeking capital that Ford Hospital was unwilling to commit. The second hospital was caught in an unusual predicament. The administration and board had been in on the negotiations, but the medical staff had not. At the moment the agreement was to be signed, the medical staff voted against it. Case's division turned down the third hospital, a 30–bed facility operating at about 40 percent capacity, because it had not been approved by the local comprehensive health planning agency.[45]

Speaking in late 1975 about future management contracts, Nelson said there were "no other real hot prospects. It's time we looked at this program. If there are no prospects, why not?" Would the hospital expand its marketing efforts into Indiana or Ohio? He replied, "Our watershed seems to go into the other direction. And there is an unrestricted resistance to Detroit by the rest of the state. Also, Ford's pattern of organization (full-time paid physicians) is not enthusiastically embraced by all medical staffs in the state's hospitals."

Despite this early negative picture of the hospital's contract management ventures, the future appeared much brighter. In late 1975 there was no other multiple-unit system with such extensive resources trying to market contract management within the lower peninsula of Michigan. Statewide, there are dozens of community hospitals in the 50 to 150 bed size that may want to buy one or more of Ford Hospital's management services.

In a report to the W. K. Kellogg Foundation covering the first year of the institutional services grant, Henry Ford Hospital was able to enumerate thirteen examples of how it was becoming involved in helping other hospitals in Michigan.[46] For example, Ford Hospital had helped Community Health Center of Branch County, Coldwater, set up an electronic data processing system in accounting; Otsego Memorial Hospital, Gaylord, review its patient charge system; three hospitals in the Holland, Michigan area with a fire and safety code project, and River District Hospital in St. Clair design and conduct a supervisory development program.

The grant launched Henry Ford Hospital into a continuing education program for nonteaching hospitals in many parts of Michigan. Also, the state's department of mental health had asked the hospital to consider providing primary care to 300 patients at two state facilities in the Detroit area.

The report to Kellogg said there had been very little interest expressed in the institution-wide management agreements, as "hospital administrators often do not consider management contracts as a topic worthy of discussion with their board of directors, and we have not considered approaching boards with the concept until we learn of a vacancy in the administrator's position...."

Outreach efforts, however, were paying off in other ways. "Many of the services ... provided to hospitals during the past year have not been available, or have been prohibitively expensive, from other sources. To the extent that individual hospitals have been strengthened by continuing medical education programs, in-service education, more effective management development, and the other programs conducted, the voluntary, nongovernmental health care system has also been strengthened."

Finally, the report said: "To our knowledge, no other Michigan hospital has yet staffed an effort to make its resources available to other institutions with more limited resources, although we are aware of at least two who are considering the possibility. A Saginaw hospital had developed management agreements with three small hospitals in the Saginaw area...."[47] Henry Ford Hospital said it appeared that the institutional services program could be self-supporting in the future. And plans were being made to expand the area of marketing into neighboring areas of northern Ohio and northern Indiana.

Nelson believes Henry Ford Hospital is improving accessibility and comprehensiveness of care in the area. And in terms of power, he said, a major confrontation occurred between Detroit area hospitals and Blue Cross in 1975. He said: "As we try to close ranks, existing systems of hospitals just carry more clout by virtue of their size."[48]

THE PEOPLES COMMUNITY HOSPITAL AUTHORITY

The Peoples Community Hospital Authority (PCHA) with main offices in Wayne is a multiple-unit hospital management system with four acute care facilities and 1,042 beds. A fifth hospital has been authorized by the voters and is scheduled to open in mid-1977.

This system has helped pioneer the authority and hospital district movement in the United States. Established in October 1955, and now just over thirty years old, PCHA is a success story marked by growth and community acceptance. This model system was authorized by a special law, Michigan's Joint Hospital Authority Act of 1945. Seven additional hospital authorities were formed in Michigan under the provisions of this law between 1960 and 1975.

The state act authorizes "two or more cities, townships and incorporated villages" to form a nonprofit corporation that can own and operate one or more community hospitals. The law provides for a board of directors as the authority's governing body, whose membership fluctuates according to the population in the area. There is one member for the first 20,000 population in each member community, and another board member for each additional 40,000 persons or fraction thereof. Population is determined by the U.S. census. These lay members, called "trustees," are appointed by the legislative bodies of the communities they represent. The law makes the construction and operation of hospitals possible by giving an authority the power to levy taxes up to a four-tenths of one mill limit.

The representative power of PCHA is concentrated in populous Wayne County, although in recent years some communities in contiguous Washtenaw County have asked to be members of the authority. Overall, there are eighteen city members, such as Allen Park, Dearborn Heights, and Ypsilanti, and five township members. The service areas include an estimated 900,000 persons.[49]

A forty-six member board of directors establishes policy. The executive director and the four hospital administrators are members of the board too. Board policy is further telescoped into an executive committee headed by the chairman of the board. The power structure is decentralized. Karl S. Klicka, M.D., who has been executive director of the authority since 1966, directs the work of the administrators and a central staff. But each hospital administrator responsible for day-to-day decisions has a strong role. The authority had no centralized medical staff depending instead on solo practitioners and small groups in the area. Licensed physicians (medical doctors, doctors of osteopathy and doctors of dental surgery) make application to the hospital of their choice. Their applications are submitted to a credentials committee and the names of those approved are sent on to the board for final approval. There are about 500 physicians on the medical staffs. The four busy emergency rooms are staffed by a group of physician specialists who are paid on a contract basis. Other than this arrangement, however, there are no full-time paid physicians.

"In the post-World War II period," Dr. Klicka explained, "there was only one major hospital in Wayne County, the public general hospital that by law was supposed to limit its services to indigent care." People in the area can be classified as primarily blue collar workers. "They are not affluent people and years ago there was no way for them to get sufficient money to get started," Dr. Klicka explained. Charles B. Cozadd, an attorney who lived in the Wayne area, got the idea of using the authority concept that would by law force the issue to be resolved by a sharing of the expenses based on ownership of property. "We now see the wisdom of the whole concept,"[50] Dr. Klicka said.

For its first decade, PCHA had only one hospital, Beyer Hospital that was leased from the city of Ypsilanti in 1948. In the early 1950s, the voters approved a $4.3 million bond offering which allowed the construction of the first two hospitals. Beyer Hospital, purchased in 1963, was replaced by a new facility in 1970. The authority's hospitals are located in four communities: 340-bed Annapolis Hospital in Wayne; 169-bed Beyer Memorial Hospital in Ypsilanti; 297-bed Outer Drive Hospital in Lincoln Park, and 236-bed Seaway Hospital in Trenton. In 1974 the 996 short-term beds then available in the four hospitals had a healthy average occupancy rate of 83 percent. There were 41,929 admissions and 4,336 births. Total expenses of $41.3 million included a four-hospital payroll of $24.2 million for 2,642 employees. In 1975 the authority had total assets of $78 million.

Annapolis Hospital in Wayne with 340 acute care beds is the largest facility. It opened in December 1957 as a full-service facility providing care in all of the major medical disciplines and general surgical care. Annapolis supports one of the largest alcoholism treatment units in Michigan—seeing 150 to 200 patients a week on an outpatient and inpatient basis. It has a unique cardiac treadmill stress tester and is one of the first U.S. hospitals to implant atomic-powered cardiac pacemakers. The outpatient service is heavy—45,000 visits to the emergency room in a recent year. A new diagnostic services unit was opened at Annapolis in 1975. Administrators estimated that it would be handling more than 40,000 tests and treatments annually.

A fifth authority hospital is under construction and scheduled to open in mid-1977. This is 232-bed Heritage Hospital in Taylor, Wayne County, a rapidly growing suburban area.

How does PCHA stack up against the arguments for multiple-unit systems?

The primary reason the authority law was passed was to allow communities to provide for their own welfare. Urban-oriented institutions in Detroit had not yet caught on to the developing needs in the suburbs, and the idea of satellite facilities was just beginning to gather a following when the authority came into existence. Over the years, authority hospitals have provided care for thousands and thousands of patients.

An authority document made a strong argument that Peoples Community hospitals were doing a good job in cost containment. Room rate per day was not considered to be a good measuring tool, but the cost of an average stay was because it includes charges for many services, including room and board. "Furthermore, a patient's total cost is affected by the efficiency with which the hospital staff schedules its patients in and out, in other words, the length of stay." Michigan Blue Cross had made a report comparing cost per stay for fifty common medical conditions in the state's hospitals. Although no specific dollar amounts were given for comparison to national statistics, the report said PCHA's four hospitals were below the state average costs per stay, both on a daily basis and on the basis of total charges.

This picture of cost consciousness was made possible because the authority's board "provides facilities needed, but doesn't over-build. Because PCHA operates four hospitals it can achieve 'efficiency of scale' not attainable by single community hospitals. For example, by pooling the needs of four hospitals it can provide advanced equipment that a single hospital couldn't afford or efficiently utilize. Through its centralized purchasing, PCHA is able to buy to better advantage...."[51]

There seems to be little doubt that the authority is accountable to the community. The forty-eight community members who make up the board are something like a "house of representatives." What the authority does, or does not do, is out there "in Macy's window," a phrase made popular by Robert M. Cunningham, Jr., long-time editor of *Modern Hospital*. If the people don't like what the authority is doing, they can either complain to their community representative or vote against the next bond issue. Over a period of twenty years, the voters have authorized five bond issues.

The human and material effectiveness of the authority can be measured by occupancy rate and patient to employee ratio. The average occupancy rate of 83 percent is considered to be good, although it might be improved through better utilization of beds. The average census in 1974 was 207 patients and the average number of employees in the four hospitals was 660. This ratio works out to 3.1 employees for every one patient, four-tenths of one percent below the national average.

PCHA can be described as a "benevolent monopoly." An opinion by the Michigan Supreme Court has held that the authority is a state agency because of its taxing power. The authority is not, however, allowed to expand into an area of the state without the invitation of the communities involved. Also, the construction of four authority hospitals has not prevented other not-for-profit hospitals from building in the same general service areas.

PCHA's central core of experts is led by Dr. Klicka, a national authority on hospital planning, administration and federal legislation, who, before he came to PCHA in 1966, managed a reorganization of another multiple-unit system, the Appalachian Regional Hospitals (see Chapter 8).

There are six central management services provided by the authority's staff in a separate building with overall staff management centered in Dr. Klicka, who explained: "My role is a typical one—keep an eye on everything. The administrators all relate to me. I play the role of picking up the best ideas. My job is one of prodding and keeping things going in the right direction."[52]

For the fiscal year ending June 30, 1975, central office operating expenses were $629,373, including $260,911 for administrative salaries and wages. These expenses are allocated to the four hospital units and are included in their operating expense statements.[53]

Other centralized functions include purchasing, architecture and engineering, public information, personnel and financial control. There is central purchasing of all food and supplies. Distribution is relatively easy because the hospitals are located within a fifteen mile radius of Wayne. This program is estimated to save each hospital at least 10 percent on its purchases each year.

There is a wide degree of standardization of routine procedures. There is an integrated system of interchange of professional personnel between the five institutions, particularly physician specialists in radiology and the clinical laboratory.

The personnel director and two assistants work in a staff capacity and handle such programs as Workmen's Compensation and insurance. Each hospital handles its own day in and day out employment program, but the central office coordinates union negotiations. About 1,000 of the 2,600 authority employees are members of unions.

A director of fiscal affairs has a staff relationship to a business manager in each of the hospitals and a line responsibility to the administrators. There is central cash management to which hospitals send in receipts and money is issued for them to operate on. The authority invests in short-term notes and certificates of deposit.[54]

Tax exempt bond financing is relatively new to most hospitals, and the Peoples Community experience is probably the most extensive in the United

States. Its first offering, for $4.3 million, was made and sold in 1955. Other offerings have been made in 1959 ($7 million), in 1961 ($1.55 million), in 1967 ($18 million) and in 1974 ($22 million). Dr. Klicka pointed out that "many states now have hospital bonding laws which are somewhat similar to the Michigan's Joint Hospital Authority Act . . . that now make it possible for all qualified hospitals to seek capital financing through the sale of tax exempt bonds."[55] Seventeen states have these laws, and in eleven other states, "authority exists for hospital financing secured by revenues and for general taxation on a local basis."[76]

PCHA has the ability to collect revenue at the rate of four-tenths of a mill per thousand dollars of assessed property valuation, which as Dr. Klicka explained, "is actually a very small charge for it amounts to only $6 to $8 annually for the average home owner residing in one of the 23 communities." The real impact comes from the amounts paid by industries. "Industry does not complain, and one can go so far as to speculate that they like it, for the assessment method assures that each manufacturer in the area will pay its fair share and the burden to provide health facilities in the community is thereby paid equitably by all industrial corporations and private businesses." Another value of this technique is the growth in property values. When the authority came into existence in 1955, the state equalized value of property in nine communities was $50 million; the value in 23 communities in 1974 exceeded $3.8 billion. The property tax in 1974 brought more than $1.5 million into the authority.[56]

The tax exempt bond financing method is not without its problems. A clear need has to be established first. Three important steps follow this determination: feasibility study, review by legal counsel and review by financial counsel. Tax exempt bonds also face an unusual hazard, Dr. Klicka explained, namely, "the role that can be played by a small community that decides to take an adversary position against a bond issue that the larger community, of which it is a part, wishes to sell."[57]

PCHA has no elaborate long-range development plan. Its expansion must relate directly to population growth and the initiative of other communities that want to become members of the authority. The new Heritage Hospital in Taylor, Michigan is fairly typical of the authority's attitude toward expansion. This facility will not contain any beds for obstetrical care, reflecting the declining national birth rate. It will, however, contain a 30-bed psychiatric unit in response to need and the national trend of providing this care in community hospitals. Taylor Hospital has the potential to be expanded to 400 beds.

The authority's strategy is one of survival. During an interview in December 1975, Dr. Klicka said the local Blue Cross plan had just placed "a 10 percent cap on [increases over] last year's costs," and although this would hurt some hospitals in the area, he felt they could adjust: "These are the kinds of things you can do if you budget well. We don't have any fat. The whole secret relates to whether you can control salary and wage benefits due to size."[58]

Survival and cost containment go hand in hand. And Dr. Klicka believes that cost containment questions evolve around three issues: the management organization, scale and control. "All of these issues get down to one thing—control—and the competence of the manager at the top. He can group the activities so that managers work as a team. He has to stimulate the group. Add all of these things together and you are going to save money. I have little or no excitement for shared services. Maybe you can show some savings, but in the final analysis, control is the essence of cost containment."

THE DETROIT MEDICAL CENTER CORPORATION

The Detroit Medical Center Corporation (DMC) is an emerging multiple-unit hospital management system with a two-part strategy. It is committed to remaining in and helping revitalize the city and to becoming one of the nation's outstanding academic health care centers. Jacques Cousin, president of the corporation, pointed out that hospitals are falling into all sorts of groupings—consortiums, shared service and affiliation arrangements. Detroit Medical Center is a combination of all three arrangements, he said, "though basically a consortium created by a group of hospitals and a university for the purposes of coordinating their planning and program development in the health field."[59] John C. Donaher, Jr., executive vice-president of the corporation, believes the center is "an emerging system" because of the scope of its programs and its potential.[60] The center includes 2,557 acute and specialty beds in six member hospitals. A seventh member of the center is Wayne State University (see Figure 7:2). The university's medical education programs are concentrated at DMC. It owns no university hospital.

Four of the hospitals that are now integrated into the center first formally met together in 1951. On the surface it might have appeared that these institutions wanted to consolidate and reallocate the city's medical resources, and Donaher admits that "one could speculate that these visionaries may have had such an objective in mind, but a review of the minutes of that meeting suggests that more immediate problems—the flight to the suburbs, the accompanying blight of the inner city, and the future of four hospitals known for their service and education very much at risk—were at issue. It was not the high sounding objectives of joint planning and nonduplication that brought together the institutions that formed the nucleus of what was ultimately to become the Detroit Medical Center of 1974."[61] A general goal of survival is what leads to mutations in organizational forms as hospitals try to adapt to environmental change.

The problem these hospitals faced was well summarized in 1954 by George E. Cartmill, then administrator of Harper Hospital, in a letter to the chairman of his board: "Basically, our mutual problem is as follows: four hospitals, each eminent in its position in the life of Detroit, now find themselves located in one of the most undesirable sections of the city. We are literally surrounded by slums." The hospitals were having trouble attracting desirable employees, because of the population flight to the suburbs and the personal danger that employees were exposed to by coming into the slum area. "Patients are reluctant to hospitalize themselves in an area where they do not wish their visitors—particularly their womenfolk—to venture after dark," Cartmill added. He said the four hospitals had two alternatives: they could either move to the suburbs or become community hospitals in the deteriorating areas. "By community hospitals within the area is meant but one course—slum hospitals caring for slum patients—practicing, perforce, slum medicine. . . . In our opinion it would be disastrous to consider the removal to another area of any of these hospitals. It would be, for the community, a cruel dissipation of already short medical time and talent. These hospitals represent a public utility whose importance cannot be reduced to financial value." The Detroit of 1980, he continued, would need one of the finest medical centers in the world, which the four hospitals, Wayne State, and other facilities could become.

The response was almost electric. The four hospitals and the medical school committed themselves to remain in the city. They began formal talks and a Medical Center Citizens Committee began hammering out a master physical plan for the center. Federal urban renewal programs came along at a fortunate time. In 1961, the Metropolitan Detroit Building Fund said it would provide $2.25 million to the hospitals to acquire land made available through urban renewal. The citizens committee reorganized as a nonprofit Medical Center Development Corporation to coordinate the physical development.

Still, the center lacked a clear focus on where it was going and what it would one day be. The Rehabilitation Institute had joined the group, making five hospitals. And the next move came primarily as a result of the August 1967 civil rights riots. Those demonstrations produced a renewed interest in moving Detroit General. But, as Donaher explained, "the corporation's attention continued to focus only on physical interrelationships, not on service interrelationships. Quid pro quo, the corporation would arrange physical relationships, and the hospitals would develop their individual programs." As these programs were being worked out, however, the hospitals began to consider shared administrative programs and developed common laundry and communications systems.

The local planning council then prodded the hospitals into a new relationship. In 1970, three of the hospitals submitted a proposed long-range plan to the council. "In response," Donaher said, "the council tabled the proposal until the hospital could obtain the corporation's endorsement of the plan and demonstrate its programmatic relation to the other institutions."

As a result, the medical center corporation began to identify medical program interrelationships and adopted this policy statement in 1971: "The acceleration and strengthening of the interinstitutional cooperation will allow the center to operate as a cohesive whole with centralized planning and coordination under a single governing body, the Detroit Medical Center," and the corporate name was changed accordingly.

The new corporation then established six written objectives that Donaher said became something of a "bible" and not a "bottom drawer document." These objectives are to: "take care of any patient, medical need being the only criterion for acceptance; design an overall service program for the center; concentrate like services; coordinate the service programs of the center with the service programs of other health care institutions; provide primary and specialty health care needs, [and] focus primary health care on specific geographical areas. . . . Staffing objectives called for a mechanism that would permit physicians to follow their transferred patients."

To rapidly transform these objectives into a workable plan and to avoid the usual lengthy process of deliberations of long-range planning committees in each hospital, DMC took a new tack. Cooperative "program panels" were set up for each of the thirty-three medical specialties. Each panel had seven members, one physician from each of the six hospitals and one physician from the medical school faculty. A hospital administrator was chairman of each panel. Each group was asked to come up with optimum programs "for prevention, detection, diagnosis, treatment, rehabilitation, health maintenance, medical education, and research. For each of these areas the panelists were asked to spell out the services, facilities, equipment, and personnel that would be required." Most importantly, the panelists were asked to identify *where* the programs should be located. "The third step was to define the relationship that should be established between the institution or organization performing certain program components and the medical center," Donaher explained.

The thirty-three panel reports were subjected to detailed examination involving the center's board. Since the reports suggested possibly new or changed roles for each institution and the medical school, a series of alternatives was also discussed between the board and a committee of each institution. In August 1973, the medical service program for the combined

DMC was adopted. Each institution had a particular role. In the process, the total bed complement was cut back from 2,557 beds to 2,257, a reduction of 300 beds.

A plan of consolidation of services was approved in late 1973 by the Greater Detroit Area Hospital Council and the Comprehensive Health Planning Council of Southeastern Michigan. That plan proposed "centers of excellence" be established at each of the institutions and "patients and physicians would be referred across institutional lines for appropriate specialized services."[62]

A presentation to the planning council noted: "By reallocation, realignment, role definition, and consolidation, the institutions of the center are developing a comprehensive system of patient care, education and research. The resulting effect of the strength of the 'sum of the parts' is to provide for an increased effectiveness of the service and care benefits through consolidation of the resources of services, personnel, equipment and finances."[63]

The "centers of excellence" are being developed in seven member institutions. The 387-bed Hutzel Hospital, formerly Woman's Hospital, is the center for OB/GYN care, but also provides medical-surgical care. All pediatric inpatient services have been consolidated at the new 310-bed Children's Hospital of Michigan. Medical and surgical services are concentrated in the two units of United Hospitals of Detroit, a merger of 377-bed Grace Hospital Central Unit and 679-bed Harper Hospital. All orthopedic inpatient care programs are centered in the 189-bed Detroit Rehabilitation Institute. Emergency and trauma care is to be located in the 498-bed Detroit General Hospital. And all outpatient care will be consolidated into a new University Clinics Building being built by the state for the Wayne State University school of medicine. In all, there were four major renovation, replacement and new construction programs under way for the Detroit Medical Center in late 1975. And the center has a huge impact on the city and the state, as Cousin points out:

> The DMC complex is the twelfth largest employer in a city where Ford, GM, and Chrysler are the top three. The general complex totals some $180 million a year in operating expenses, $120 million a year in payroll, and $500 million in assets when it completes its present construction program. Payrolls represent at least $1.5 million in taxes to the City of Detroit and some $5 million to the State of Michigan. Nearly 10,000 employees represent significant purchasing power throughout the area. In payroll taxes alone there is generated many times over the real estate taxes lost by the urban renewal of 100 acres. We are an economic asset to the community, an integral part of rebuilding Detroit.[64]

Cousin adds that "the medical center's presence has influenced others and therefore created jobs. In or adjacent to our 100 acres the Red Cross has built a new $3.5 million blood bank, there is a new $5 million cancer center, the Kresge Eye Institute, the C. S. Mott Center for human development, two banks have established new branches and a third will open next month [November 1975]. Apartments for 400 persons are starting ... just outside my office and some 1,600 [apartments] have been recently completed directly across our campus. Two new churches have been dedicated."65

The corporate organization is headed by a twenty-two-member board of trustees, three members from each hospital and the university, plus Cousin. Each hospital retained its identity as a separate corporation with its own board and medical staff. Wayne State has similar autonomy. "They [the hospitals and university] are totally autonomous from us and from each other,"66 Donaher said. The small central staff is headed by Cousin, Donaher and a comptroller. There are also a few second level managers and secretaries.

The staff has been delegated some rather large responsibilities— negotiations with governmental and third-party agencies and other segments of the power structure, for example. These duties are handled by Cousin and Donaher. All requests for state-approved certificates of need involving over $100,000 must come through their office. This control over major capital expenditures "places a good deal of responsibility upon the DMC and is an indication of how far the institutions have gone toward mutual cooperation," Cousin said.67

The DMC institutions probably provide as wide a range of clinical services as can be found anywhere in the United States. And the hospitals are known throughout the world for several firsts, which include use of a mechanical heart on a human, closed circuit television for surgical teaching, open heart surgery on a hemophiliac, discovery of Cooley's anemia, use of xeroradiography to diagnose breast cancer and identification of methadone poisoning in children.68

In 1974 the six medical center hospitals showed these totals: beds, 2,535; admissions, 72,180 and patient days, 721,180. The average length of stay was ten days and average census was 1,978 for an overall occupancy rate of 77 percent. There were 328,364 outpatient visits and 244,736 emergency room visits. There were 1,500 physicians on the various medical staffs backed up by 6,012 full-time employees. The overall medical center objective is to stabilize the occupancy rate at around 90 percent, a difficult and worthy goal.

About half of the center's 1,500 physicians have an appointment at two or more hospitals. The center's interns and residents are consolidated into a single medical center education program. Donaher said the ramifications of the early planning are "fairly obvious. A unified medical staff is no longer an interesting academic conjecture; it is a necessity."69

But this objective is not easy to reach. Donaher explained that the DMC board of trustees has passed a resolution "urging the medical staffs to get on with it." He said that the doctors were reminded that centers of excellence could not be developed to the exclusion of patients and that patients could not get access to the proper care unless their doctors could get access to the proper hospital.[75]

A common medical record for the seven-member institutions would help bring about the unification. In a "one-bite-at-a-time" approach to this objective, Donaher said, "we're trying to get a uniform medical index—that's non-threatening." The approach to the staffing issue is one of gentle prodding, not pushing, because the ultimate objective, he explained, is a complete integration of the medical staff, a uniform, interchangeable staff arrangement whereby every doctor would have a primary hospital and affiliate status at all other hospitals and be able to follow patients wherever they need services.

Cousin pointed out the obvious advantages in admissions, consultations, discharges, record-keeping, finances, teaching and policies that a unified staff could mean for the DMC; but, he found that "professional interest, referral patterns, fear of corporate medicine, fear of loss of autonomy—all of these very real fears (some more deserved than others) make difficult attempts to weave medical staffs into the fabric of so complex a project as the DMC. But we must and I am certain we will."

Attempts with some successes at medical staff unity have spilled over into administrative areas. Patient reservations, medical records, the discharge department, data processing, central transcribing, and central communications have been developed and turned over to a subsidiary organization—DMC Cooperative Services Corporation. This organization, which has its own bylaws and board (a representative from each of the seven DMC units), is charged with operations and policy of administrative services. Another subsidiary, DMC Shared Services Cooperative, was set up with the same membership to coordinate group purchasing and shared services programs within the center and for other hospitals in the region.

As Donaher commented: "These changes quite obviously have an impact on the usual financial mix that exists in hospital operations; the exact ramifications are under study. . . . One can surmise that with the exclusion of fixed costs through loan repayments and depreciation the collective effect may not be significantly different from what it is now. However, the individual impact may be still another matter."

Despite this positive record of accomplishment, Donaher wondering whether the center could adjust to the change—especially the exodus of doctors and patients to the suburbs—said that "one step that the center took to meet this challenge of change was consolidation of services. Consolidation provides a greater base for subspecialization than can six hospitals providing essentially similar services. Now, quite simply, the center is in a better position to ask the excellent hospitals that surround it if there are any services, medical or administrative, that they would like the center to perform either for them or in conjunction with them."

Donaher added: "A cooperative allows the possibility to offer a service to institutions outside our membership. This might be a program in personnel, financial consulting, or in management contracts. We are going to step back in a couple of years and ask: Is this organization still appropriate? If not, how do we adjust? We [the DMC Corporation] can do practically anything ... everything a hospital can do."

Within the center, he said, "We are getting more and more into operations and services, but we don't have to do everything under the sun."[80] For example, DMC tied in with the Hospital Bureau, Pleasantville, New York, for group purchasing. The center pays the salary of a fulltime Hospital Bureau employee who works from Detroit. "We leased their expertise," Donaher said. He feels that management contracting may be several years away, "but we are thinking 'outside', which is not necessarily a response to competition." He gave this example: "I don't necessarily view Henry Ford Hospital as competition—it has a closed staff and is a fine institution. Competition is not all bad. Detroit institutions may be able to get together and collectively work in one area, say personnel services to other hospitals. The Macy versus Gimbles syndrome is disappearing."

Cousin stated his multiple-unit philosophy well in a speech to the top management group of Samaritan Health Services, Phoenix, Arizona: "What you are doing here and what we are doing in Detroit places us in the forefront of some unique developments which are inevitably coming down the pike and which will place these multi-institutional organizations in a much better position to cope with governmental interference, with unionization, with social and economic changes, and a whole host of other outside influences. Individual institutions cannot cope with many of these outside influences."[70]

NOTES

1. Map of Hospitals in Metropolitan Chicago, Prepared by the Chicago Hospital Council, December 1974.

2. A. Merridew, "Doctors Seeking Greener Suburb Pastures, Flee City," *Chicago Tribune Metro/North,* November 20, 1975, p. 1.

3.

4. 1975-1976 AAMC Director of American Medical Education.

5. Telephone interview with an Evanston Hospital public information representative, January 12, 1976.

6. A.J. Snider, "Med School Moving Out of Chicago," *The Chicago Daily News* (April 15, 1974), p. 1, 20.

7. "Rush-Presbyterian-St. Luke's and Mount Sinai Expand Cooperation," a joint news release, December 18, 1975.

8. While in early 1976 most of the Health Systems Agencies had been agreed to, there were fights between competing groups in many large metropolitan areas, including Chicago.

9. Rush University System for Health, an unsigned proposal and description, revised October 1972.

10. "A Report of Stewardship," Rush-Presbyterian-St. Luke's Medical Center, 1975.

11. "Medical Delivery, A Hospital System Responds," Evangelical Hospital Association report, undated, p. 8.

12. J.A. Campbell, et. al., *Education in the Health Fields for State of Illinois Board of Higher Education*, Vol. I, June 1968.

13. "A Report of Stewardship," op. cit., note 10.

14. Rush managers often use this term in their conversation to designate the medical center as the "hub" of the network of hospitals and educational institutions.

15. From a telephone interview with Nathan Kramer, vice-president for prepaid health plans.

16. "A Report of Stewardship," op. cit., note 10.

17. "A Statement on Branch Hospital Policy," Rush-Presbyterian-St. Luke's Medical Center, February 24, 1975.

18. NewsRounds (January 1976). A monthly publication of Rush-Presbyterian-St. Lukes' Medical Center.

19. "Chicago Medical Center Aids Downstate Illinois Hospital," news release, RPSLMC, September 9, 1975.

20. This material is from a draft of an "agreement of association" between RPSLMC and associated and affiliated hospitals in Illinois, undated.

21. "Hospital Corporation of America," a prospectus, Merrill Lynch, Pierce, Fenner & Smith, Inc., October 23, 1975.

22. "Rush-Presbyterian-St. Luke's and Mount Sinai Expand Cooperation," a joint news release by the two institutions, December 18, 1975.

23. R.C. Jelinek, T.K. Zinn and J.R. Brya, "Tell the Computer How Sick the Patients Are and It Will Tell How Many Nurses They Need," *Modern Hospital* (December 1973), pp. 81-85.

24. "Medicus Systems Corporation Announces Acquisition of Spectra Medical Systems," news release, December 4, 1975.

25. A letter from Gail L. Warden to the Rush Health Services Development Institute Task Force, July 26, 1975, p. 4.

26. G.L. Warden and M.E. Sinioris, "Medical School Based Sharing—The Rush University System for Health," to be published in the June 1976 issue of *Topics in Health Care Financing*.

27. Confidential interview with the authors.

28. Medical Delivery, op. cit., note 11.

29. N. Goldstein, "EHA Puts Hospitals Into Operation," *Suburban Week* (October 22-23, 1975), p. W3.

30. "Challenge," a publication of the Evangelical Hospital Association, Winter/Spring 1975.

31. Articles of Incorporation and Bylaws of the Evangelical Hospital Association (United Church of Christ), undated, p. 1.

32. Medical Delivery, op. cit., note 11.

33. S.F. Kasbeer, "The Emerging Age of Systems," a paper presented to the Council for Health and Welfare Services, United Church of Christ, March 10, 1975.

34. Telephone interview with The Rev. Paul F. Umbeck, January 30, 1976.

35. The World Almanac & Book of Facts (New York: Newspaper Enterprise Assoc., 1976), p. 210.

36. "Summary Description of Detroit Quadrangle Corporation, The Metropolitan Northwest Detroit Hospitals Corporation," excerpts from a paper by Sr. Gertrude Bastnagel delivered at St. Louis University, April 4, 1974.

37. Telephone interview with Stanley R. Nelson, December 16, 1975.

38. "The Unique Reality," 1974 Annual Report, Henry Ford Hospital.

39. Pattern of Administrative Function, Henry Ford Hospital, January 1976.

40. "Proposals for Support to Initiate a Program for the Development and Improvement of a Health Care System," submitted to the W.K. Kellogg Foundation, October 10, 1974. Subsequent quotations are from this report until noted otherwise.

41. 1974 Annual Report, op. cit., note 38.

42. S.R. Nelson, op. cit., note 37.

43. Proposals to the W.K. Kellogg Foundation, op. cit., note 40.

44. A.R. Case, "Ford Hospital to Offer Health Care Management Services," Michigan Hospitals (May 1975), pp. 4-5.

45. S.R. Nelson, op. cit., note 37. Subsequent quotations are from this interview unless noted otherwise.

46. Henry Ford Hospital, Report to the W.K. Kellogg Foundation, January 31, 1976.

47. Ibid.

48. S.R. Nelson, op. cit., note 37.

49. "Questions and Answers," Peoples Community Hospital Authority, November 1973.

50. Telephone interview with Karl S. Klicka, M.D., December 10, 1976.

51. "Questions and Answers," op. cit., note 49.

52. K.S. Klicka, op. cit., note 50.

53. Ibid.

54. Ibid.

55. K.S. Klicka, "Tax Exempt Financing for Hospitals," a paper presented at the American Hospital Association's annual meeting, August 20, 1975.

56. Ibid.

57. Ibid.

58. K.S. Klicka, op. cit., note 50. Subsequent quotations are from this interview until noted otherwise.

59. J. Cousin, "OK—We've Merged—Now What?" A presentation to Samaritan Health Services, Inc., Phoenix, Arizona, October 22, 1975.

60. Telephone interview with John C. Donaher, Jr., December 22, 1975.

61. J.C. Donaher, Jr., "The Changing Anatomy of an Academic Health Center," a presentation before the American Hospital Association's third annual invitational conference on shared services, April 29-May 1, 1974. All subsequent quotations are from this report until noted otherwise.

62. Ibid. Also see "Institutions in the Detroit Medical Center Agree to Shared Medical Services Plan," *Modern Hospital,* (December 1973), pp. 31-32.

63. The Detroit Medical Center's presentation to the Greater Detroit Area Hospital Council's Planning Committee, October 16, 1973.

64. J. Cousin, op. cit., note 59.

65. Ibid.

66. J.C. Donaher, Jr., op. cit., note 60.

67. J. Cousin, op. cit., note 59.

68. Presentation to the planning committee, op. cit., note 63.

69. J.C. Donaher, Jr., op. cit., note 60. All subsequent quotations are from this interview until noted otherwise.

70. J Cousin, op. cit., note 59.

Chapter 8
East South Central States

The East South Central census division includes the states of Kentucky, Tennessee, Alabama and Mississippi. The 1975 nationwide study of system activity shows that these states have at least 123 nonfederal hospitals and 35,686 beds involved in hospital systems of all types.

Appalachian Regional Hospitals has its corporate headquarters in Lexington, Kentucky. It operates ten hospitals in Kentucky, West Virginia and Virginia, and is discussed in detail.

This census area also is the headquarters for three of the largest for-profit multiple hospital systems in the United States. Their influence spreads far beyond the four-state region into other states.

Nashville, Tennessee, is the headquarters city for two of the best-known investor-owned, proprietary systems of hospitals—Hospital Corporation of America and Hospital Affiliates International. These two systems, giants in the field, are also described in detail, to illustrate how this field has grown.

Years ago, James A. Hamilton reported: "Proprietary hospitals are privately owned and managed institutions which are operated on a 'profit,' as opposed to a 'nonprofit' basis. In other words, they are private business ventures and all or a portion of any operating surplus may revert to their owners."[1] He thought proprietaries had been wrongly condemned for having "mercenary and ulterior motives in a field that is normally benevolent in nature." The criticism applied to the few, and in many rural areas they were the only source of care. Data available in 1956 showed 1,208 proprietary hospitals with a total 50,447 beds. Average bed size was 42, but nearly 37 percent of the facilities had less than 25 beds.

The situation in 1974 was drastically changed. Between 1956 and 1960, according to AHA data, 352 proprietary hospitals either went out of business or were sold to community-based or other organizations. In 1960, bed capacity had decreased to 37,000. The single doctor owner of a hospital, and

Table 8:1 The Nine Largest Chains of Investor-owned Hospitals

Name	Facilities owned		Facilities managed on a contract basis in U.S.	
	Number	Beds	Number	Beds
American International Beverly Hills, Calif.	41	5,094	3	433
American Medicorp Bala Cynwyd, Penn.	34	6,996	7	859
Beverly Enterprises Pasadena, Calif.	9	941	1	85
Charter Medical Macon, Ga.	11	1,440	7	962
Hospital Affiliates International Nashville, Tenn.	30	3,531	34	4,713
Hospital Corporation of America Nashville, Tenn.	60	9,508	7	992
Humana Louisville, Kentucky	60	7,372	—	—
Hyatt Medical Enterprises Encino, California	5	588	10	929
Mendenco Houston, Texas	12	1,644	2	444
TOTALS	262	37,094	67	9,435

Source: *Federation of American Hospitals Review,* June—July 1975.

to a lesser degree group doctor ownership of a hospital, is going the way of the mastodon. Current data show 841 investor-owned (for-profit) hospitals with a total 73,769 beds. These facilities break down into three categories: 743 short-term general (68,355 beds), 66 psychiatric (4,169 beds) and 32 facilities in an all-other category (1,245 beds).

The greatest proportion of investor-owned hospitals are managed by thirty-two corporate chains that have appeared on the American scene, particularly since the passage of Medicare and Medicaid. The thirty-two chains own 379 hospitals (51,044 beds) and are prime examples of multiple-unit management systems. They are involved in a considerable export business too. Chains also contract manage more than 100 hospitals in the United States and foreign countries. The table summarizes statistics available in mid-1975 for the nine largest investor-owned corporations. These organizations own 262

U.S. hospitals, 37,094 beds, and through contract management they have a significant influence over another 67 U.S. hospitals with 9,435 beds.

APPALACHIAN REGIONAL HOSPITALS

John L. Lewis, the bushy-browed, long-time president of the United Mine Workers of America, was one of the most powerful labor leaders of this century. He ruled the UMW with an iron hand and was able to negotiate unprecedented benefits for miners in the coal fields of the Appalachian Region, and elsewhere. By the early 1950s, Lewis was unhappy with the quality of medical care that union members and their families were receiving in the proprietary hospitals of Central Appalachia. Out of that discontent the Miners Memorial Hospital Association (MMHA) was organized to provide a system of hospitals in areas of need. In 1953-1954, Lewis presided at the dedication of five hospitals that became the nucleus of one of the most interesting and innovative multiple-unit systems in the United States.[2] In the late 1950s, five more facilities were added to MMHA building a system stretching from Beckley, West Virginia, in the north, and running on a zig-zag course southwest to Middlesboro, Kentucky.

Lewis never really wanted the UMW to get into the business of building and owning hospitals. He supposedly asked the industrialist, Henry J. Kaiser, to develop something like an "Appalachian Kaiser System" to serve the medical needs of his miners. But Kaiser didn't go along with the idea.[3]

The UMW through its Welfare and Retirement Fund made policy and essentially ran the hospitals from its central office in Washington.[4] While the hospitals were open to non-UMW-supported patients, the facilities of the MMHA were always looked on in their communities as either "the miners' hospital" or "the UMW hospital." In addition to absentee ownership and management, therefore, there was no community focus.

A decade after Lewis opened the hospitals, UMW said its fund could no longer support four of the hospitals. The communities or another organization would have to take them over within a year or the hospitals would be closed. The demand for care had not gone down, but the demand for coal had. The intertwining problems of (1) rising cost of care and (2) hospital deficits threatened the fiscal integrity of the UMW fund.[5]

A Presbyterian minister in Harlan, Kentucky, recognized the futility of the situation. The communities had neither the money nor the management know-how to run the hospitals. He appealed to the Board of National Missions of the United Presbyterian Church. The board set in motion a number of events that culminated on October 1, 1963, when Appalachian Regional Hospitals (ARH), a nonprofit, nonchurch corporation began operating the five hospitals. The remaining five hospitals were added to the system in 1964.[6]

The ARH system today includes ten hospitals with a total of 1,036 short-term (intermediate) beds and 173 long-term beds (see Figure 8:1). The AHA 1975 *Guide Issue,* which includes statistics for the year 1974, had available information on all of the system's hospitals except Morgan County. These data show that nine ARH facilities had 33,862 admissions, an average census of 698 patients and an average occupancy rate of 61.2 percent. During the reporting year, there had been 6,772 births while total expenses came to $35.8 million for 2,290 full-time employees.

But this is only part of the story. The comprehensiveness of the ARH system is almost unique in the United States. Each hospital has an emergency room and outpatient clinic. Eight of the facilities provide home health care services and there are extended care facilities at four hospitals.

The very fact that the system is comprehensive and responsive to the needs of its patients has meant that ARH has been in something of a crisis situation ever since its founding more than twelve years ago. The three presidents of

Figure 8:1

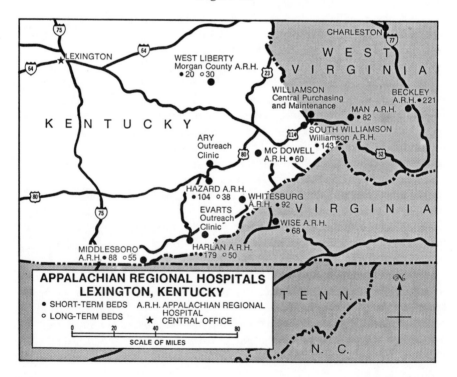

ARH have faced massive problems related to the same continuing issue: reimbursement from the federal government, four state governments, Blue Cross and other third parties.[7]

Nine months after ARH took over, the five hospitals had run up a deficit of $630,385 because they were serving people who could not pay. But the ARH board went ahead and bought the remaining five hospitals. A total investment of $8 million bought ten hospitals worth more than $30 million. The State of Kentucky, the UMW fund and a Kentucky insurance company helped stave off financial disaster with direct support for indigent care and short-term loans.

Karl S. Klicka, M.D., the first president of the ARH, spent much of his three years with the system trying to alleviate the financial crisis and reorient the hospitals toward their communities. ARH, Dr. Klicka said, "accepted an organization that had been directed by a strong central authority. The operational manual and personnel policy manual left very little flexibility to the unit hospital administrators. These hospitals had not cultivated the interest of the lay leadership in their communities. The hospitals were owned by the Welfare and Retirement Fund, UMW, and all important administrative decisions were made in Washington, D.C. My trustees instructed me to re-organize the system and to begin by establishing these hospitals as community hospitals in the truest sense."

Dr. Klicka, now executive director of Peoples Community Hospital Authority, Wayne, Michigan (see Chapter 7), pointed out that the ARH board of trustees had legal authority over the hospitals; central management offices were established in Lexington, Kentucky, about seventy miles west of the closest ARH hospital. In an attempt at local autonomy, advisory councils for the hospitals were established in each of the ten communities. As Dr. Klicka explained, "They [the council members] recognized and fully accepted our intention to have them work through the individual hospital administrators who in turn would be responsible to me, the president and chief executive officer of the corporation, who in turn would be responsible to the trustees." Two members of each advisory council were elected to the ARH board of trustees in an attempt to tie the system together.

The early ARH management faced similar problems to those encountered by Alfred P. Sloan, because "Sloan ... had the responsibility of creating the organizational pattern for General Motors. He faced, and dealt with, the question of balance between centralization and decentralization." Dr. Klicka said the ARH objective was "to maintain the type of working relationship between the units and the central office that will stimulate the individual communities to maximum levels, while at the same time retaining sufficient control centrally to assure compliance with trustee policy in all matters."[8]

Dr. Klicka was convinced that by 1966 the hospitals had been converted to a community orientation.

The second president of ARH, T. P. Hipkens, served the system from September 1966 until his resignation in September 1973. Under Hipkens' direction, ARH underwent rapid development into intensive, extended and home health care. He established three special units for rehabilitation, a stroke center, three emergency care centers, a mental health unit and other pioneering programs. ARH developed mobile transportation units. Land was made available at six of the hospitals for the construction of doctors' office buildings. A division of continuing education was established, and ARH began experimenting with the use of paraprofessionals.[9]

By June of 1968, the ARH deficit had been reduced to $60,000 and many of the short-term loans had been paid off. But by early 1973, the rapid development program and inadequate third-party reimbursement policies had ARH seriously in the red. When Hipkens resigned, the chairmanship of the thirty member board of directors had just been turned over to David K. Heydinger, M.D., a surgeon and associate professor of clinical anatomy at Ohio State University, chief of general surgery at Riverside Methodist Hospital and heavily engaged in basic and clinical research.

Dr. Heydinger, a board member since the inception of ARH, traveled throughout the system to see what should be done. Based on his assessment, the board asked Dr. Heydinger to take over as president and he accepted, saying: "I was so enmeshed in illness care at Columbus that I had gone as far as I could go; the ditch I was digging was getting deeper and deeper. I assume one-thirtieth of the responsibility for what happened."

After two years in the job, Dr. Heydinger believes he has some, but certainly not all, of the answers. He has moved to restructure the ARH system in several ways. "We have been highly centralized—now we are going just the other way. Our idea is to get away from ARH as the owners of the hospitals; the people who use the hospitals own them."[10] The advisory councils that Dr. Klicka established have been replaced by local boards of trustees. This new approach was outlined in the board's statement of operating policy in February 1974. That statement also referred to the crises over the past decade and related the system's problems to

first, its commitment to keep the original MMHA hospitals open and operating; second, its ongoing commitment to the principle of providing quality health care for all, regardless of ability to pay; and, third, the inadequacy of government health insurance and other sources of revenue to cover the costs of services rendered to ARH's predominantly poor and elderly service population.

Notwithstanding these financial crises, what began as a rescue operation [ARH] has evolved into a nationally recognized model of health care delivery. The period of growth and change has seen traditional acute-care hospitals, linked by centralized management and strengthened by the concomitant sharing of resources, evolve into a system of health care with greatly enhanced capacity for service and greatly expanded potential for the future. The system provides a network of coordinated services and levels of health care in a rural, mountainous region which is unique in the United States.

The board statement said the future offered many challenges and that those challenges "require the adoption of changes in the governance of the ARH system as a means of realizing and honoring its fundamental principles." The board statement noted seven values of the centralized support services: (1) new programs can be developed and implemented rapidly; (2) The use of systems financial planning and forecasting, and systems accounting procedures can relieve individual hospitals of the burdens imposed by the complexities of health care financing mechanisms. Moreover, since the system as a whole represents a regional service capacity, the system can speak with greater authority and representation to governmental and private health insurors, and to other sources of capital for the financial needs of services and programs; (3) a logistical value in volume buying of supplies and pharmaceuticals and scheduled maintenance of plant and equipment; (4) system wide coordination of personnel recruitment, training and development; (5) a shared management pool of experts and modern business tools, such as electronic data processing, and (6) advantages in public affairs because "the system ... brings to bear on outside audiences the individual community attitudes and requirements, and in a forceful way expresses their needs in such areas as seeking changes in public policy in health financing."

The board underlined the purpose of the system—to serve the individual hospitals and their patients, and not the system. The board must ensure that it doesn't stifle flexibility and initiative at the local level, the statement added, and the way to do this was "to establish parameters for each level of capacity, and to establish the means for delegating authority to the local level." Each of the hospitals was evolving into a community health center, and "quite simply, the provision of health services with its attendant social and financial ramifications, especially in a regional area of Appalachia, is too important to be the sole province of either administration represented by the hospital administrator or medicine represented by the physician. Lay people must be more involved, in a responsible way, in order to reconcile the considerations of medical science and business functions with the needs of the people."[11]

The central board could not delegate its *responsibility,* the statement said, but it could delegate its *authority.* And that's what has been done. Ten local governing boards now have a considerable amount of authority—medical staff privileges, management of local operations, quality of care and utilization review, planning of facilities and services, development of local financial support, cooperative efforts with other providers in the area and public affairs and public awareness of the ARH health care system.

Dr. Heydinger says that the central board, a prestigious group of individuals including former governors of Kentucky and West Virginia, is "performance-oriented while the local boards are operations-oriented." And the central board is no longer self-perpetuating; members may serve a maximum of two, three-year terms. The current (1975-76) chairman is James H. Harless, a coal and lumber businessman from Gilbert, West Virginia.

The ARH system has also continued to expand its outreach efforts. "We have about 150 four-wheeled vehicles traveling the mountains all the time," Dr. Heydinger said. These mobile units contain home health aids, pediatric nurse practitioners, physicians assistants and health education specialists. Central Appalachia presents a tremendous challenge because of the distances involved, distances that in Dr. Heydinger's opinion, "make cost benefit determinations almost impossible."[12] In 1975, Dr. Heydinger traveled about 30,000 miles by car—usually the only way to get from one place to another. Interstate highways and the new Mountain Parkway will improve the area's gross transportation system, but not the need to drive on the gravel and dirt roads that snake up and down the creeks and hollows of ARH's service areas.

The rapid development of the ARH system has also included pioneering programs now being duplicated in other areas of the United States. The Hazard Children's Service Program, for example, "is a comprehensive preventive health and ambulatory care program for infants, children, and pregnant women in the Hazard-Perry County area of eastern Kentucky." It was originally begun by a board-certified pediatrician at the hospital in Hazard and was restricted to preventive health outreach programs in the homes of children born in a five-county service area. Through a Robert Wood Johnson Foundation grant, it has been expanded to include hospital-based services. The grant also provided for an evaluation of the effectiveness of the program. "The long-range goal," according to ARH, "is to maximize sound physical, mental, and psychosocial functioning of children and their families who live in the area.[13] Dr. Heydinger explained that this program is staffed by pediatric nurse practitioners and specialists in OB/GYN. The program "is having an apparent impact of kinds when [the children] get to school, but trying to assess it is difficult."[14]

At the ARH hospital in Beckley, West Virginia, there is a comprehensive alcoholism and mental health crisis intervention treatment center. But the most critical need, services for the elderly, is still only a dream in Dr. Heydinger's mind: "I don't know a group more forgotten than the elderly, unless it is the dying. The people are totally overcome with apathy... they have a sense of total helplessness. And many of them are living in 10 by 12-foot rooms." Hospitals need to try everything to help solve this problem, he believes, "from day care and yoga to transcendental meditation and biofeedback."[15]

Other innovative programs include two primary care centers that have been organized out of the hospital in Hazard. These centers, Homeplace and Hindman, include holding, obstetrical, and emergency beds. Each center employs a wide range of specialists and primary care physicians, and there is a strong emphasis on dental care.

The ARH system has permanent facilities in eighteen communities (see Figure 8:1), including the ten hospital locations, the corporate office in Lexington, Kentucky, a central management services group in Williamson, West Virginia, and "outreach stations" in Wheelwright and Phelps, Kentucky.

The Office of the President is responsible for development and fund raising, public information, planning, budgeting, and personnel and labor relations. Dr. Heydinger has three other main divisions reporting to his office: support services, hospital operations and fiscal affairs. The support services include: a mail out pharmacy with average volume of 1,200 to 1,500 prescriptions a day; central pharmacy services, including a unique computerized drug interaction monitoring system; purchasing; material management and central maintenance. The fiscal affairs division includes such functions as accounting, payroll, electronic data processing and accounts payable.[16]

The central office staff was faced with a tough problem less than two months after Dr. Heydinger was named president: a strike at all of the hospitals that lasted almost four months and temporarily crippled the system. The central issue was wages. "The hospitals are political because they are big employers," Dr. Heydinger said. The April to July 1974 strike went to arbitration and a decision was handed down in September granting retroactive pay increases. But the decision came so late in the year that it was impossible to adjust prospective rate formulas with third-parties. An estimated 1,800 of the system's 2,000 nonprofessional employees are union members.

Late in 1975 Dr. Heydinger said, "All of the units are running deficits on their hospital operations." The 1975 deficit was about $2.1 million, compared to $556,000 in 1974.   The strike had an impact, he said, but the primary problem was "overexpansion of program.   The extended care facilities have killed us, and there are still two new facilities under construction."

The Appalachian Regional Commission "has been of great help to us in the past six or eight months," Dr. Heydinger said, "by providing deficit financing. This system out-paced itself, but the ARC demanded that." What's badly needed he feels is some decision on a more equitable means of reimbursing the ARH system, its ten hospitals and dozens of outpatient and outreach efforts. Fifty percent of the system's patients are reimbursed through Medicare and Medicaid, 27 percent through the UMW Welfare & Retirement Fund, 11 percent are self-pay, and the remaining 5 to 6 percent of care is delivered free.

The system doesn't have a tax base to draw on as compared to a county or regional hospital authority.   Local philanthropy is practically nonexistent, although the new community focus of boards may help that situation. Kentucky passed a coal severance tax in 1975 designed to return money to the communities where the coal was mined.   ARH should receive some benefits from that tax, even though Dr. Heydinger said the impact would be slight. None of the four states in ARH service areas allows for tax-exempt bond financing.   The system was able to borrow $6 million in the money market several years ago, but its bonds received a BB medium grade rating by Standard & Poor's.

Running a system that is about 80 percent cost reimbursed is the continuing critical issue that Dr. Heydinger and his associates face.   If the reimbursement formulas can't be brought in line more nearly to costs, the only option will be to cut services.

"The basic problem of just getting to the next town is where you get caught in cost:benefit," he said.   The system's hospitals are on a prospective, all-inclusive rate system with no itemization of bills for patients.   Blue Cross has complained about the average daily cost, he said, "and it was high.   But we argued for a comparable, per incident cost.   We have peer review in all of our hospitals and the length of stay is so much lower than the national average—around 5.8 to 5.9 days.   So we worked up a system of relative value units that is a much more equitable way to look at what you charge."

What he called the "horrendous drain" of low occupancy rates in the ECFs will take a different kind of initiative, however.   The key to solving this problem, he believes, is to educate the system's physicians on how to use the units and to ensure them they will get paid.   ARH has around 350 physicians who work in the ten hospitals and dozens of outpatient units.   After the issue of reimbursement, physician manpower is the most critical problem.   The turnover of doctors is rapid.   Most of the physicians are foreign medical graduates.   The sixteen doctors who provide care at the Man, West Virginia, hospital are all foreign medical graduates.   Rural physicians are not reimbursed on the same level as their counterparts in urban areas because usual and customary fees are lower.

Dr. Heydinger says he was not really able to devote full attention to the system and its problems until September 1974—after the long and disturbing strike. He believes it takes "about two years to filter through a system." But he has moved on four fronts: board structure; physician recruitment; potential systems objectives that are described in his document "Objective Total Health: A Request for Funding,"[17] and a new marketing plan.

The 33-member central board, he said, is "no longer a 'yes' board. It is about equally composed of 'movers and shakers, and bottom-liners.' "[18] The local governing boards, he believes, are showing more initiative in their own communities and are beginning to plan for the future. The local board members are no longer members of the central board. The administrator and one or two physicians on the medical staff must be members of the local board, but they cannot become president. His document on recruitment of doctors readily identifies needs by specialty and geographical area. It also lists external forces "that hinder the overall physician recruitment programs: lack of adequate housing; lack of modern shopping centers; isolation, and distance from university medical centers."[19] There is neither a university medical school nor large nonprofit teaching hospital-medical center located within ARH's service areas. The University of Kentucky and the West Virginia University medical centers have some teaching programs within systems hospitals and the National Health Service Corps has supplied a few doctors. Dr. Heydinger hopes a four-year medical school that may develop around Marshall University, Huntington, West Virginia, through a new program by the Veterans Administration, may one day bring more U.S.-trained doctors to the area. One answer, he believes, is to educate the M.D.s in the area so that they get caught up in the thread and fabric of life in Central Appalachia and don't want to leave. Younger and middle age people are returning to the hills of Kentucky, West Virginia and Virginia. As manufacturing industries have slacked off in the upper midwest, coal is booming back home.

"Objective: Total Health" is a combination of Dr. Heydinger's philosophy and observations on the world of health care together with a review of potential political developments in the United States.[20] He argues that quality health care must be based on outcomes and not the process of providing care in acute hospitals. He proposes that the doctors of Central Appalachia band together and become a living test laboratory for delivery system models and innovative approaches to care. "I needed to get to 1,500 to 2,000 physicians. I got to lots of them, but not that many. My new idea is a different way to this same approach," Dr. Heydinger said.[21]

Early in 1976, Dr. Heydinger proposed to the central board of ARH that a new corporation be formed and called Appalachian Health System. "We've got to get some profit," he said, "in order to do what needs to be done, establish an aging center for example, and fill in the chink holes within the system." All of the ARH shared service and management services programs would be transferred to the profit-making arm. The system already provides group purchasing and various management and consulting services to other institutions.

A second proposal will be made to the board to move the corporate headquarters from Lexington to a community closer to the geographical center of the system, perhaps Whitesburg, Kentucky, or Williamson, West Virginia.

ARH managers have prepared detailed shared services marketing plans, including an analysis of the competition in the service areas of the four states. And the competition can be rough. In Beckley, West Virginia, for example, Hospital Corporation of America has opened a new 135-bed Raleigh General Hospital; most of the doctors on the OB/GYN staff once practiced at the ARH facility in Beckley. "We are in direct competition with the facility in Beckley," Dr. Heydinger said, "and HCA has made proposals to take over the whole ARH system." In other communities, the competition is of a different type: other hospitals taxi indigent patients who are out of benefits to the ARH facilities. Meanwhile, Dr. Heydinger said: "We are already getting some proposals from other hospitals in the area that want us to take them over."

HOSPITAL CORPORATION OF AMERICA

Thomas P. Frist, M.D., had a very successful medical practice in the Nashville, Tennessee area. Five of the state's governors had been his patients. By the late 1950s, his practice was so successful and beds were in such short supply that he decided to build his own hospital. In 1960, he opened Park View Hospital.[22]

One of Dr. Frist's patients was Jack C. Massey, a pharmacist, successful businessman, and long-time chairman of the board of Baptist Hospital in Nashville. Massey owned his own surgical supply business, the sale of which made him a multimillionaire. Using that capital, Massey bought a company called Kentucky Fried Chicken from a man who went by the name of "Colonel Sanders." Along with his friend John Y. Brown, Massey nourished the company along and Kentucky Fried Chicken went public. The success of Colonel Sanders' special recipe of herbs and spices, a formula that turned ordinary fried chicken into a "finger lickin' good" product, made Kentucky Fried Chicken a glamour stock of the 1960s.

Dr. Frist, meanwhile, saw that his hospital was operating at costs and charges less than those of competing hospitals in Nashville. A doctor at a hospital in Lewisburg, Tennessee, was experiencing a bed demand problem too. He asked Dr. Frist for help. Based on this business potential, Dr. Frist, his son (Thomas P. Frist, Jr., M.D.), Henry Hooker and Massey formed Hospital Corporation of America (HCA) on August 9, 1968, by changing the corporate name of Park View Hospital.

By the end of the decade, more than 100 companies had been formed in the United States to provide health care in hospitals and nursing homes. In late 1975 there were thirty-two major for-profit multiple-unit management corporations that owned and operated hospitals.

The formation of HCA was a pioneering venture. It occurred a little over three years after Medicare and Medicaid became law. There was a high demand for new beds. Comprehensive health planning agencies were relatively weak. State certificate of need laws were an idea whose time had not quite come. And consumer pressures about the rising cost of care had not generated enough concern in the state capitals for rate-setting and rate-regulation programs to convince legislators that these concepts should become law.

The voluntary hospital sector reacted with emotion to the formation and growth of the chains. The most frequently heard criticisms were that the proprietary chains "skim the cream," don't provide free care, don't offer high-cost and low-income services, and don't absorb the costs of medical education.[23]

More than seven years after HCA was formed, most of these criticisms are still being heard, but the voices are neither as loud nor heard as often. And the criticisms have meant very little to the ability of the chains to grow. Voluntary hospitals are now looking more and more to the for-profit chains, their management systems and techniques, for guidance in forming not-for-profit hospital systems.

Some of the emotion is seeping out of the arguments against the chain hospitals. There is a detente of sorts in light of events of the early 1970s. Through their trade organization, the Federation of American Hospitals, for-profit facilities have mustered quite a lot of political muscle in Washington. Through a good public relations program, for-profit chains now have some of their peers thinking of them as investor-owned facilities. Through their trade organization and its legal staff, the chains are willing to fight some of the biggest battles of all: the need for adequate reimbursement formulas from the federal and state governments and the need for economic freedom without the constraints of bureaucratic-ridden state regulatory and rate-setting agencies.[24] Meanwhile, the chains have continued to grow.

By the end of June 1975, HCA owned or leased fifty-nine U.S. hospitals and

managed another six—some 10,112 beds in all.   The corporation had
negotiated two other management contracts for hospitals under construction
in the United States, in addition to contracts to manage three foreign
hospitals (see Figure 8:2).   By the end of 1976, HCA planned to open six
more new hospitals in the United States and wrap up negotiations on
additional domestic management contracts.   The HCA's domestic goal is to
build four or five hospitals a year and add three to five other facilities through
management contracts.   The yearly foreign goal is to add one or two
managed hospitals to the chain.[25]

Figure 8:2

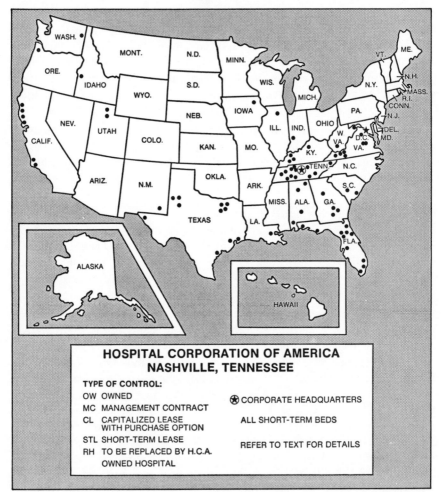

HOSPITAL CORPORATION OF AMERICA
NASHVILLE, TENNESSEE

TYPE OF CONTROL:

OW OWNED
MC MANAGEMENT CONTRACT
CL CAPITALIZED LEASE
     WITH PURCHASE OPTION
STL SHORT-TERM LEASE
RH TO BE REPLACED BY H.C.A.
     OWNED HOSPITAL

⊛ CORPORATE HEADQUARTERS

ALL SHORT-TERM BEDS

REFER TO TEXT FOR DETAILS

State, City, and Hospital	Beds	Control
ALABAMA		
Hartselle: Hartselle Hosp.	123	CL
Huntsville: Crestwood Hosp.	147	CL
Mobile: Doctors Hosp.	216	CL
Selma: Medical Center Hosp.	150	OW
CALIFORNIA		
Vallejo: Broadway Hosp.	90	OW
Ukiah: Ukiah General Hosp.	45	OW RH
Thousand Oaks: Los Robles Hosp.	220	OW
Sebastopol: Palm Drive Hosp.	44	OW RH
Ross: Ross General Hosp.	193	OW
Downey: Rio Hondo Memorial	146	OW
FLORIDA		
Fort Pierce: Ft. Pierce Memorial Hosp.	240	MC RH
Gainesville: North Florida Regional Hosp.	170	OW
Lakeland: Lakeland Manor Hosp.	66	OW
Ocala: Marion County Community Hosp.	126	OW
Palatka: Putnam Memorial Hosp.	120	MC RH
Pensacola: West Florida Hosp.	317	OW
Plantation: Plantation General Hosp.	258	OW
St. Augustine: St. Augustine General Hosp.	115	MC
Tamarac: University Community Hosp.	209	OW
Panama City: Bay Hosp.	150	CL
Miami: Bascom Palmer Eye Institute, University of Miami	115	MC
GEORGIA		
Albany: Palmyra Park Hosp.	223	OW
Atlanta: West Paces Ferry Hosp.	342	OW
Macon: Coliseum Park Hosp.	258	OW
Rome: Redmond Park Hosp.	149	OW
IDAHO		
Caldwell: Caldwell Memorial Hosp.	148	RH
ILLINOIS		
DeKalb: Kishwaukee Community Hosp.	172	MC*
INDIANA		
Terre Haute: Terre Haute Regional Hosp.	290	STL
IOWA		
Dyersville: Dyersville Community Hosp.	88	MC
KENTUCKY		
Bowling Green: Greenview Hosp.	157	OW
Frankfort: Kings Daughters Memorial	130	OW
Mayfield: Smith County Hosp.	116	CL
Morganfield: Union County Hosp.	52	OW
LOUISIANA		
Metairie: Lakeside Hosp. for Women	97	OW
NEW MEXICO		
Carlsbad: Carlsbad Regional Medical Center	127	MC
OREGON		
McMinnville: McMinnville Hosp.	78	OW

State, City, and Hospital	Beds	Control
South Carolina		
Charleston: North Trident Regional Hosp.	220	OW
Aiken: Aiken Community Hosp.	190	OW
Tennessee		
Athens: Athens Community Hosp.	118	CL
Brownsville: Haywood Park General......................	50	CL
Carthage: Smith County Hosp.	43	OW RH
Donelson: Donelson Hosp.	182	OW
Erin: Trinity Hosp.	38	OW
Humboldt: Humboldt Cedar Crest	62	CL
Kingsport: Indian Path Hosp.	196	OW
Lawrenceburg: Crocket General Hosp.	106	CL
Livingston: Lady Ann Hosp.	55	STL RH
McMinnville: River Park Hosp.	60	OW
Nashville:		
Miller Hosp.	97	OW
Parkview Hosp.	313	OW
Parthenon Pavilion (psychiatric).......................	100	OW
Smithville: DeKalb General Hosp.	54	OW
Texas		
Arlington: Arlington Community Hosp.	73	OW RH
Big Spring: Malone Hogan Hosp.	153	OW
El Paso: Sun Towers Hosp.	219	OW
Grand Prairie: Great Southwest General...............	98	OW
Houston: Diagnostic Center Hosp.	297	OW
Levelland: Cook Memorial Hosp............................	67	OW
Lubbock: University Hosp.	99	OW
Pasadena: Pasadena Bayshore Hosp.	469	OW
Plano: Plano General Hosp....................................	193	OW
Victoria: DeTar Hosp..	191	OW
Fort Worth: Medical Plaza Hosp.	334	OW
Utah		
Brigham City: Cooley Memorial Hosp......................	60	OW
Bountiful: South Davis Community Hosp.................	150	OW
Virginia		
Alexandria: Circle Terrace Hosp.	124	OW
Blacksburg: Montgomery County Community Hosp..	100	CL
Martinsville: Memorial Hosp. of Martinsville and Henry County...	223	MC
Pulaski: Pulaski Community Hosp.	129	CL
Richmond:		
Chippenham Hosp...	201	OW
Tucker Pavilion (psychiatric)............................	100	OW
Johnston-Willis Hosp.	352	OW
Salem: Lewis-Gale Hosp...	322	OW
Washington		
Spokane: Holy Family Hosp.	228	MC

State, City, and Hospital	Beds	Control
WEST VIRGINIA		
Martinsburg: King Daughters Hosp.	180	MC
Beckley: Raleigh General Hosp.	166	OW

* Cancelled 1976.

HCA's domestic operations are concentrated in the South, although new expansion has taken the company into all census divisions of the United States except the New England and Middle Atlantic states. Fifteen of its hospitals are located in Tennessee, but in recent years the corporation also has looked north, west, and southwest for expansion into Indiana, Illinois, Utah, New Mexico, California and Texas.

The contract managed foreign hospitals are a facility owned by Banco Nacional de Mexico in Mexico City, a doctor-owned hospital in Panama City, Panama, and the King Faisal Specialist Hospital and Research Center in Riyadh, Saudia Arabia.

The fundamental strategy difference between for-profit and voluntary hospitals is the profit motive. The rationale for the for-profit approach is straightforward: This is a free enterprise economy—patients pay a profit to their physician and their pharmacist, so why not to their hospital? Quality of care is a nebulous thing, making answers to these questions almost impossible: Is the quality of patient care any better in a nonprofit hospital than a for-profit hospital? Do patients really care?

HCA says it "is the world's largest hospital management company. The company was founded with the fundamental belief that private enterprise can deliver a superior quality of health care at a reasonable cost using private capital, paying all property and income taxes and providing the finest facilities and equipment available. In pursuing this policy, the company is consciously working to contain the rising cost of health care and to return its shareholders a fair return on their investment."[26] At the end of September 30, 1975, HCA had operating revenues of $287.4 million and a net income of $16.1 million. The more than 9,000 stockholders were paid $1.73 a share. At the time, HCA had $13.6 million in working capital, total assets of $415.7 million, and liabilities of $217.7 million.

The source of HCA's 1974 operating revenues from patients worked out this way: Medicare, 29 percent, Medicaid, 3 percent; Blue Cross, 8 percent; and all other sources, 60 percent.

As of the end of 1974, HCA hospitals counted 7,200 licensed physicians as members of their medical staffs. A few of the doctors were salaried and employed to staff emergency rooms. The company had about 16,000 full-time employees, including 2,700 registered nurses. HCA also had about 4,000 part-time employees, including over 1,000 RNs, available to meet fluctuating demands.

Like other hospitals, HCA facilities noted a decline in occupancy in 1975 compared to 1974. Total average occupancy for sixty-one hospitals in 1974 was 79 percent; the rate for sixty-five hospitals up into the fall of 1975 was 77 percent. According to a prospectus, this decline was attributed to "several factors including a general decline in average length of inpatient stay, the opening of new hospitals, competitive conditions in three locations, and general economic conditions."[27]

The HCA corporate structure is one that combines centralization and decentralization. The top managers and supporting personnel and the major central office functions and services—financing, data processing, purchasing, architectural and engineering development, and management systems are concentrated at Nashville.

There are four regional offices where vice-presidents direct the overall management operations in the hospitals although the objective is to give the day-to-day administrator a high degree of local control. In 1973, HCA allowed each administrator an average $800 per bed for a discretionary capital expenditure program. The administrator was free to spend this money as he wanted, but items costing $5,000 or more were reviewed in Nashville.

John C. Neff, HCA's president and chief executive officer, said the company's management development system aims at taking new hospital administration course graduates and working them up in the corporate organization. "They like the idea of working for the same group all the time and being able to grow professionally to the extent of their ability. And our problem is that we're always looking for administrators to move on up—to give them additional challenges, and responsibilities. He gets well paid—we probably pay him a *little* bit more than the average not-for-profit hospital. He's got more authority. He's treated much more like a professional businessman and he's got some stock options, usually, and so he likes this business. . . ."[28]

There is a fifteen-member board of directors of HCA led by John A. Hill, chairman, including three physicians. Eight of the directors are inside the corporation and the remaining seven are outside of the board. Management control is further concentrated in a five-member executive committee.

The top management team also includes twelve vice-presidents who are not members of the board of directors. These individuals are either in charge of the four geographical divisions and international operations or support functions such as planning and construction, treasurer, purchasing, controller, real estate and management services.

In an interview, Neff discussed HCA's philosophy and the rationale of for-profit chains.   The original idea was an attempt "to build a blue chip organization that delivers a quality of health care at a reasonable price, and, using private capital, still providing a reasonable return to our investors." Neff said that since the advent of Medicare "all hospitals decently run will make money.   We don't call them (other hospitals) non-profit, you understand; we call them non-tax-paying."   HCA and the other for-profit chains use this argument persuasively as the reason they do not provide charity care and engage in major teaching programs.   In 1974, HCA paid $14.5 million in income taxes based on operating revenues of $297.7 million.

Each HCA hospital has its own board of trustees; the corporate representative on the board is the administrator.   Doctors are also on the board of each hospital, Neff said, to put the doctor "on the same level as the trustees so that he's not in a subservient position."   Doctors are not allowed to run the business end of the hospital, "but they should have continuing input into the ethical, professional, and medical aspects of the hospitals," such as adding new services.   Boards are not crucial to HCA's management approach, but they do provide a bridge between Nashville and the staffs of the individual hospitals.   There is no attempt made to obtain business leaders in the community as board members, because HCA wants total management control of the hospital.

HCA retains strict financial control over each hospital by reserving the right to approve operating, capital and people budgets.   "The key to our business, in one sentence," Neff said, "is flexible staffing—staffing your hospital in accordance with the occupancy requirements—not too few, not too many.   Something like 60 percent of our expenses are labor."

Most of HCA's acquisitions have been of for-profit hospitals and the main criteria looked for are quality of the medical staff and quality of the physical plant.   New hospitals are another matter.   As Neff said: "We have to decide: Is this an attractive place?   Is there really an honest to goodness need?   Do the people want us?   Do the townspeople want us?   Does the medical staff want us?   Does the Chamber of Commerce want us?   Do the newspapers want us?   Does everybody want us to come in?"

If HCA can determine that it's wanted, a critical look is taken at such factors as bed need versus population.   "An awfully lot of hospitals in this country are technically and physically obsolete.   They are in downtown areas with no parking. . . and people are moving out to the suburbs. . ."

Neff, when asked how he acquired doctors, replied: "We start with them. We start usually with a nucleus of a medical staff that has expressed an interest.   I don't mean they sign a contract, but we don't go into a town just by saying . . . we'll go build a hospital.   We are usually approached by a group of doctors or by the town . . . by someone who comes up and says, 'We need a hospital and here's why.' . . . The basic point is that we don't go cold into a town. We've started into towns and found out that the atmosphere wasn't attractive for one reason or another." Ft. Meyers, Florida, provides an example, Neff said. "We bought a piece of ground down there. We were all set ... had a whole doctor group and ran into a lot of bad publicity. The newspapers decided to run a bunch of articles about profiteering bastards trying to make money off the sick and all that jazz. So we said, the hell with it. We'll go some place else with our money."

HCA's efforts to gain acceptance on the local, state and national levels have involved top management in continuous public relations programs. In HCA's early days, money lenders in the East were turned off by a negative image of for-profits, Neff said, "and we had to start out in an educational program that goes on constantly." The grassroots educational program includes efforts to educate members of service organizations, hospital managers, physicians, bankers, lenders, security analysts, governors, state legislators and members of the Congress. In 1975 it also included an extensive advertising campaign in news magazines.

In HCA's short history of a little over seven years, the lenders have really come around. The corporation has been able to sell its bonds with relative ease—including a $33 million mortgage bond issue offered in October 1975 that was rated A.

HCA was able to start out big in 1968—eight or so hospitals obtained from people who would take letter stock before the company went public, Neff said, for there was confidence in the stock market in those days. Today, he believes, all of the major hospital management companies are already in the business: "First of all, you can't gather up the hospitals; secondly, you can't run out and build hospitals." Comprehensive health planning agencies won't allow it, he said. Neff did project a bullish outlook for HCA—an estimated 15 to 20 percent growth in earnings each year. He predicted expansion of existing hospitals, construction of new hospitals, additional domestic and foreign management contracts and new areas of growth—health maintenance organizations, multiphasic screening centers, and clinical laboratories.

Calling hospitals a stable business, Neff added: "A hospital running 75 percent occupancy, a reasonable size hospital under reasonable management, throws out money. This is a terrific cash flow business. This is a service business with a large brick and mortar base ... very unusual, the only business you've ever heard of that has no sales campaign, no public relations, no advertising. We don't have any salesmen, any quotas—all we do is open our doors seven days a week, 365 days a year, and stand back. It's a very peculiar business, and a very stable business. People who run hospitals with an 80 percent occupancy and tell me they are losing money are either lousy managers or a bunch of damn liars."

HCA hospitals tend to be located in communities of medium-size population; in many locations HCA has the only hospital in town. By staying with the medium-sized hospital, HCA can make the argument that more specialized services belong in the university hospital or the larger hospitals that *choose* to play the research, development, and training role. The smallest HCA facility is 38–bed Trinity Hospital in Erin, Tennessee; the largest is 469–bed Pasadena Bayshore Hospital, Pasadena, Texas. Six of the corporate hospitals have over 300 beds. HCA has fifteen hospitals in Tennessee. Based on information available from ten of the hospitals, nine provide organized emergency services but none of the hospitals operate an organized outpatient department. A 1975 bond offering prospectus noted: "The company follows accepted areawide health planning concepts and usually does not engage in extensive research or educational programs or offers services which unnecessarily duplicate those offered by neighboring hospitals."[29]

While HCA sees moderate growth ahead in domestic management contracts, there are no signs that the company will jump in with both feet as has Hospital Affiliates International. HCA had a bad experience with the medical staff at North Shore Hospital, Miami, Florida, and canceled its agreement. But in a little over a year, HCA turned around 228–bed Holy Family Hospital, Spokane, Washington. "The whole problem of a management contract," said Sam A. Brooks, Jr., vice-president and treasurer, "is that it usually isn't too hard to turn a hospital around, and once you do it is easy to run. Then you have to hustle to prove to the hospital that you can do something for them."[30]

HCA has taken an interesting tack in its real estate acquisitions, perhaps as something of a hedge against the future. Its 1975 hospital building programs included the construction of three physicians' office buildings on adjacent property, a long-evident trend being seen in the not-for-profit field too. HCA tends to buy much more land around its hospitals than is needed. This additional land provides space for other ventures—gas stations, motels, pharmacies, restaurants, and middle income housing, for example.

The outlook for HCA is bullish, depending on what the federal government and the state governments do in terms of laws and regulations to control beds, services, reimbursement rates and utilization. Thomas M. McGinnis, Jr. of the institutional department of F. Eberstadt & Co., New York financial analysts, did an extensive research paper on HCA in August 1975. He gave HCA a good report, even during times of high domestic inflation, because of its "ability to offset cost increases with (i) price adjustments and (ii) operating efficiencies." McGinnis said: "Because management reviews expense trends in the company's hospitals quite closely, price increases are effected promptly when necessary. Given the general absence of government controls (very few states require prior approval of hospital rate increases) the inelastic demand for hospital services, and a lack of price competition among hospitals, there is no significant external restraint on any cost-supported price increases by the industry. . . ."

McGinnis also said that the biggest threat to the stock would be government price controls. He believed that HCA could offset any negative impact of new government programs "through a combination of (i) operating efficiencies, (ii) price increases, (iii) gains in market share, and (iv) anticipated growth of the medical services market. Also, HCA, through its vice-president for government relations, is expanding company efforts to influence regulatory change, particularly at the state and local levels. Finally, we anticipate that hospital trade associations will rely increasingly on the courts to obtain relief from unsatisfactory rulings by government agencies; already some preliminary victories have been won through litigation by the industry."

McGinnis added that Public Law 93-641, which mandated the establishment of Health Systems Agencies, "clearly will make it more difficult for hospital companies to grow by adding bed capacity and services; on the other hand, it considerably enhances the franchise of existing hospitals." The HSAs should reduce competition, he believed, and HCA should have a better prospect of "obtaining its fair share of expansions. . . ."[31]

HOSPITAL AFFILIATES INTERNATIONAL

A third large multiple unit hospital system that has its headquarters within the East South Central states is Hospital Affiliates International (HAI), Nashville, Tennessee. Like HCA, it was also founded in 1968. By early November 1975, HAI owned twenty-five U.S. hospitals and operated thirty-seven other domestic facilities through management contract arrangements. Overall, HAI had control and influence over 8,067 beds in the United States. It also is in the management contract business overseas at the 187–bed American Hospital in Paris, France, where HAI also is helping plan a new complex, and the new 150–bed Medical Center of the Marianas, a Catholic hospital on Guam.

In the year ending December 31, 1974, HAI had net revenues of $68.1 million and net earnings of $3.9 million. Its sixty-two U.S. hospitals are located in twenty states. While HAI reveals the locations of its wholly-owned hospitals, the public relations director said, because of competition it does not reveal the names and locations of its contract-managed facilities and occupancy rates.[32] Without such information it is not possible to give a comparative picture of HAI in terms of average census, occupancy rate, total expenses, payroll expenses, number of employees and extent of services.

The two physicians and two businessmen who founded HAI, Irwin B. Eskind, M.D., Herbert J. Schulman, M.D., Baron Coleman and Richard J.

Eskind, had the same motivation as the founders of HCA: they believed a profit could be made through managing hospitals on a business basis. Hospital Affiliates had no base to start from and it took persuasive arguments to gain its first affiliate in 1968—the 108–bed Spring Branch Memorial Hospital in Houston, Texas, a facility owned by sixteen doctors. A second Texas hospital was soon added and a hospital in Haverford, Pennsylvania became the third affiliate. The chain grew rapidly and went public in 1969.

Other for-profit chains have expanded through acquisitions and new construction. HAI has used that route to grow too, but has concentrated on managing hospitals owned by others. Many of these facilities are nonprofit. It claims the distinction of being the first chain to go into the domestic management contract business. HAI's 1971 annual report said: "For the long term, an area of great potential for our industry is contract management. Contracts will become a major factor in the hospital industry in the coming years as more hospitals seek to apply more efficient and more effective management systems in the delivery of maximum quality health care."[33] The first opportunity to try out this approach came in 1971 when HAI stepped in to manage a bankrupt nonprofit hospital, the new 105–bed Medical Center of Independence, Missouri, that was still under contract in late 1975.

Further strengthening its management contract focus, HAI in late 1975 reincorporated in Delaware as Hospital Affiliates International. The company also had a headline-making announcement on November 26, 1975 when it said it would transfer ownership of its twenty-five hospitals to a real estate investment trust (REIT) to be administered by many of the same board members of the original corporation. The stockholders of the trust would be the same as those who held shares that day in HAI. At the same time, HAI said nineteen of the hospitals in the trust would be leased to American Medicorp of Bala Cynwyd, Pennsylvania.[34] American Medicorp already owned thirty-four hospitals (6,996 beds) and managed another seven facilities (859 beds) under management contracts. Lease rentals would be paid into the equity trust for distribution to stockholders.

With that announcement, the old HAI corporate organization would have ceased to exist. A new public company would be formed and the stock would be traded over the counter. HAI would orient itself in one central direction: contract management. One objective was to open up new areas for expansion in, for example, the Northeast and Middle West.[35]

An observer within the for-profit field interpreted the November 1975, developments this way. "HAI was sitting there on an equity position of about $20 million compared to our $150 million. We have a bigger base and can go to the debt market to finance a continuing hospital building program of $50 to $60 million a year. They couldn't build any more hospitals. They probably thought ... we might as well form a real estate investment trust.

Their investment is held in equity and they don't have to be active in the management of the hospitals. Under the REIT, they can make a payout of about 90 percent of earnings; Uncle Sam won't get half . . . so they create dividends, wind up getting 90 percent of earnings flowing back as dividends."[36]   But HAI's effort to concentrate solely on contract management was blocked by the Internal Revenue Service.

Jack R. Anderson, president of HAI, said in a letter to stockholders dated January 23, 1976:

> Our intent in entering into this transaction in November was to benefit shareholders through payment of substantial cash dividends, while at the same time giving them the opportunity to participate in an ongoing newly-created company which would continue to manage hospitals owned by others. Although we had investigated to a substantial degree the viability of such a concept, sufficiently adequate assurances that the needed tax rulings and other approvals could be obtained were not forthcoming. Such rulings would have been necessary to assure that the proposed exchange of stock would have been tax-free, and to permit present Hospital Affiliates shareholders to acquire a pro rata interest in the new management company. Consequently, we decided that it was in the best interest of our shareholders for Hospital Affiliates to terminate the reorganization plan.[37]

HAI was emphasizing management contracts early in its history. Just six years after the company was formed, HAI's 1974 annual report said: "As national trends in health care and hospital services continue to burden the non-profit and public hospitals, the importance and need for professional management and development services will expand. Anticipating this demand, Hospital Affiliates is developing its capacity to provide management contract services to an expanding number and variety of medical institutions. Working with hospitals, boards and administrators, Hospital Affiliates is providing an appealing and profitable alternative to charity and public subsidy of inefficient hospital operations."

Later in the same report, HAI said: "Historically, hospitals have operated as single, independent units in a protective environment fostered by cost reimbursement, contributions, and grants. Volunteer hospital boards made up of concerned, professional people from the community have been unable to devote enough time to the operations of the hospital. Often, there has been little incentive to exercise rigorous controls in the nonprofit facility. Frequently, expenses have been inadequately controlled, and occasionally unnecessary services have been created."[38]   The management contract should also be attractive to the nonprofit hospital, the report added, because the hospital would retain its tax-exempt status.

Of its 37 managed U.S. hospitals, most are in the 75 bed to 150 bed size and they are located in rural and suburban areas. HAI has a first to its credit—a contract to manage the new 310–bed University Hospital and Ambulatory Care Teaching Facility at Tulane Medical Center, New Orleans, when it opens in 1976.

The Tulane contract is unusual because it is the first U.S. university teaching center to be managed by a for-profit company. A professor of hospital administration who is familiar with the contract interpreted it as "a redressing of the university power structure; it alters the traditional balance of power. The university wanted financial talents beyond the capabilities of the usual hospital administrative structure."[39] The project is being financed through $37.5 million in revenue bonds issued by the Health Education Authority of Louisiana (HEAL). Tulane will pay HEAL rent on the new structures and this income will be used to amortize the bonds.

The seventeen officers of HAI are led by Jack R. Anderson, president, who is also the author of *The Road to Recovery*. Anderson argues persuasively that (1) not-for-profit hospitals are in serious need of help, basically in the area of good management, and (2) for-profit chains can provide that expert management through contract arrangements. His book also attempts to accomplish several other things: (1) defend the for-profit hospital industry by answering criticisms that have been heard since 1968; (2) show that the chains are more efficient in all areas of management; (3) push the HAI management approach by explaining detailed procedures, and (4) argue that the "road to recovery" that failing voluntary hospitals should take will lead them to good for-profit management companies, i.e. HAI.

Some of Anderson's concepts are controversial. He argues that there are only two types of hospitals: nonprofit and tax-paying. He justifies the limited service component of for-profits as due to their bed size and the desire to stay away from duplication. HAI has concentrated on building in rural and urban areas of need, Anderson said, and therefore sees its management contract potential as the 2,000 or so U.S. hospitals of 70 beds or more. For-profits are assuming a proper role in educational programs for managers and para-professionals equal to community hospitals of comparable size. The chains have not chosen to get into medical education for that is the role of the teaching hospitals.

Anderson says that most non-profit hospitals have an employee to patient ratio of 3.0 or more to 1 while the ratio in for-profit facilities is 2.0 to 2.5 to 1. Also, he says, nonprofits' labor costs are 60 to 70 percent of expenses while in for-profit facilities they are around 50 to 55 percent. Part of the for-profit saving occurs through more equitable staffing related to specifically defined needs and through the use of part-time personnel. Anderson also believes that nonprofits waste money in construction by not using standardized approaches. He cited a Blue Cross and Blue Shield study that projected the per bed construction cost at $67,000. He compared this to a cost of $34,000 per bed in a group of hospitals built by Humana. Anderson also argued that the for-profits take "their share" of Medicare and Medicaid patients, but he did not elaborate.

And Anderson says: "It has been argued that since healing of the sick is the hospital's sole purpose, businesslike efficiency must take a back seat. . . . It has been suggested that the two concepts—efficient operation and the social role of hospitals—are almost mutually exclusive. Delivering the best patient care, however, is certainly not related to inefficiency. Obviously, the more efficiently a hospital is run, the better it is able to serve its patients. Poor care does not result from a hospital being in the black but, rather, from one being in the red. . . ."[40]

The Road to Recovery skims over several major issues. The tremendous charity load carried by many voluntary nonprofit hospitals. The push for outpatient care and organized clinics, a trend that may radically change the character of the for-profit chain business. Anderson also glosses over the inner-city health problems and the tremendous need in those areas. And he fairly well avoids the continuing problem of how to pay for medical education. Anderson's book is valuable, however, for it lays out some national issues in detail. It provides something of a handbook for not-for-profit managers, particularly those who are managers in multiple unit systems.

Another issue not faced in any detail in his book is the competitive situation created in many communities where nonprofit hospitals must compete with for-profit facilities for patients and doctors. Head-on-head competition has already had an impact on occupancy rates of both types of hospitals. As more emphasis is placed on outpatient care, inpatient census figures will undoubtedly go down, at least until more demand is created through new programs that provide coverage to more Americans. Underused capacity and duplicate services were created in a time of weak planning agencies and the absence of certificate of need laws. The Health Systems Agencies mandated under Public Law 93-641 have the potential for mediating this overbuilding and duplication. For these reasons, HAI may have made a wise move de-emphasizing the new hospital construction business.

Robert L. Parker, a vice-president at Beverly Enterprises, owner of six hospitals and manager of one, commented to a *Business Week* reporter late in 1975: "For companies that want to stay in the hospital business, the most desirable way to survive the current government reimbursement and regulation climate, is management contracts. There is just no longer any adequate return from tying up investor capital in brick and mortar."[41]

NOTES

1. J.A. Hamilton, *Patterns of Hospital Ownership and Control,* Minneapolis: University of Minnesota Press (1961), p. 92.

2. "The ARH Story," adapted from an article in *The Post-Herald and Register,* Beckley, West Virginia (December 15, 1968).

3. Interviews with David K. Heydinger, M.D., November 21, 1975 in Atlanta, Georgia, and January 4, 1976 in Chicago, Illinois.

4. K.S. Klicka, "Multi-Unit Hospital Operations," a presentation before the American Hospital Association's Annual Meeting, August 31, 1966.

5. "The ARH Story," op. cit., note 2.

6. Ibid.

7. D.K. Keydinger, op. cit., note 3.

8. K.S. Klicka, op. cit., note 4.

9. D.K. Heydinger, op. cit., note 3.

10. Ibid.

11. "Statement of Operating Policy, Appalachian Regional Hospitals, Inc.," February 1974.

12. D. K. Heydinger, op. cit., note 3.

13. "Hazard Children's Services Program," a descriptive paper dated November 1974.

14. D.K. Heydinger, op. cit., note 3.

15. Ibid.

16. D.K. Heydinger, op. cit., note 3. Until noted otherwise, all quotations are from the interviews.

17. D.K. Heydinger, "Objective: Total Health—A Request for Funding," undated and unpublished.

18. D.K. Heydinger, op. cit., note 3.

19. "Physician Manpower and Recruitment Plan for Appalachian Regional Hospitals," September 4, 1975, p. 51.

20. D.K. Heydinger, op. cit., note 17.

21. D.K. Heydinger, op. cit., note 3. All subsequent quotations are from the interviews until otherwise noted.

22. Telephone interview with David G. Williamson, Jr., January 12, 1976.

23. For a general discussion of these criticisms see J.T. Foster, "Proprietary Hospitals Go Public," *Modern Hospital* (March 1969), p. 80 and "What's Good for the Common Stock is Good for the Common Duct," *Modern Hospital* (March 1969), p. 79.

24. "Associations: FAH Documents Its Muscle and Takes Swings at Government," *Modern Healthcare,* Short-Term Care Edition (May 19, 1975), pp. 16b, 16c.

25. D.G. Williamson, Jr., op. cit., note 22 and "Hospital Corporation of America," a prospectus, Merrill Lynch, Pierce, Fenner & Smith, October 23, 1975.

26. HCA 1974 Annual Report.

27. HCA prospectus, op. cit., note 25.

28. M. Brown and W. Money, taped interview with John C. Neff, Nashville, Tennessee, November 17, 1973. Until otherwise noted, all quotations are from this interview.

29. HCA prospectus, op. cit., note 25.

30. "How Outsiders Manage Hospitals for Profit," *Business Week* (November 24, 1975), p. 56.

31. Research Notes, HCA, New York, N.Y.: F. Eberstadt & Co., Inc., August 19, 1975.

32. Telephone interview with Lanson J. Hyde III, January 15, 1976.

33. Hospital Affiliates, Inc., 1971 Annual Report.

34. Hospital Affiliates International, Inc., press release, November 26, 1975.

35. L.J. Hyde III, op. cit., note 32.

36. Confidential interview with the authors.

37. HAI letter to shareholders and a joint press release with American Medicorp, Inc., both dated January 23, 1976.

38. HAI 1974 Annual Report.

39. Confidential interview with the authors.

40. J.R. Anderson, *The Road to Recovery*, Nashville, Tennessee: Rich Publishing Co., 1976.

41. Op. cit., note 30.

Chapter 9
West North Central States

The seven West North Central States begin as a huge block of land starting at the U.S.-Canadian border on the north. They sweep down the belly of the United States and sit on top of the northern borders of Oklahoma and Arkansas. This huge area contains 343,877 square miles of land and is generally rural with a low population density. The main industries are farming, dairying and businesses related to the production of food. This is the nation's breadbasket, the Great Plains. This area of small town, rural America is also characterized by small hospitals, as shown in Table 9:1.

Table 9:1   Hospital Statistics of West North Central States

State	Number of Community Hospitals	Beds	Hospitals Under 100 Beds
Iowa	135	16,523	89
Kansas	143	12,536	111
Minnesota	172	23,157	105
Missouri	144	24,765	68
Nebraska	94	8,975	72
North Dakota	53	4,261	40
South Dakota	51	3,562	40
TOTALS	791	93,779	430

Source: Hospital Statistics, 1975 Edition. 1974 Data from the American Hospital Association Annual Survey, pp. 30, 31.

The 1975 study by the American Hospital Association and the Health Services Research Center of Northwestern University shows that there are at least 251 nonfederal hospitals and 57,240 beds in the West North Central States that are members of multiple hospital systems. This area shows the third highest level of systems activity in the nation after the Pacific States and the East North Central States.

There are several notable exceptions to the rural character of this census region, such as the Twin Cities of Minneapolis-St. Paul, a booming region of hospital systems activity.

Six multiple hospital systems are discussed here in some detail: (1) The Lutheran Hospitals and Homes Society of America, Fargo, North Dakota; the systems in the Minneapolis-St. Paul area, (2) Fairview Community Hospitals, (3) Health Central, (4) Minneapolis Medical Center, and (5) United Hospitals of St. Paul, and (6) the Great Plains Lutheran Hospitals, Phillipsburg, Kansas.

The West North Central States have long been a scene of other religious-sponsored health care activity. In addition to the systems that have developed through the efforts of Lutheran congregations, Catholic-sponsored hospitals are spread throughout every state in this census division.

And in Wichita, Kansas, a system is beginning to develop around the 697-bed Wesley Medical Center (WMC). Roy C. House, president and chief executive officer of the WMC, explained that thirty-five hospitals in the area are now involved in group purchasing, and eight of the hospitals are involved in a cooperative relationship. The Cooperative Association for Shared Services, located in a separate building on the Wesley Medical Center campus, was initially funded through the Kansas Regional Medical Program. Through the cooperative, House said, "we are getting ready to make our first moves."[1] About eighteen areas of managerial expertise have been developed by the co-op members and are ready for "export" to other hospitals.

LUTHERAN HOSPITALS AND HOMES
SOCIETY OF AMERICA

The Lutheran Hospitals and Homes Society of America (LHHSA), Fargo, North Dakota, is the largest nongovernmental, not-for-profit multiple hospital system in the United States. In March 1976 the Society was operating ninety institutions.[3] This figure included fifty-seven hospitals, twenty-four skilled nursing homes, six intermediate care facilities, two homes for the aged, and a school for crippled children. These facilities are located in sixty-five communities in thirteen western and midwestern states from Alaska to Arizona, from Montana to Illinois (see Figure 9:1). Twenty-nine of the institutions are owned by the Society and the remainder are operated through lease agreements with the ownership body—counties, cities, hospital districts and nonprofit corporations. All of the facilities are managed as though they were owned.

This system, one of the oldest in the United States, was established in 1938 by a group of Lutheran laymen led by Frederick R. Knautz who served as its executive director for thirty years.[2]

Harry M. Malm, president and chief executive officer of LHHSA, explained the environment that led to the formation of the society this way:

> When the first crisis hit the hospital field after 1929 the few and inadequate institutions, already struggling for resources to serve rural and small-town America, nearly were wiped out. Their way to salvation was the adoption of better business methods; yet, where in rural America could the individual hospital find manpower with the business expertise to accomplish such a task? Many hospitals had no full-time management. In various institutions the job of administration was relegated to community members who provided leadership on a part-time, voluntary basis. How, then, were hospitals to recruit full-time professional, knowledgeable in modern business methods, to take them out of the red and into the black?
>
> The answer: through a joint effort. The men responsible for seven health facilities in the Great Plains formed a corporation and imposed the principle of central management, borrowed from the world of commerce. The man [Knautz] chosen to supervise the activities of the newly-related facilities had a wealth of prior experience as business manager for the New Guinea mission outposts. He quickly applied those group management principles to the failing hospitals. The techniques included group purchasing, centralized accounting, and central financial management.[3]

What Knautz started in 1938 Malm is continuing today as the Society continues to innovate and take on new challenges in additional states. Malm, who has been very active in American Hospital Association activities and a member of the Perloff committee, is nationally respected within hospital and financial groups for his knowledge and skill. A low-keyed jolly man, he is more like a friendly country storekeeper who will sit and play checkers with the customers than a Wall Street banker although in 1975 he was responsible for an annual volume of earnings of $82 million. This ability of Malm's and other members of the central administrative staff to function in varied environments has been a key to the Society's success because its managers understand the needs of rural communities and are able to deal with urban bankers and money lenders.

Although the word "Lutheran" appears in the corporate name, the Society has no ties to and receives no financial support from the church. The sixteen member board of directors of Lutheran laymen and pastors is drawn from the Society's service areas. The board has a lot of power and is independent of the administrative staff; Malm is not a member and likes it that way.[4] The board includes two physicians and the 1975 chairman was an attorney in Fargo. Members serve three-year terms. Board power is further concentrated in a six-member executive committee.

The central office staff in Fargo includes Malm, two vice-presidents, treasurer, secretary, controller, ten specialists in various areas of health care administration, and a clerical staff of thirty. The specialists are a field administrator, assistant director for legal affairs, insurance assistant, chief accountant, purchasing agent, functional planner, construction administrator, facilities engineer, internal audit specialist and special projects supervisor. Three corporate officers serve as field representatives—two for specific geographical areas and the third for the larger institutions now involved in major construction projects.

All of the institutions are under complete management control during the duration of the lease. Malm explained that "this means that the centralized services of the Society's home office ... are applied to each institution following identical procedures. The Society exercises strong management control over each institution. The organization has found through experience that the best way for a multiple system to function is by assuming complete responsibility for the operation."

The largest single central function is accounting, which as a section "performs all but the most basic accounting and bookkeeping tasks for each institution. This again eliminates the need for additional personnel in each institution. It has the more important advantage of offering each institution accounting expertise that would not otherwise be available to the small hospital or nursing home."[5] The accounting staff receives daily and monthly recap sheets from each institution and provides the information for day-to-day operation of each institution. These data are also used in long-range planning. Accounting systems are computerized. The Society has been buying EDP time but will convert to its own computer operation and have computers in Fargo and Mesa, Arizona.

Malm, the two vice-presidents, and the field administrators spend quite a lot of time traveling to and from the institutions and Fargo. The distances are great: the closest facility is in Lisbon, North Dakota, some eighty miles from Fargo; the most distant is in Fairbanks, Alaska, several thousand miles away. The cost of centralized management is prorated among member institutions based on the number of occupied beds. All 7,000 employees in the ninety facilities are employed by the Society and receive their paychecks from Fargo.

Most management agreements are ninty-nine-year contracts. In Valdez, Alaska, however, the Society is managing the fifteen-bed general hospital for the city through an agreement that goes to 1980. The Society is paid $2,500 a month.[6]

Every attempt is made to retain the community focus of the institution, a philosophy inherent in the Society's expansion policy. It will not go to a community unless formally invited to come. And then, it will not add a health care institution to its membership unless the central staff and board of directors are convinced that a genuine need exists for the institution and that it is supported by its community. Nine out of every ten requests for assistance are turned down.

"In many instances," Malm said, "Society investigations have revealed that the particular community requesting services is adequately provided for by a hospital or home in a neighboring town within reasonable distance. In these cases, the community often is seeking to perpetuate its hospital not because it is necessary to meet the health needs of the community, but rather because it has some influence on the economic life of the community. In these instances the request for assistance is refused, and the responsibility for disposition of the institution remains within the community."[7]

And the Society has taken on the role of helping sift out the health care delivery system in parts of rural America. From 1970 through 1974, the Society terminated its relationship with ten facilities either because the institutions were no longer needed in the service areas or the community's attitude toward the Society had changed. Twice in recent years, in Clear Lake, South Dakota, and Syracuse, Nebraska, Malm's organization has turned over its nursing homes to a competing long-term care system—Good Samaritan of Sioux Falls, South Dakota.

Malm has taken an optimistic view toward Public Law 93-641. In March 1975, he told a conference in Pennsylvania: "It is a bill with considerable promise and if we put our heads together with government and the consumer public, it could provide wonderful opportunities for innovation and for taking the right steps in reorganizing our delivery system.... The consumer has all too often been left out of the planning process and this situation has promoted the consumer antagonism that has so vigorously attacked our health care delivery system."

The new law does not emphasize one area of need at the expense of others, Malm said, and much of what was outlined in the law "parallels closely what we have been doing on a smaller scale as a systems operation for almost 40 years. And we know it can work effectively." As the scene is set for reorganization, still other forces have been at work. "In the last few years the financial pressures of the Economic Stabilization Program, rampant inflation, and a continuing commitment to maintaining and improving the quality of care delivered, have forced health care provides to expand their horizons. The advantages of cooperative efforts began to overshadow the competitive atmosphere that had existed in many areas."

Many people thought it was impossible to organize a rural health care system and make small hospitals survive and flourish; but as Malm said:

> By providing substantial cost-savings and offering managerial expertise to the smallest institutions, our experience has done what many thought was impossible. Our rural areas have frequently been neglected by the planning processes of the past. Failure to consider the impact of many of the federal regulations on the small, rural institution has forced many rural health care institutions to close their doors. In some instances this resulted in the natural elimination of some institutions which no longer were needed.
>
> In other cases, however, the demise of rural hospitals has led to tremendous medical hardships for the people living in the area. In the states in which the Society operates population density is low and distances are great. Admittedly every small community cannot justify its own hospital or nursing home. On the other hand good planning would not justify traveling many, many miles, often over inferior roads, to reach medical care in a distant city.

The emphasis on local identity comes through in another way. Each institution has its own community board of directors appointed by the Society's board of directors. The medical staff of each institution is directly responsible to the Society's board of directors, but the local board processes applications, outlines privileges and other medical staff business, and makes recommendations for action to the Society's board of directors. The Society also encourages participation in local programs which may provide better services or lower costs than similar programs within the organization. Society institutions are free to enter local purchasing systems if they can effect savings by such an arrangement.[8]

There seems to be no rhyme or reason to the geographical spread of the Society's facilities and institutions that are located in such small communities as Soldotna, Alaska; Choteau, Montana; Clayton, New Mexico; and Durand, Wisconsin. The Society says "their location in no way indicates inferior facilities or second-rate patient treatment.... The Society's emphasis on concern for the patient's well-being is more than just a medical interest. The Society was founded on principles of human care and compassion—of service to fellow man. It has implemented these goals by enabling institutions that

Figure 9:1

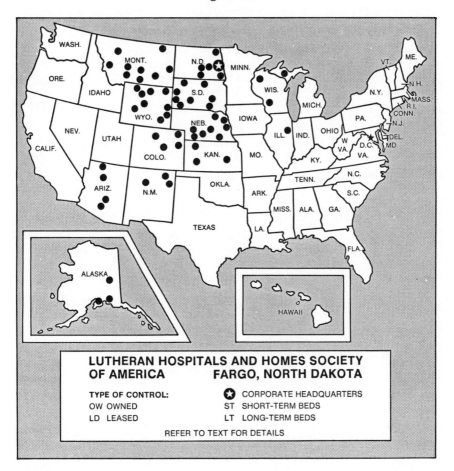

LUTHERAN HOSPITALS AND HOMES SOCIETY
OF AMERICA   FARGO, NORTH DAKOTA

TYPE OF CONTROL: ⭐ CORPORATE HEADQUARTERS
OW OWNED   ST SHORT-TERM BEDS
LD LEASED   LT LONG-TERM BEDS

REFER TO TEXT FOR DETAILS

		Beds		
State, Community, Hospital or Nursing Home		ST	LT	Control
ALASKA				
Fairbanks:	Fairbanks Memorial Hosp.	116		LD
Soldotna:	Central Penninsula General Hosp.	30		LD
Valdez:	Valdez Community Hosp.	15		LD
ARIZONA				
Chandler:	Community Hosp. in Chandler	42		LD
Mesa:	Mesa Lutheran Hosp.	250		OW
Page:	Page Hospital	25		LD
Williams:	Williams Hosp.	27		LD

State, Community, Hospital or Nursing Home	Beds		Control
	ST	LT	
COLORADO			
Akron: Washington County Public Hosp.......	19		LD
Nursing Home Unit............................		24	LD
Brush: East Morgan Community Hosp..........	29		LD
Loveland: Loveland Memorial Hosp...................	49		LD
Sterling: Logan County Hosp............................	98		LD
ILLINOIS			
Hoopeston: Hoopeston Community Memorial Hosp.	44		OW
Nursing Home Unit............................		50	OW
KANSAS			
Hugoton: Stevens County Hosp.	22		LD
Pioneer Manor...................................		56	LD
Marion: St. Luke Hosp.....................................	25		LD
Nursing Home Unit		18	LD
Oberlin: Decatur County Hosp.........................	24		LD
Long-Term Care Unit		33	LD
Satanta: Satanta District Hosp.........................	14		LD
Senior Citizens' Home		26	LD
MICHIGAN			
Crystal Falls: Crystal Manor		90	OW
MONTANA			
Choteau: Teton Memorial Hosp.	22		LD
Deer Lodge: Powell County Memorial Hosp..........	35		LD
Hardin: Big Horn County Memorial Hosp......	16		LD
Nursing Home Unit............................		34	LD
Harlowton: Wheatland Memorial Hosp.	25		LD
Nursing Home Unit............................		31	LD
Livingston: Livingston Memorial Hosp................	54		LD
Red Lodge: Carbon County Memorial Hosp..........	28		OW
Nursing Home Unit............................		24	OW
Roundup: Roundup Memorial Hosp.	17		LD
Roundup Memorial Nursing Home ...		16	LD
Scobey: Daniels Memorial Hosp......................	11		LD
Daniels Memorial Nursing Home......		28	LD
Wilbaux: Wilbaux County Nursing Home.........		40	LD
NEBRASKA			
Cambridge: Cambridge Memorial Hosp.	31		LD
Long-Term Nursing Care Unit..........		30	LD
Heritage Plaza....................................		50	LD
Creighton: Lundberg Memorial Hosp.	38		LD
Grand Island: Lutheran Memorial Hosp....................	74		OW
Bauman Home.....................................	74		OW
Hebron: Thayer County Memorial Hosp.........	22		LD
Lexington: Lexington Community Hosp.	40		LD
North Platte: Great Plains Medical Center	100		LD
Oakland: Oakland Memorial Hosp.	21		LD

State, Community, Hospital or Nursing Home	Beds		Control
	ST	LT	
Pender: Pender Community Hosp.....................	47		LD
NEW MEXICO			
Clayton: Union County General Hosp.	38		LD
Los Alamos: Los Alamos Medical Center...............	88		OW
Raton: Northern Colfax County Hosp...........	52		LD
NORTH DAKOTA			
Cavalier: Pembina County Memorial Hosp.......	53		LD
Fargo: Fargo Nursing Home	102		OW
Jamestown: Central Dakota Nursing Home..........		100	OW
Crippled Children's School.................		94	OW
Lisbon: Community Memorial Hosp...............	25		OW
Nursing Home Unit		20	OW
Valley City: Sheyenne Memorial Nursing Home ...		78	OW
Sheyenne Manor................................		80	OW
Wishek: Wishek Community Hosp.	31		LD
SOUTH DAKOTA			
Custer: Custer Community Hosp.	16		LD
Eureka: Lutheran Home..................................	64		OW
Gregory: Gregory Community Hosp..................	32		OW
Rosebud Nursing Home......................	58		OW
Hot Springs: Southern Hills General Hosp.	49		OW
Lutheran Nursing Home		50	OW
Lemmon: Five Counties Hosp............................	30		OW
Five Counties Nursing Home.............		32	OW
Philip: Hans P. Peterson Memorial Hosp......	20		OW
Philip Nursing Home		30	OW
Spearfish: Lookout Memorial Hosp....................	20		OW
Wessington			
Springs: Jerauld Co. Memorial Hosp.	37		LD
WISCONSIN			
Durand: Chippewa Valley Area Hosp..............	31		LD
Nursing Home Unit	45		LD
Hayward: Hayward Area Memorial Hosp.	44		OW
Nursing Home Unit		57	OW
WYOMING			
Buffalo: Johnson County Memorial Hosp........	26		LD
Amie Holt Mem. Nursing Home Wing......................................		40	LD
Gillette: Campbell County Memorial Hosp.....	31		LD
Lander: Bishop Randall Hosp..........................	56		LD
Lusk: Niobrara County Memorial Hosp......	12		LD
Nursing Home Unit	12		LD
Powell: Powell Hosp......................................	47		LD
Powell Nursing Home		73	LD
Riverton: Fremont County Memorial Hosp.......	56		LD
Torrington: Goshen County Memorial Hosp.........	46		LD
Nursing Home Unit		30	LD

		Beds		
State, Community, Hospital or Nursing Home		ST	LT	Control
Wheatland:	Platte County Memorial Hosp...........	43		LD
	Nursing Home Unit		24	LD
Worland:	Washakie Memorial Hosp....................	36		LD

otherwise would have found management difficult to function effectively in their communities and by bringing quality medical care to areas otherwise deprived."[9]

As Figure 9:1 shows, the LHHSA operates hospitals, skilled nursing home units and intermediate care facilities in Alaska, Arizona, Colorado, Illinois, Kansas, Michigan, Montana, Nebraska, New Mexico, North Dakota, South Dakota, Wisconsin and Wyoming. Most of the nursing home units are attached to hospitals. The Crippled Children's School in Jamestown, North Dakota, provides medical and therapeutic care and education; and in Alaska, the Society has cooperated with the Indian Health Service to offer quality care to Alaskan natives.

There are 1,420 physicians (550 active, 420 courtesy, and 450 others) who are members of the medical staffs of the hospitals. Most of these doctors also provide medical supervision in the skilled nursing homes. All of the hospitals provide primary care and offer medical, surgical and OB/GYN services. They are equipped to do routine laboratory and x-ray work. Clinical and pathological laboratory services and radiology are provided by hospital-based physicians through contracts negotiated by the local administrator and approved by the central office. Most of these contracts are based on gross revenues from test fees although some contracts are for specific dollar amounts. All of the hospitals have emergency rooms.

The average size of the fifty-seven hospitals is forty beds. Sixteen of the hospitals are accredited by the Joint Commission on Accreditation of Hospitals. In all but two instances, the Society operates the only hospital in the community. In early 1975 the Society employed 647 full-time and 541 part-time registered nurses, 311 full-time and 157 part-time licensed practical or vocational nurses, and 3,211 full-time and 1,619 part-time other personnel. There are sixty-one administrators and seven assistant administrators for the facilities and their average length of service is ten years. Some of the administrators in small hospitals are registered nurses and others have master's degrees in hospital administration.

In 1974, the Society's fifty-five hospitals had 84,041 admissions and provided 471,108 patient days of care. There were 2,239 beds in operation. The average length of stay was 5.6 days and the overall average occupancy rate was 57.8 percent. This rate varied from 48.3 percent in facilities with 25 or fewer beds to 77.5 percent in hospitals of over 100 beds. The hospitals had a total income of $55.7 million. In that same period, the Society's gross operating revenue was $64.3 million and net revenue was $2.6 million. The mix of patient days by payor or type worked out in 1974 as: 41 percent Medicare, 20 percent Blue Cross, 5 percent Medicaid, 25 percent commerical insurance and 9 percent private payment.

A large building and renovation program is under way. In early 1976, the Society had $60 million in new construction in progress. This program will extend through February 1977 and involves nine major projects located in six states. These projects include replacement hospitals in Loveland, Colorado; Torrington, Wyoming; Gregory, South Dakota; Hayward, Wisconsin, and Lisbon, North Dakota. The most expensive projects are an addition to the 250-bed Mesa Lutheran Hospital in Mesa, Arizona, $9.4 million, and $6.6 million for a new 80-bed Loveland Memorial Hospital in Loveland, Colorado.

Some of the service areas are experiencing tremendous industrial and population growth. In Wyoming, for example, where the Society operates one-third of the acute care facilities, there is a boom in energy development. In Alaska, there is another energy boom and demand for beds and services because of the Trans-Alaskan pipeline. And at Mesa, Arizona, the population immigration is continuing, particularly of the over-65 population. The Society grew slowly in the 1940s, had a rapid growth during the 1950s and moderate growth in the 1960s. Malm said the Society now has "the heaviest load of major construction projects the organization has known."[10]

The capital to finance this growth was obtained from Hill-Burton grants and loan guarantees, current and projected revenues, and other sources. The Loveland project is partially financed by $5.5 million in tax-exempt revenue bonds issued by the county under the provisions of a new Colorado law. Standard and Poor's rated the bonds A+ and they were sold in a day and a half. The Society guaranteed payment of the bonds and was, as Malm said, "the first multiple hospital system to back the issuance of bonds with the financial strength of the system itself."[11]

The Society has had an excellent record of financial stability over the years. In 1974 there were net operating revenues of $2.49 million. Malm makes money with money through central office investments in short-term securities. The Society's financial record is so solid that it has a $14 million line of credit with a consortium of banks.

MINNEAPOLIS—ST. PAUL'S HOSPITAL SYSTEMS

Between the 1960 census and the 1970 census, Minnesota had a population gain of almost a half million persons. Today the state has a population estimated at 3.833 million spread over a land area of 84,068 miles. A high proportion of this population—1.87 million persons—is located in southeastern Minnesota in the Twin Cities of Minneapolis-St. Paul and their suburban areas. These areas are hospital-rich. Minnesota has 173 short-term, general hospitals with 23,157 beds. According to the American Hospital Association's 1974 accounting, 7,055 of those beds are concentrated in 14 acute care hospitals of Hennepin County or Minneapolis. Another 3,202 beds are located in 11 facilities in Ramsey County or St. Paul.

Some of the most significant facts about Minnesota's hospitals are their number, size and location. One hundred and five of the state's hospitals contain less than one hundred beds. The state average occupancy rate is only 71.2 percent. Some comprehensive health planners are willing to accept this uneconomical utilization and its inflationary impact on hospital costs in rural areas. However, the average occupancy rate for Minneapolis hospitals is 73.6 percent. And the average rate in St. Paul is 68 percent. Along with Dade County, Florida; Atlanta, Georgia; and Orange County, California, the Minneapolis-St. Paul region is generally recognized as one of the most over-bedded areas in the United States.

Low occupancy rates are symptomatic of several things: (1) a lack of comprehensive health planning, (2) competition between hospitals for patients and doctors, (3) problems in gaining and maintaining good referral patterns and (4) population shifts to the suburbs where patients receive care in other hospitals.

These are some of the characteristics bothering hospitals in the Twin Cities despite the healthy picture of a busy commerce in manfacturing, wholesaling, retailing, finance and education. There are twenty-five industri-al parks in Minneapolis. And the city is trying to revitalize its downtown area through such projects as Gateway Center. St. Paul has a busy commerce in electronics, printing and publishing. Its Capital Center project is an attempt to upgrade the urban area.

Meanwhile, overbedding, competition, and need for referrals—these rea-sons and others are pushing many Twin Cities hospitals into adopting the multiple-unit hospital system strategy as a way to survive and grow.

In some ways, the University of Minnesota hospitals are a system. Certainly the university's influence in medical education has a huge impact on the hospitals. Besides the 748 beds in its Health Sciences Center, the university sends its students to the following hospitals for educational experience: Hennepin County General, Saint Paul-Ramsey, and the Veter-ans Administration and Mount Sinai in Minneapolis.[12]

METROPOLITAN MEDICAL CENTER

One of the most interesting trends in Minneapolis is the unusual relation-ship that has developed between a public hospital and a private hospital. Hennepin County General Hospital is a 405-bed facility that is more than eighty years old. Like many public hospitals it has suffered in recent years from a deteriorating physical plant. It was built just a few blocks from two of the city's oldest hospitals: Swedish Hospital, established in 1898, and St. Barnabas Hospital, which opened its doors in 1871. These two institutions consolidated in 1970 into 736-bed Metropolitan Medical Center (MMC).[13]

Three projects were under way in early 1976 to bring Hennepin County General and MMC into closer physical and operational relationships. The old Hennepin County General was being replaced by a 305-bed hospital estimated to cost $36.7 million. MMC was being remodeled and a new 156-bed addition added at an estimated $29.1 million, including some refinancing of debt.

A new 238-bed Center Hospital is being built upon air rights between the county hospital and the medical center. This $21.1 million project is being financed by revenue bonds sold by a corporation set up for that specific purpose.[14]

The resulting medical complex will provide a total 1,182 beds—461 designated for Hennepin County General Hospital and 721 as MMC beds, a reduction of 132 beds from the previously licensed complement. In Center Hospital, 156 beds will be for Hennepin County General and 127 for MMC The two hospitals will lease space in the building.

There are about twenty shared service programs between the two hospitals including pediatrics, material management, library and cafeteria facilities and communications. Technological devices are shared too, such as radiation therapy and a new EMI scanner. These services are being managed through a series of "provider" and "manager" relationships. This degree of public-private cooperation is unusual. And the two hospitals, retaining their identities and separate corporate structures, do not profess to be a multiple-unit system.

Nonetheless, the Twin Cities have become something of a cradle of multiple-unit systems during the last decade. (See Figure 9:2) In 1965 Fairview Community Hospitals reorganized as a system when it opened a satellite facility. Health Central became a system in 1970. That same year another system was born in Minneapolis when Abbott Hospital and Northwestern Hospital consolidated their resources and efforts in health care. The systems efforts are carried out through an association called Minneapolis Medical Center. And in St. Paul, a new system came into existence in 1973 when St. Luke's and Charles T. Miller Hospital formed United Hospitals.

As a strategy for survival, managers of the four systems are trying to increase referrals into their center city hospitals with more emphasis on outpatient care and community outreach programs. They are also looking beyond the Twin Cities marketing area to hospitals in rural areas of

Figure 9:2

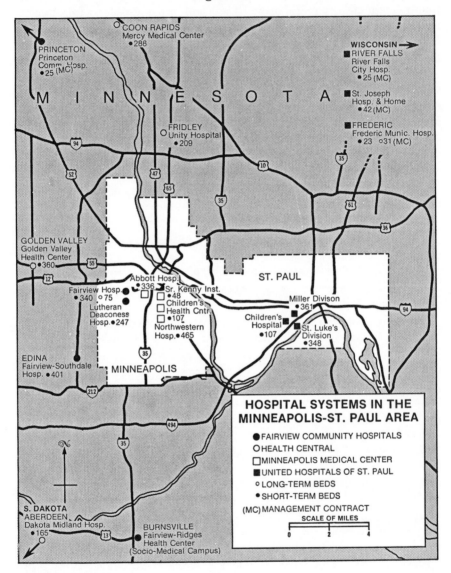

Minnesota and Wisconsin. These managers are trying to put together the interlocking pieces of larger multiple-unit health care systems. Their strategy is also one of growth.

The only Catholic hospital in Minneapolis, 503-bed St. Mary's, is planning to enter the systems competition too. Whether by contract management, lease or merger, St. Mary's says it is willing to help out struggling Catholic hospitals [in the area] so they can survive and carry out their religious mission.[15]

FAIRVIEW COMMUNITY HOSPITALS

Fairview Community Hospitals, Minneapolis, Minnesota, is one of the best-known of the nonprofit, multiple-unit hospital management systems. Although the Fairview system is only ten years old, it has received much attention in the health care literature. Fairview's aggressive president and chief executive officer, Carl N. Platou, has become something of an evangelist for the systems concept.

Some of Platou's philosophy came out during a workshop on multiple systems in Atlanta. After comparing the mission of a hospital to that of a church or a school, he said "You make a system go through a human understanding of the other fellow's needs. . . . A hospital in transition must be able to change its habits. This calls for personal change, but there must be freedom of action. And that doesn't mean that hospitals don't coordinate." What Platou fears is that a single hospital administrator will end up being involved in "the management of decline" for he doesn't have time to look at the broader issues and "is going to be usurped by the regulatory people." And, Platou says, "Boards are going to have to look beyond the psychology of the single roof. If they don't look at the total community health care needs, they will default and the proprietaries will move in. It has become the responsibility of the metropolitan institutions to go out and extend themselves to the rural institutions."[6]

Platou's approach to systems management is based heavily on the holding company concept. Discussing this organization structure in an article for the *Harvard Business Review*,[17] Platou and James A. Rice, an associate at Control Systems Research of St. Louis proposed that multihospital holding companies be widely developed as an organization form, because holding companies could help managers meet consumers' health care needs while preserving local autonomy, the wide variety of services and unit stability that a central management company can offer.

They define a bank holding company "as any company that has ownership control over a bank or group of banks. It has a central corporate office, board, and management, while its individual member banks are operated by their own boards of directors, made up of the civic and business leaders of their given community. The vital characteristics of the bank holding company, so far as the present debate is concerned, are the local board of directors and local management, and, therefore, its responsiveness to local community needs."

Platou and Rice then made a valuable distinction: "In these respects, the bank holding company organization can be sharply distinguished from branch banking. Like branch banking, the holding company organization provides strength to its member banks in a broad geographic area, enabling them to draw on the superior managerial services and capital resources of the group. But, unlike branch banking, which is decentralized in a geographical sense only, the holding company maintains community integrity through local directors and managers." Platou and Rice also strongly argued for preserving the hospitals' mission as an institution to "provide compassionate care. . . . Yet, while we need to retain the ethical principles on which hospitals were first organized, we also need to eliminate any inherited management limitations. The holding company concept is a vehicle for getting the best of both worlds—a strong ethic and a sophisticated management."

Platou, a member of the board of a Minneapolis bank, has pointed out that the First National Bank system of Minneapolis now includes ninety-seven units located in seven states. He sees direct relationships between health and wealth.

Another concept that drives Platou and other top managers of the Fairview system is something called the "consector theory," a concept described in an article for *Hospital Administration*. Minneapolis and St. Paul are generally recognized as highly over-bedded areas. Platou and his associates proposed that Twin Cities health care institutions adopt the new theory. Consector theory is vertical integration. It says that health care resources should "be developed on a service area basis, with one hospital management assuming responsibility for the health care of residents within a specific service area." (A similar concept is contained in Public Law 93-641.) Platou and his colleagues added: "The ultimate test for a health care delivery system, as in any service industry, must be described in terms of consumer satisfaction. The premises of the Consector Theory—pinpointed responsibility, planned growth, and community identity—all work toward that end."[19]

Under the holding company approach, hospitals have three flexible levels of participation within the Fairview Community Hospitals system: (1) ownership, (2) total management agreements and (3) shared services affiliations. These are the three ways that autonomous hospitals can either marry into the system, become engaged, or establish some continuing relationship.

The Fairview system traces its early history to 1905 when a group of Norwegian pastors and laymen formed the Norwegian United Church Hospital Corporation. By 1907 they had acquired a 19-acre site on the lush banks of the Mississippi River. Construction began that year on Thomas Hospital, a tuberculosis facility. In 1914, the corporation had changed its name to United Church Hospital Association and had enough money to build two wings to the hospital. In 1916 Fairview Lutheran Hospital opened its doors and it has been growing ever since. The word "Lutheran" was dropped from the hospital name in the early 1970s.

Today's 415-bed Fairview Hospital is located in a highly institutionalized community called Cedar/Riverside on the West Bank, an area that includes 493-bed St. Mary's Hospital as well as a new town development and the University of Minnesota's business and social science campus. Fairview serves a diverse community of senior citizens, college students and local residents. The hospital jointly operates two family practice clinics in conjunction with St. Mary's and the university medical school.

Fairview's active medical staff includes 285 physicians and 945 full-time employees. There are residency programs in family practice, urology, OB/GYN, orthopedics and oral surgery. The Twin Cities Scoliosis Center is headquartered there. Fairview also operates an extensive rehabilitation center, a 75-bed extended care facility, and is building an eight-story medical office building in conjunction with St. Mary's. Joint purchasing, the West Bank Radiation Center and a heating plant also are shared with St. Mary's.

As early as 1954 several community groups visited Fairview to discuss the possibility of building a hospital in the growing Southdale suburban area, an area southwest of central Minneapolis. A few years later the hospital was given a fifteen-acre tract of land and announced plans to build a satellite. Ground was broken in 1963 and in 1965 Fairview-Southdale Hospital was opened. It was expanded just three years later to keep up with population demands. This hospital now has 401 short-term beds and provides a full range of acute medical and surgical services. Ancillary services were expanded in 1974. There are 410 physicians on the staff.

Fairview-Southdale serves a relatively young and rapidly expanding population. More than 70 percent of the area residents are under 45 years of age. More than 60 percent of the families earn between $10,000 and $25,000 a year. The hospital's special programs are a unique blend of religion and health care, which include marriage counseling, family counseling, alcoholism, death consultation and patient education.

The opening of Fairview-Southdale marked the birth of a new multiple-unit system. Eight years later in January 1973, a third unit joined the system when Lutheran Deaconess Hospital consolidated its efforts with the other two hospitals. This decision was explained as due to a "realization that Lutheran Deaconess could be far more effective in the delivery of health care services and could actively participate through a broader corporate base.... There has been the opportunity to share a wide variety of services resulting in improved patient care at more economical costs."

Lutheran Deaconess, which traces its history to 1919, is located in the inner city. About half of its patients come from five neighborhoods around the hospital and its physicians are scattered throughout Hennepin County. Deaconess supports and participates in fourteen programs which provide a wide range of services created primarily to help residents of the inner city, many of whom are American Indians. Outpatient care is emphasized through an Early and Emergency Care Program for the immediate neighborhood and there were nearly 40,000 patient visits logged through this program in a recent year.

When Lutheran Deaconess joined the system, the present Fairview corporate name was adopted. In 1974 the three hospitals owned and operated 1,064 beds, including 75 long-term beds, owned and operated assets worth $34 million, and had 38,962 admissions. The three hospitals had an average census of 791 and an average occupancy rate of 74.3. They employed 2,394 persons in paraprofessional and support jobs, and had combined expenses of $36.5 million, including $20.3 million for payroll. But the reach and influence of the Fairview system is much greater than these statistics show.

Even before the consolidation with Lutheran Deaconess, the system was beginning to grow in influence outside the Twin Cities area. In 1970 Fairview began selling its computer service to 115-bed Naeve Hospital of Albert Lea, Minnesota. This was the corporation's first shared service affiliation. A few years later the board president of Naeve Hospital said: "Our ability to draw upon consultants from the Fairview management team benefited us significantly as we planned our new building program." The computer network now reaches to nine Minnesota hospitals.

This type of growth is fairly typical of many systems. But in 1974 Fairview trustees launched into a new venture when they signed a three-year management services affiliation agreement with 25-bed Princeton Community Hospital, Princeton, Minnesota, a small town fifty miles northwest of Minneapolis. The board chairman of Princeton Hospital commented, "This relationship ... gives us access to the management expertise of all the hospitals involved in the system without submerging our individual identity and community responsiveness."[20] The holding company concept was beginning to be accepted.

And shared services affiliations have been developed within the state with: Naeve Hospital, Alberta Lea; St. Olaf Hospital, Austin; Divine Redeemer Memorial Hospital, South Saint Paul; Northwestern Hospital Services, Thief River Falls; Bemidji Hospital, Bemidji; Northfield City Hospital, Ebenezer Society, Nursing Home, Minneapolis, and Miller Dwan Hospital, Duluth. One affiliate is in Wisconsin—the St. Croix Valley Memorial Hospital.

Fairview also put the consector theory into practice in 1974 when plans were announced for development of a 140-acre site further south of Fairview-Southdale in another growing suburban area. This so-called Ridges Medical Socio-Educational Campus is twenty-five miles from the center of Minneapolis. The development of this site will take place over a period of fifteen years. The campus will include $100 million in facilities, including a new Lutheran church, an outpatient clinic, a major facility for the aging population in the area and a doctors' office building. This site will also become the home for a fourth Minneapolis inpatient facility owned by the system. The development of this huge complex couldn't have been accomplished without a broadly-based system management. As Platou said, "We had to deal with many different community groups. And the Fairview organization had credibility."[21]

The Fairview system has a prestigious twenty-five member board of trustees. The chairman in 1975 was H. P. Skoglund, chairman of the board of North American Life and Casualty Company, and the board is dotted with representatives from business, industry, banking and education. Platou and the administrators of each of the corporate owned hospitals also are members of the board. The board makes overall policy for the system and most of the decisions are made through an executive committee.

Fairview, Fairview-Southdale and Lutheran Deaconess also have retained separate community boards that make local policy. The three systems hospitals also look for continuing guidance from the American Lutheran Church; they list dozens of congregations as associated with their hospitals. Many of the congregations have appointed delegates to the hospitals.

Medical staff organization follows similar patterns. Fairview, and Fairview-Southdale share a common medical staff and Lutheran Deaconess have a separate medical staff organization.

Through long-range planning the Fairview system had done a considerable amount of soul-searching about its mission in the Upper Midwest. An April 1974 internal document titled, "Strategy for External Corporate Growth" [24] listed a number of strengths: strong board, leadership capability, size, growth experience, financial and management resources, multiple-unit experience and a positive image. That document also addressed itself to the system's weaknesses, noting: "Our strategy for continued hospital growth must take into consideration those areas where we have relatively little experience or demonstrated capability."[22]

Systems planners noted, for example, that Fairview really had no experience with contract management even though a contract had been signed to manage Princeton Hospital. By early 1974, after discussions in late 1973, several Fairview managers had visited the small facility and assessed the problems. These problems were poor external and internal communications, external and internal pressures to hold down costs, low census, competition from ten other hospitals in a forty-mile radius to the town, and poor employee morale related to the benefit structure. On March 31, 1974, the hospital had a net loss on operations of about $2,000 for the previous year. A year later, the hospital had a net gain on operations of about $2,000. In terms of service use and volume of care, however, the hospital had not made such progress.

In April 1975, a planning committee document noted that while morale and communications problems had greatly improved, there was serious doubt that Princeton Hospital could remain in business as an inpatient facility unless aggressive steps were taken. But in December 1975, Platou said, "Princeton Hospital is doing beautifully. It is $70,000 ahead on net revenue this year as compared to a similar time last year. The community is involved. The medical staff is involved in all sorts of conferences and seminars. And the hospital has applied for a survey by the Joint Commission on Accreditation of Hospitals."[23]

The planning statement noted two other system weaknesses: Fairview hadn't "organized [its] managerial resources to pursue a growth strategy."[24] And the system would have to provide a broader range of shared services in order to offer a more complete program to its affiliate hospitals. Despite these limits, the planners recommended that in the next three years (1974-1977) Fairview expand its base of operations 15 percent a year, achieve management or ownership relationships with another 8 to 12 hospitals, expand the shared service program 200 to 250 beds each year, analyze the potential for developing a major health maintenance organization, and study the increased need for human service programs, particularly in primary care and geriatrics.

The growth goals may not have been met. But by late 1975, Fairview was expanding its services to affiliated hospitals. All twenty-one service departments were involved in one or more shared service programs. Platou said, "The department heads all go out, but the doctors only to a minimal extent. Our idea is that we don't steal patients." One of the biggest shared service expansion areas would be into a whole gamut of fiscal and financial areas. Fairview is also looking toward increasing its management contract affiliations. Platou said two other hospitals are under active consideration as management contract members of the Fairview Community Hospitals System.[25] Platou is oriented to growth. For that reason, he and Robert Van Hauer, the president of Health Central, another multiple-unit system in the Minneapolis region, have been engaged in merger discussions for several years.

HEALTH CENTRAL, INC.

Health Central, with offices in north Minneapolis, Minnesota, is a multiple-unit hospital management that traces its history to a doctor-owned hospital built around the turn of the century. While only a little over five years old, Health Central is a system growing in power and influence, which now operates four short-term, general hospitals in Minnesota and one in

South Dakota (see Figure 9:2). Its influence spreads to another thirty-seven hospitals and four nursing homes through affiliate agreements for shared services.[26]

Robert Van Hauer, "the old Dutchman," is the president of Health Central. A dynamic person with an individualistic style, he manages Health Central and a staff of thirty-five persons from an office complex far removed from any of the systems hospitals. Fundamentally a money-manager and an expert on board and medical staff relationships, he has seen, in the last twenty-five years, the bits and pieces of a multiple-unit system fall into place.

Health Central's early history, although hazy, supposedly began when a doctor built a small general hospital for his patients in north Minneapolis around the turn of the century. Early in the Depression the hospital went bankrupt. A businessman named Raymond T. Rascop picked up the deed. He had a difficult time in the mid-1930s running Homewood Hospital until the medical profession's penchant against psychiatrists provided a solution. The city's four psychiatrists couldn't gain admission to any medical staff. They had patients, however, and that's what Rascop needed for his empty beds. So the for-profit facility was converted to a psychiatric hospital.

By the late 1930s Homewood Hospital was out of space and had no place to expand. Rascop and his associates, purchasing an abandoned greenhouse and other buildings on a large plot of land in the Glenwood Hills section of the city, converted one of the buildings to a 20-bed inpatient unit. Glenwood Hills Hospital opened in 1937. By the end of 1966, the hospital had changed its service status to that of a general hospital, although a psychiatric building was included in the complex, and had grown to 204 general beds and 158 specialty beds. Glenwood Hills was always known as a hospital for the mentally ill despite the range of general care services offered. The board, realizing this problem, changed the name to Golden Valley Health Center in 1973.

The colorful history of Health Central is a story of overcoming one obstacle after another. A citizens group in Coon Rapids, Minnesota, wanted to build a hospital but they were blocked by a state attorney general's interpretation of their right to do so under a hospital district law. The citizens withdrew from the hospital district and approached Van Hauer for help. Out of that relationship came Mercy Hospital, now the 288-bed Mercy Medical Center in Coon Rapids, which opened in 1965.

A third institution was added to the system in 1966. Unity Hospital, Fridley, Minnesota, was able to secure financing because the Glenwood Hills organization agreed to operate it for the community. The fourth hospital in the Health Central system is Dakota Midland Hospital in Aberdeen, South Dakota, some 290 miles from Minneapolis, which came into the system in 1974.

Strictly speaking, Van Hauer explained, Health Central owns only Golden Valley Health Center and Mercy Hospital. "The other two facilities are leased and we have the option to acquire them. But we, and the government agencies, view these arrangements as delayed purchase contracts. We own and operate them and carry them on our books as assets." A fifth hospital acquisition presently under consideration "is now leased to a Catholic order and they want out . . . don't have the personnel to operate it. We have an option to buy." Health Central is also considering the purchase of one or more non-profit nursing homes, because as Van Hauer commented in December 1975, "We want to get into that business too."

The period between 1966 and 1970 was something of a shakedown time. Assistant administrators at each of the three hospitals were reporting to Van Hauer, who felt that "as an exercise in management, it wasn't worth two whoops; it just didn't work."[27] Each of the assistants was promoted to administrator and Van Hauer was put into the newly-created post of executive vice-president of Glenwood Hills Hospitals.

By 1970, however, the joint venture wasn't working too well. Van Hauer explained,

> It was extremely tedious to have to take any major piece of business before three boards . . . in order to get any action taken. And, then there always was the threat that one or more of these boards might refuse to participate in the action and upset the applecart, and there were other reasons too.
>
> There has been some difficulties with respect to the fund drive at Anoka [a reference to the county where Mercy Medical Center is located] that didn't pan out as well as it should have and there were some residuals of debt that had accrued and caused some problems. So in order to resolve these internal problems, remove these causes of difficulty and to prepare us to move more swiftly and more effectively in the future, it was decided to terminate the existence of Glenwood Hills Hospitals, Inc., and Anoka Community Hospital, Inc., and consolidate them into a new Corporation. . . .[28]

Health Central came into existence on October 1, 1970, "We decided that health was central to our purpose and that's where the name came from,"[29] Van Hauer stated. Each hospital retained its own board, but a new sixteen-member corporate board was also created with representatives from each of the hospitals. Also represented on the corporate board are representatives of Health Central's Education and Research Division. Each hospital is considered to be a division, although Dakota Midland has not been in the organization long enough to reach that status.

Physicians on the medical staffs of the four hospitals are all in the service areas. They apply to the credentials committee of the medical staff. If the request is approved, it then goes to the board of Health Central.

There is little doubt that Van Hauer is the major driving force at Health Central. The articles of incorporation are routine. They allow the corporation to carry out the usual activities that any organization would need to do to provide health care: buy, lease, own, operate and construct. They state that the system may also set up a pre-payment system.

The central board sets policy, determines goals, reviews divisional budgets, determines the scope of operations, enters into new agreements with other health care organizations and can establish other divisions and subsidiary corporations. The role of each division is: "1. To assess the needs of the service area of the division; 2. To plan to meet the needs of such service area; 3. To translate such plans into capital budgets for necessary maintenance and expansion and into operating budgets for the conduct of the division, and 4. To make all decisions necessary to administer such budgets."[30]

The central office staff is composed of thirty-five persons, about half and half professional managers and clerical support persons. This staff is located in north Minneapolis in a separate, seven-story office building owned by a separate Health Central entity called 2010 Corporation.

Central staff functions include purchasing and procurement, accounting, management engineering, architectural and drafting services and management consulting.

Health Central negotiates purchasing contracts for forty-one facilities—thirty-seven relatively small hospitals and four large, non-profit nursing homes. These institutions have about 3,000 beds so buying is accomplished for over 4,000 beds. The system office does not handle billing, collections, warehousing or delivery. Materials and supplies are drop-shipped. Van Hauer indicates that "this works good for us and for the hospitals. They maintain billing relationships with suppliers, and they maintain their identity. If they want to pull out they are immediately back in contact with suppliers."[31]

The accounting office handles every function related to cash flow, which is provided as a shared service to some of the affiliate institutions and includes: patient accounts, accounts receivable, payroll, general ledger and development of budgets. This section is also responsible for the corporate-wide budget and long-range financing. Van Hauer is the lone management consultant. Affiliate hospitals that want the purchasing service pay an annual fee based on bed size; all other services are billed on the basis of time and a percentage of the salary of the person involved.

Just two years after the system was formed, Van Hauer, speaking as Health Central's executive vice-president, told board, medical staff and management representatives: "I see our hospitals beginning to move outside their walls to develop other services. I think that eventually we are going to see some sort of first aid station or neighborhood health centers, some sort of establishments operating at some distance from the home base and providing some group of services yet to be determined. I don't think this is going to be peculiar to our organization—I think it is going to be true of other hospitals as well—so I think we should include it in our view of our future."[32]

Van Hauer, looking for a bright future, predicted that each hospital complex would soon have a doctors' office building. Health Central was supplying shared services (purchasing and procurement) to several hospitals and more than a half dozen other facilities "are contemplating applying to us for some sort of assistance."[33] Health Central has growing in-service education programs. Other facilities may seek help in this area. Health Central was launching an EKG telephone-reading system and he felt shared service hospitals would buy this too. The system was also seriously considering self-insurance in areas such as malpractice, public liability, and workmen's compensation.

Health Central once operated a computer center but phased it out in the early 1970s and tied in with a Blue Cross program. And Van Hauer then made a passing reference to merger discussions that had been going on with Fairview Community Hospitals: "We are also in conversations with another hospital who may want to affiliate with us and that hospital happens to be possessed with a fantastic computer center of their own that is only being partly utilized. They may decide to join with us and we may be very happy to have them. . . . Why should we be doing all of these things? We need to expand, to grow, to provide leadership, *if* the role of the hospital in the future is to be safeguarded and *if* the hospital is to be the center of health services in the future."[34]

This 1972 speech began to point the Health Central system toward a rapidly developing future. And as 1975 ended, the Health Central statistical picture showed: 1,022 beds; 31,167 admissions; an average census in the four hospitals of 156 patients; an average occupancy rate of 66.7 percent; expenses of $20.3 million, including $10.7 million for payroll, and 1,806 employees. Total assets were $51.5 million.

MINNEAPOLIS MEDICAL CENTER, INC.

A third major multiple-unit hospital system based in Minneapolis has grown up around 801-bed Abbott-Northwestern Hospital, a single corporate unit that came about through a consolidation in 1970.[35] This system grew by another 48 beds in 1974 when the American Rehabilitation Foundation, better known as Sister Kenny Institute, merged its resources with the consolidated hospitals and became a division of Abbott-Northwestern. A fourth separate and highly independent institution, the 107-bed Minneapolis Children's Health Center and Hospital, is located in close geographic proximity to the other three institutions. These four institutions were linked together in 1966 into an association called Minneapolis Medical Center, Inc. (MMC) (see Figure 9:2).

MMC is what Raymond E. Seaver, executive vice-president, calls "a broker's office." The medical center umbrella organization doesn't own or control any of the hospitals, yet it is a mechanism for coordination of services within the downtown campus. Its primary mission, however, is to bring about economies of scale and sell the hospitals' clinical and management expertise to rural institutions in Minnesota and nearby areas of Wisconsin. The four hospitals of MMC have 956 beds. The influence of this center spreads far and wide in the state through group purchasing and shared services programs. In all, MMC has an impact on about fifty other small and medium size hospitals in Minnesota, North Dakota and Wisconsin.[36]

The major power base within MMI is at Abbott-Northwestern, where Gordon M. Sprenger is president and chief executive officer.

A table of organization shows these fourteen job titles reporting directly to Sprenger: assistant to president; administrative resident, medical staff liaison; directors of finance, medical education, professional activities, and fund raising and public relations; chaplain; president of Sister Kenny Institute; associate administrator and director of administrative affairs; administrators of the two hospital divisions; director of personnel, and the executive director of nursing. Sprenger, in turn, reports to the board of directors through its executive committee. The board is huge—eighty members in all. The executive committee is large too—twenty-eight members.[37]

Statistically, the impact of Abbott-Northwestern and Sister Kenny Institute is extensive: 27,574 admissions; $30.4 million in total expenses, including $17.4 million for payroll; 2,090 employees and total assets of $42 million. In 1974 Abbott-Northwestern's occupancy rate was 78.2 percent, higher than the average for short-term care hospitals in over-bedded Minneapolis, but Sister Kenny Institute had a low occupancy rate of 56.3 percent. Children's Health Center and Hospital handled 4,604 admissions; the average census was 67 for an average occupancy of only 62.6 percent. Expenses were $5.9 million with payroll for 320 employees accounting for $2.6 million of the total. An estimated 85 percent of the center's patients come from Hennepin County.

Northwestern Hospital was founded in 1882. Abbott Hospital, named for its founder, Dr. Amos Abbott, commenced operations in 1902. Left to Westminster Presbyterian Church when the doctor died, the church in 1964 deeded the property to the hospital trustees. Sister Kenny Institute originally began operations to treat polio victims. Children's Health Center opened in January 1973 as a new hospital. This hospital had had an interested citizens group and board for almost twenty years, but no inpatient facility. When MMC was formed in 1966, Children's Health Center became a charter member. And when Abbott and Northwestern agreed to give up their pediatric services and consolidate them in a new hospital, MMC became a reality.

Abbott-Northwestern and the Children's Health Center, a tertiary care center and major educational resource for the Upper Midwest region, offer an impressive array of specialty and subspecialty services. Pediatric care is concentrated at the new Children's Health Center and rehabilitation at the Sister Kenny Institute. The charge system is broken down into ten categories, ranging from medical/surgical care and cardiac care to charges on the mental health and minimal care units. The most expensive care in 1974 was that for chemotherapy—$224.50 day, while the nursery cost was lowest—$35 to $40 a day.[38]

Since the turn of this decade, the two hospitals have branched out into pioneering programs. In 1970 the Northwestern Hospital division established an alcoholism and chemical dependency unit and by 1975 the unit had treated about 2,500 patients. Another nonprofit corporation, Abbott-Northwestern Hospital Foundation for Living, was formed in 1971 to provide assistance in fund-raising and distributing educational materials for this program. This foundation also operates a 65-bed treatment center on a lease basis.

In 1973 the Abbott Hospital division established and began conducting a new kind of senior citizen's program in cooperation with the Minneapolis Age and Opportunity Center. Under this unique program, which has had favorable nationwide publicity, the hospital and its doctors provide services for Medicare-eligible patients who can't afford to pay the deductible and nonreimbursible costs under Title 18. Abbott and its physicians absorb these costs. About 10 to 15 percent of the hospital's patient days are accountable for by referrals through the MAO program.

A new community mental health center with emphasis on providing services for adolescents and young adults was placed in full operation at the Abbott Division in 1974. This hospital is also expanding its inpatient mental health beds to 100.

Minneapolis Medical Center is a not-for-profit corporation formed under the provisions of Chapter 317 of Minnesota statutes. MMC is fundamentally a shared service organization that draws heavily on the expertise available within the two sponsoring corporations. There are fourteen directors, the salaried executive vice-president, and a small staff. Abbott-Northwestern Hospital and the Children's Medical Center each appoint five of the directors and three directors are elected from the community at large. The fourteenth member is the executive vice-president.   MMC's budget is derived in approximately equal parts from (1) fee income from users of its service, and (2) research and development support of sponsor organizations.

The MMC organization has three primary divisions: Central Planning, Core Services and a program called Services To Other Institutions (STOI). Until the fall of 1975, the umbrella organization was also responsible for another division called Life Institute, established in June 1973. Closely allied with Medtronics, a Minneapolis-based major manufacturer of electronic devices such as implantable cardiac pacemakers, the Life Institute had been formed to identify "factors which impede acceptance of known bio-engineering technology into private medical practice, followed by the pursuit of educational efforts to eliminate or reduce such factors."[39]

Central Planning is a very active division of the center because of the building and renovation program under way.   In 1974, MMC sold $4 million in taxable bonds to finance an office building and other projects.   The Abbott Hospital unit is being relocated to the Northwestern campus.   The hospital board was to decide in January, 1976, whether to go ahead with the project, estimated to cost around $35 million, but Sprenger was confident that the board would give the go-ahead.   This project will be financed by tax-exempt bonds, a new financing route that just opened up through a Minnesota law. The new hospital will contain about 800 short-term beds; construction would begin in 1977 with completion planned for 1980.   The objective, Sprenger said, is to bring all of the units together into manageable configurations, because the people duplication is unreal. . . . They don't like being shuttled around."[40]   The separation of units is not acceptable to patients.

The Core Services division handles such functions for all four hospitals as purchasing, warehousing, data processing, printing, laundry, courier service and consultation with Children's Health Center.   They also relate directly to MMC's third major division, STOI (Services To Other Institutions).

Hospitals that use these services have no official corporate ties to the center.   But STOI's objectives are systems oriented, namely, "To build a strong base of patient referrals to MMC sponsor institutions by: (1) providing continuing education and health care information services to physicians and health care providers throughout the region;   (2) sharing the benefits of higher quality services at lower operating costs achieved by: (a) concentrating and managing volumes of material and program needs;   (b) avoiding unnecessary duplication of costly human, space, material, and financial resources, and (c) pooling needs and resources to attract and implement up-to-date systems, technologies and top quality management expertise."   A third objective is "providing leadership in the development of optional systems of health services delivery throughout the region."[41]

Several programs fall into the category of health care information and education services. These include continuing education programs to rural hospitals and county medical societies and in-service education programs in clinical nursing subjects. Other programs fall into the category of clinical support, which include a laboratory and pathology reference and consultation service and a daily courier service to and from the hospitals to pick up patient samples that can't be analyzed in the local laboratories. The center is also providing computer analysis and cardiologist interpretation of electrocardiograms and pulmonary function test analysis and interpretation.

The most widely used STOI programs fall into the category of administrative support services. Fifty-five hospitals are participating in a shared materials distribution service in which MMC does the group purchasing and then makes weekly, biweekly or monthly shipments to the hospitals. The center also offers a program in consultation on financial systems. But the Facilities Management Service seems to have the most potential for providing a base on which the system can grow through acquisitions. When this program was announced, MMC said in a marketing brochure:

> Managing a health care facility is a very complex job. The day-to-day operation of an institution which strives to provide optimum care to all patients at a reasonable cost is demanding enough; innovations are coming to the field at a staggering pace. But today's administrator must also be able to deal effectively with planning and funding agencies at all levels of government. In many instances the job has grown beyond the capacity of the stand-alone administrator in a small hospital, where revenues cannot support the specialized assistants.

An on-site administrator would be furnished to the participating institution, who would function "in the traditional way—responding to the needs of the board, the medical staff, and the employees of the institution and serving as the community member of its family." The on-site manager would have valuable management expertise available in Minneapolis as back-up, the statement promised. "The net effect of the program is to give the participating institution—no matter how small—a staff of qualified personnel in all phases of health care administration without the enormous payroll burden this staff would impose under traditional patterns."[42]

By mid-1975 a total of seven hospitals—ranging in bed size from 13 to 150—were being managed by MMC. But Sprenger said because the program was not producing the desired effect—increasing referrals into the four-hospital, regional complex in Minneapolis—"... we may drop it."[43] Indeed, in November 1975, this modification was announced: "This service is being modified to provide administrative *consultation* and support service on a 'pay as you use' item-by-item basis and away from the current responsibility for management basis of the facilities management agreement. All seven hospitals will be converted to the corresponding affiliate arrangement by the end of December, 1976."

This statement also pointed out that STOI "service fees are designed to cover costs of providing services." Stated another way, there was no out-and-out profit motive behind the program. Volume of services might result in some economic gains for the sponsoring organizations and there might be some economic gain "realized indirectly through margins of income over expenses associated with patients referred as a result of the medical center exposure through STOI. In view of the fact that these are largely tertiary levels of care, fixed costs are fairly stable. This results in significant marginal net income for sponsor institutions."

STOI would benefit Abbott-Northwestern and Children's Medical Center in other ways by: "(1) positive visibility in the regional market from which significantly import levels of patient referrals are necessary to build a growing medical center; (2) lowered cost of providing some educational and management services to sponsor institutions through sharing the cost over a broader base of users, and (3) positive political and social implications resulting from our demonstrated willingness to share our strengths and leadership to help remedy maldistribution problems in the health care delivery industry."[44]

When the management contract program began, the concept was for MMC to recruit and hire the administrator for the hospital and the individual would be employed by the center. Seaver said,

We'd be responsible and provide the management expertise and back-up. These were three-year contracts. We were paid a fee based on the salary and benefits of the administrator plus a $6,000 per year supervisory over-ride fee.

This program was of good benefit to them, but the contracts are being concluded and all of the hospitals will be converted to a new system by the end of 1976. We won't extend ourselves further into full management authority. We had the responsibility, but not the clout to make things go ... the local boards still made the policy decisions. There were power problems—too many workers down the line who were worried about their jobs. And some hospital boards are just not in step with what's going on. We hoped to get tertiary care referrals—and referrals are up. But this is not profitable in terms of the risk involved. If we were really interested, the thing to have would be lease or purchase agreements.

> We launched this program in response to a request for help from a small hospital . . . and it just grew. It was a way for us to reach out.

Seaver does not label the experiment a failure, however. All seven hospitals are being switched to an "affiliate, administrative consultation basis."[45] And an increased emphasis will be placed on in-service education programs in medical and nursing subjects.

Rural Minnesota hospitals, even though they need help, are concerned about systems expansion and development in the state. Sprenger says that "some hospitals see the systems as vultures sitting in the Twin Cities ready to eat them up."[46] There is competition between systems within the city and throughout the state, and "Minneapolis is a competitive town medically . . . the fact that it is slightly over-bedded does make it competitive and is the reason for so many cooperative ventures." The health board has made all kinds of projections for the city and called for an over-all medical/surgical occupancy rate of 85 percent, 75 percent in obstetrics and pediatrics and 90 percent in psychiatry. In 1975 Abbott-Northwestern boosted its over-all occupancy rate to 85 percent in medical/surgical beds and to 81 percent for all beds.

Abbott-Northwestern and MMC are working on accessibility problems within the city and in the out-state areas, but Sprenger believes that "some of those small hosptials should die. We would like to convince them that's what should happen—because they are located so close to each other and are competing for the same patients." At the same time, the outreach programs have given the center new "power in a constructive way. When we go before the health board we can say—look at all those hospitals we relate to out-state. They're very impressed with that. This gives us added clout to get what we need and want. And a captive insurance program is now possible by using our economic power."

In terms of accountability, Sprenger believes systems offer definite advantages to health care consumers because there are fewer organizations to deal with. There are also definite economies within systems, Sprenger added, "but don't oversell systems on that basis. Computer manufacturers used to sell their products on the basis of economy. But no more. Their pitch now is, 'You get a better quality product.' The real argument for multiple unit hospital systems is one of survival."

UNITED HOSPITALS OF ST. PAUL

United Hospitals of St. Paul, Minnesota, is a multiple-unit system established January 1, 1972 by consolidation of St. Luke's Hospital and the Charles T. Miller Hospital. This system is a "saving" influence in its center city location, an area of urban decay, and in its neighboring regions of western Wisconsin (see Figure 9:2).

"We are on the edge of a real dying area," commented William N. Wallace, president of United Hospitals, "even the whore houses have moved away."[47] His organization had made a commitment to the city and to excellent medical care, Wallace said. "Patients will have to seek us out, as they have before. We've always had a program for the worthy poor, through our Miller Outpatient Department. And we've always attracted the very, very rich too because of our highly specialized care."

United Hospitals, according to Wallace, came into being for three simple reasons: "One, this is the 'land of the cooperatives,' particularly in private college associations. Two, there was a question of the downtown survival of the core city of St. Paul. Three, the two hospitals had falling censuses, and a desire to muster their resources. In St. Paul we are the only real system." But the systems idea is spreading, because "the two Lutheran hospitals are now talking to each other for the first time. A system is the answer for survival, whether we have national health insurance or not. In planning programs, size is a hell of a factor. So is financial strength."

St. Luke's Hospital traces its history to 1855 when St. Paul was only a village of 5,000 people at the head of navigation of the Mississippi River. Miller Hospital, much younger, opened its doors in 1920. United Hospitals offers just about every specialty in medical care available in the United States, such as the 600 heart procedures done in 1973. And it is continuing to add new services. As Wallace dryly remarked, "We now look for specialists of the *left* lung."

At the same time, a considerable effort has been made to provide community outreach services. Current programs include nurse clinics for the elderly at two St. Paul high-rise complexes, a congregate dining program for elderly high-rise residents, an emphysema-asthma clinic, health education programs for the deaf and for the elderly and a health education center for young adults. And the Miller Outpatient Department, locally known as MOD, continues to provide service as a primary care facility for the medically indigent. There were almost 6,000 outpatient visits in 1974.[48]

The decision to consolidate came as the result of in-depth studies by management consultants E. D. Rosenfeld Associates, of New York City and hospital consultants Souder, Clark, Griffin and Associates, Encino, California. The study, completed in 1971, charts a master plan for development of health care in the city. It had been commissioned by Associated Capital Hospitals, a shared services group composed of five Saint Paul hospitals.[49]

The United Hospital organization provides that a single Board of Directors operate two acute care units: Miller Hospital division, and the St. Luke's Hospital division. Construction work is scheduled to get under way in mid-

1976 for a replacement facility for these hospitals on the St. Luke's site. Acute care beds will be reduced to 600 when the new facility opens in 1979. Also to be constructed through an estimated $70 million program is a new 110 to 120-bed St. Paul's Children's Hospital. This facility will share common walls with the two United Hospitals and a whole range of support and clinical services. It is now being managed by United Hospitals on a contract basis. Wallace calls the coming relationship one of a "physical consolidation. Pediatricians on the staff of Children's have said we'll merge in a few years. My comment is—we're waiting for you baby."

United Hospitals was to go into the money market with an offering of tax-exempt bonds in 1976 that will be issued through state authority. Investment houses and management consulting companies don't doubt that the money will come through, because of the size of the offering. Another reason that the future looks good may be the fact that United Hospitals can help create a more rational system in the St. Paul area, a system that helps increase inpatient occupancy rates and holds the line on costs.

In 1974, the 636 beds in United Hospitals were used to serve 19,027 patients. The average census was 485 and the occupancy rate 75.7 percent. Expenses were $22.6 million, including a payroll of $12.9 million for 1,656 employees. There are 415 active and courtesy appointments to the combined medical staff. The present (1975) Children's Hospital is located just a few blocks from St. Luke's. In 1974 Children's had 107 beds and 4,155 admissions. The average census was only 63 creating an occupancy rate of 58.9 percent. Expenses were $4.5 million and payroll for 310 employees was $2.8 million. Wallace said in late 1975 that "expenses at this facility are approaching $300 per patient per day."

United Hospitals is also making other moves in an attempt to increase referrals into the St. Paul specialty center and help along lagging occupancy rates. Three hospitals and three nursing homes in eastern Wisconsin are being managed on a year-by-year contract basis. Support services, such as advice on medical records, accounting and clinical services are charged on the basis of 140 percent of costs; the facilities pay for administrative/ management services on the basis of 125 percent of costs. (This same charge structure is applied in the management of Children's Hospital.)

The Wisconsin facilities involved in these arrangements are 25-bed River Falls City Hospital, River Falls, 42-bed St. Joseph Hospital and Home, and nursing homes owned by each hospital; and the 54-bed (including a 31-bed long-term care unit) Frederic Municipal Hospital, Frederic. Wallace explained "We are merging the four units in River Falls into the River Falls Area Hospital.... The city asked us to put the pieces together. These small hospitals face competition from other facilities just a few miles away.

Wallace believes that United Hospitals can be a force for growth, stability and even the elimination of some facilities in the nearby Wisconsin area.

In other external programs, United Hospitals does the purchasing for twenty nursing homes in the rural Wisconsin region. He hopes that the system can eventually get as many as twenty small hospitals together through management contracts. One way to accomplish this may be through St. Croix [Wisconsin] Valley Shared Services, an organization Wallace is trying to spawn. "This is a small, local trade area that includes 14 hospitals due east of St. Paul. They range in size from 25 to 60 beds."

Wallace said United Hospitals is interested in permanent arrangements: "We want to go either the merger route or to contract management; we're not anxious to just hold hands." But he believes in a community focus for the facilities, and community control and initiative that will provide the bricks and mortar—"We're not interested in building or ownership."

As United Hospitals looks to the future, it is undergoing a management reorganization. When St. Luke's and Miller Hospital consolidated, they inherited a seventy-five-member corporation. A twenty-member Board of Directors was elected from this group; Wallace is one of two representatives from administration on the board. Each hospital has seven members, the combined medical staff has three members and the auxiliary has one member. Executive vice-president positions will be filled in the areas of medical staff relations, operations (including responsibility for administration of the two hospital divisions), finance, and personnel. Emphasis will be placed on financial control; as Wallace said, "The source of our power is in the till."

In a little over three years, United Hospitals consolidated into single entities the corporate membership from the two hospitals, the board of directors, medical and dental staff, administration, auxiliary, OB unit and all support departments—such as fiscal, personnel, medical records, dietary and purchasing. This was accomplished although the two divisions remained geographically separated.

United's Board of Directors has adopted a detailed and comprehensive statement of long-range objectives with six principal aims: quality of care consistent with lowest possible cost, education and training of physicians and allied health personnel, research aimed at illness and health maintenance, an improved health care delivery systems, improved health and welfare of the community, and a fiscally responsible management.[51]

THE GREAT PLAINS LUTHERAN HOSPITALS, INC.

The Great Plains Lutheran Hospitals (GPLH), Phillipsburg, Kansas, is an unusual hospital system born as a result of the Hill-Burton program. This

Figure 9:3

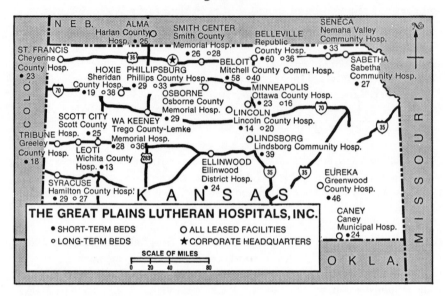

THE GREAT PLAINS LUTHERAN HOSPITALS, INC.

system includes twenty-one small hospitals (see Figure 9:3) that are managed on a lease basis by a group of rural health care experts.

The Hill-Burton program was established by federal law in 1946 to meet the need for additional hospital beds, particularly in rural areas. This federal program pumped millions of dollars of construction money into small towns and communities all across the United States. In some ways, Hill-Burton created the rural health care problem.

In the late 1940s, said Curtis C. Erickson, executive director of GPLH, "many counties in Kansas were building hospitals that had never had them before. They were struggling along and asking, How do we run our hospitals?" What the communities needed were good managers. Catholic orders were asked to take over the operations, he recalled, but they couldn't handle any more hospitals.[52]

From a recommendation by The Reverend C. F. Schaffinit, Erickson recalled, the American Lutheran Church by resolution at a convention in 1950 created a Central District committee to study the problem. This committee considered as a pattern the Lutheran Hospitals and Homes Society of America, Fargo, North Dakota, primarily because Rev. Schaffinit had at one time been employed by the Society, but the final operational plan developed was quite different. LHHSA, established in 1938, was already a success story in health care delivery (reviewed earlier in this chapter).

Schaffinit's central district committee became the core of leadership that formed GPLH and he became the organization's first executive director. The new corporation with offices set up in Phillipsburg began in 1951 to manage its first institution—the 26-bed Smith County Memorial Hospital at Smith Center, Kansas, a town thirty miles from Phillipsburg. Seven other small hospitals came under the GPLH umbrella before the decade was out; another five hospitals were added during the 1960s, and eight other facilities joined the system from 1970 through 1975. One of the hospitals—Harlan County Hospital—is located just north of the Kansas border at Alma, Nebraska.

The 21 hospitals have a total of 612 short-term beds. Nine of the institutions also have contiguous long-term care units and these facilities add another 274 beds to the system. All of the hospitals are voluntary, not-for-profit, owned by either a city, county or district governmental unit and leased to GPLH for management on terms of up to fifteen years. All of the hospitals are certified to treat Medicare patients; six are also accredited by the Joint Commission on Accreditation of Hospitals.

Most Kansas and Nebraska Lutherans trace their ancestors to Germany although a few immigrated to the United States from Scandinavian countries. They began to settle in Kansas in the 1870s and 1880s. Although Kansas has growing metropolitan centers such as Kansas City, Wichita, and Topeka, it is still basically an agricultural state. The primary crops are wheat and milo, and a considerable industry has built up around feed lots for cattle.

Kansas had a population of 2.26 million in the 1970 census. The state's 82,264 square miles are only sparsely populated in Great Plains' primary service areas of central and western Kansas. Most of the hospitals are located in counties with a population of 10,000 or less. An analysis of patient service patterns shows a small number of births, predominately middle-aged and older patients, and a high proportion of the population over age 65. In most of the communities, Medicare-eligible patients make up 20 percent or more of the population.

There are 152 short-term general hospitals in Kansas with a total of 14,804 beds. Of these hospitals 82 are nongovernmental, not-for-profit; 4, for-profit, and the remaining 57, owned by state or local government. The significant thing about Kansas' hospitals, however, is their small bed size. Only 11 facilities have 200 or more beds. There are 21 hospitals in the 100-199 bed category, 46 in the 50-99 bed category, and 65 hospitals in the 49 or fewer beds category.

Considering their small bed size, the GPLH hospitals' service programs are quite diverse. All facilities except one are equipped for routine and general surgery, x-ray, basic clinical laboratory procedures, obstetrical care and emergency rooms. Only one hospital does not provide surgery or obstetrical service because of its closeness to an urban area. Most provide inhalation therapy and six of the facilities have their own physical therapists. Erickson points out that the Great Plains hospitals have helped pioneer shared clinical services in pathology and radiology, the well-known circuit riding concept.[53]

An analysis of the Great Plains Lutheran Hospitals, based on 1974 short-term general care statistics, shows that 20 of the hospitals had an average length of stay of 6.78 days, an average daily census of 16.48 patients, and an average occupancy rate of 54 percent. The hospitals recorded 18,496 admissions, 1,145 births, and provided over 126,000 days of care. A day of care costs $58.46 to $90.47, with the average being $72.90. Long-term care statistics show an average length of stay of 307.9 days, an average census of 254.1 patients, and an average occupancy rate of 92.7 percent. An average day of care costs $22.45. The 21 hospitals employed 2,436 persons, an employee to patient ratio of 2.8:1. Total expenses were $10.25-million with more than $6-million going for payroll.

Overall control and direction of the Great Plains system is vested in a thirteen-member board of directors that is elected from an association membership of Lutherans. Board members may serve two, three-year terms. This organization is the operating agency for the hospitals. While overall policy is established by the directors, each community retains its local board of trustees that serves as the liaison between the corporation and the community.

Each hospital organizes its medical staff separately. Some physicians practice only at the Great Plains-managed hospital. Other doctors also have courtesy privileges at nearby hospitals. None of the hospitals employ full-time physicians. Typically, they depend on doctors in the community as their medical staff. Five of the hospitals have one physician; four have two physicians; nine have three; one has four, and two, seven. Most of the physicians are in their forties, or older, and there are good signs that a few family physicians will be setting up practice in the Great Plains hospital areas in the near future.

Under current guidelines established by the board of directors, the corporation does not own any health care facilities. "We are strictly a managing agency," Erickson said. "We do nothing in capital financing. We lease or manage. The communities provide the bricks and mortar."[54]

The central office in Phillipsburg consists of Erickson, five area directors, three accountants, an educational director, a registered record administrator and two secretaries—thirteen persons in all. This office is linked to the 21 hospitals by a WATS line, that has been quite valuable in day-to-day consultation and problem-solving. The central office staff spends a lot of time on the road, however, and in 1974 they logged 284,896 miles by car. The closest hospital to Phillipsburg is only a 30-mile drive; but 24-bed Caney Municipal Hospital, Caney, Kansas, is 370 miles away.

The primary services provided by the central staff are those of administration, accounting, computer services, medical record department supervision and educational programs. Key administrative responsibilities are vested in the executive director and the five area directors. Three area directors are each responsible for four hospitals; and three for three hospitals each. These administrators work directly with superintendents in each hospital, all of whom are registered nurses. "In practice," Erickson said, "we have six administrators taking a look at one hospital and its problems. Many small hospitals really can't justify a fulltime, qualified administrator. All of the area administrators are college people, most with a background in business, and none of us are [hospital administration] course people. Not many of the courses train people for this type of administration."[55]

Great Plains' three accountants travel often to the hospitals and work directly in training office personnel to handle billing, charges and collection. The central staff uses a uniform chart of accounts system. But no money is handled by the central staff. Each hospital handles its own revenue, expenses, buying and banking locally. The central organization has made available batch processing computer service for accounting and payroll functions.

The central office budget for 1975 was $283,320. Each hospital is charged a monthly operating fee, which currently works out to $550 for an acute care facility of twenty-four beds or less. Hospitals of larger size are charged another $5 per month per licensed acute bed. And those facilities with long-term care units pay another $3 per bed per month. The shared service programs, in accounting and computer services, education and medical records, are billed on the basis of minimum and maximum fees per month at a rate per patient day.

In a report to the 1975 annual meeting, Erickson said the central staff was a minimal one for the number of facilities being managed: "The central office program through the years has expanded from what originally started as only administration to the other areas of accounting, education, and medical records. In a number of our hospitals we now have an ongoing educational program.... The emphasis is on continuing education for all categories of employees which makes the task ... a large one when you consider the fact that we have such a large number of different types of workers.... We are continuing to add to the accounting program ... and have increased the computer services, and will continue to add other programs to the computer in the coming years. Our central office core method of management has been used for many years and is now being studied and used in other areas of the country...."[56]

Another role of the central office is to work with members of the U.S. Congress, such as Rep. Keith G. Sebelius, Republican from the First District of Kansas. Erickson researched, prepared and wrote a statement for Sebelius that was presented before the Subcommittee on Health of the House Committee on Ways and Means in June 1975. That statement contained a strong pitch for relief from the problems the federal bureaucracy is creating for small, rural hospitals. An example of a problem was the government's insistence on a peer review structure that would be almost impossible to use in small hospitals. Erickson and Sebelius asked: How can you perform peer review in a hospital that has a medical staff of only one or two doctors?

GPLH has shown a steady growth in a quarter century of operations. The corporation does not seek growth; it goes to the community on the basis of a plea for help. As Erickson said, "In recent years the organization has been approached when the hospitals are in difficulty. It seems that's when we're asked to come in." Over the years, for example, the organization has taken over three Catholic hospitals which the Sisters no longer wanted to operate and four faltering county or city operations. The corporation's twenty-first hospital was added in 1975 when the 13-bed Wichita County Hospital at Leoti, Kansas was reopened after the community obtained a new physician. A new $1,300,000 structure is being built with community funds through the issuance of county general obligation bonds, the most often used capital financing method in Kansas rural communities. GPLH has no marketing plan as such. It does, however, have a proven track record.

According to a policy statement, "In each locale, GPLH strives to assist the community in meeting its changing health needs by continually adding health services to the local hospital. Therefore, a community health center is developing from the traditional acute general hospital." The corporation said it "is making every attempt to keep abreast of the changing patterns of health care in order to continue to provide their communities the types of services to meet the health needs."

In a report to association members in 1975, Erickson said: "We sincerely ask for your continued support ... through your membership—not for the money involved, but for your support of the principle that a church-related organization is an asset in the health field through sound and concerned Christian management." This philosophy may be best summed up by the Great Plains motto taken from Matthew 20:28, "Not to be ministered unto, but to minister."

"There's no question that there's going to be a continuing need for our kind of services," Erickson said in an interview. "As government brings more pressure to bear on hospitals, I see no other answer. The institutions are not going to go away, and certainly it is more economical to group together. So, I guess we've got a future."[57]

NOTES

1. Interview with Roy C. House, Atlanta, Georgia, November 21, 1975.

2. Lutheran Hospitals Homes Society of America, an undated brochure. The number and type of facilities were revised through correspondence with the Society.

3. H.M. Malm, "Multi-Hospital Management; Analyzing an Example,"*Hospital Administration* (Spring 1974), pp. 31,32.

4. Taped interview with H.M. Malm by W. Money, Fargo, North Dakota, November 14, 1973.

5. H.M. Malm, op. cit., note 3.

6. Explained in a prospectus, "$5,500.00 County of Larimer, Colorado Hospital Facility Revenue Bonds (Lutheran Hospitals and Homes Society Loveland Project) Series 1975," August 6, 1975, p. 16.

7. H.M. Malm, op. cit., note 3.

8. H.M. Malm, "The Hospital Challenge: Putting it All Together," a paper presented to a conference on the National Health Planning and Resources Development Act of 1974, Harrisburg, Pennsylvania, March 24, 1975.

9. LHHSA brochure, op. cit., note 2.

10. H.M. Malm, "System Wide Capital Financing," a paper presented to a Fairview Hospital System seminar, Minneapolis, Minnesota, November 8, 1975.

11. Ibid.

12. 1975-1976 AAMC Directory of Medical Education, pp. 305-326.

13. "Five Years After Consolidation," a special progress report of the emergence and development of the Metropolitan Medical Center, 1972 to 1975.

14. A Preliminary Official Statement (February 15, 1974) on a $19.5 million first mortgage hospital revenue bond offering by Hennepin County, Minnesota and Metropolitan Medical Center.

15. Personal letter to the authors.

16. C.N. Platou, "Multi-Hospital Affiliations," a paper presented to an American Hospital Association workshop, Atlanta, Georgia, November 20, 1975.

17. C.N. Platou, J.A. Rice, "Multihospital Holding Companies," *Harvard Business Review* (May-June 1972), pp. 3-8.

18. Ibid.

19. C.N. Platou, D.C. Wegmiller, W.H. Palmer and J.G. King, "The Consector Theory of Hospital Development," *Hospital Administration* (Spring 1973), pp. 61-75.

20. Fairview Community Hospital, 1974 Annual Report, p. 4.

21. Telephone interview with C.N. Platou, December 4, 1975.

22. "Five Year Operating Plan, Goals and Objectives," Fairview Community Hospital, a 1973 draft document.

23. C.N. Platou, op. cit. 21., note 21.

24. "Five Year Operating Plan," op. cit., note 22.

25. C.N. Platou, op. cit., note 21.

26. Telephone interview with Robert Van Hauer, December 16, 1975.

27. Ibid.

28. "The History of Health Central, Inc.," a Non-Profit Health Care Corporation, founded October 1, 1970, Minneapolis, Minnesota, p. 12.

29. R. Van Hauer, op. cit., note 26.

30. By-Laws of Health Central, Inc., adopted August 30, 1972, p. 2.

31. R. Van Hauer, op. cit., note 26.

32. "The History of Health Central, Inc.," op. cit., note 28.

33. Ibid.

34. Ibid.

35. Explained in a letter from Gordon M. Sprenger, December 2, 1975.

36. "Minneapolis Medical Center, Inc., A Coordinated Approach to Health Care," a general descriptive brochure, undated.

37. Abbott-Northwestern Hospital Corporation Organization, a chart dated July 24, 1975.

38. These figures were included in a prospectus for a bond offering made in 1975.

39. General descriptive brochure, op. cit., note 36.

40. Telephone interview with Gordon M. Sprenger, November 26, 1975.

41. "STOI Programs," a brochure published by MMC, undated.

42. "MMCI Shared Services Profile," a statement dated November 28, 1975.

43. G.M. Sprenger, op. cit., note 40.

44. Shared Services Profile, op. cit., note 42.

45. Telephone interview with Raymond E. Seaver, December 29, 1975.

46. R.E. Sprenger, op. cit., note 40. All subsequent quotations are from this interview until otherwise noted.

47. Telephone interview with William N. Wallace, December 9, 1975. All subsequent quotations are from this interview until otherwise noted.

48. "A Responsibility Report to Our Community," United Hospitals, Inc., Saint Paul, Minnesota, 1974.

49. "A Report on the Consolidation of Two Major Hospitals," an undated statement by United Hospitals.

50. W.N. Wallace, op. cit., note 47.

51. All other quotations until otherwise noted are from the interview with W.N. Wallace.

52. "Statement of Long-Range Objectives," by the Board of Directors of United Hospitals, Inc., March 2, 1972.

53. Telephone interview with Curtis C. Erickson, November 25, 1975.

54. C.C. Erickson, "How a Group of Smaller Hospitals Provides a Full Range of Medical Specialty Services," Hospitals (June 16, 1963), pp. 68-70, 73, 74.

55. C.C. Erickson, op. cit., note 53.

56. Ibid.

57. C.C. Erickson, an untitled statement furnished to Great Plains Lutheran Hospitals members, May 27, 1975. Until otherwise noted all quotations are from this statement.

58. C.C. Erickson, op. cit., note 53.

Chapter 10
West South Central States

In the four states of the West South Central census division—Arkansas, Louisiana, Oklahoma and Texas—the study of nationwide hospital system activity, undertaken as part of the American Hospital Association's annual accounting for its 1975 directory, shows that 199 nonfederal hospitals and 48,638 beds in this large geographical area can be counted as members of systems. As the first survey of its type to locate and document hospital system activity in this area, it was undoubtedly limited. These four states contain many Catholic-sponsored hospitals that were not reported in the survey because the motherhouse was located in another state. And Texas, in particular, is a hotbed of for-profit hospital system activity and expansion—one major chain is headquartered in Texas. System hospitals may have been counted in the corporate office state.

It is believed, however, that most systems activity is concentrated in Texas. But there are exceptions in terms of trends, such as the Rural Health Care Alliance in southeastern Oklahoma and north central Texas, which was formed by fifteen hospitals in a relatively poor area of the United States. According to one report, "It is the purpose of the Alliance to get specialized care and current medical information to the rural area it serves without expensive duplication of equipment and personnel. The use of shared services largely accomplishes this purpose." The 171-bed Valley View Hospital, Ada, Oklahoma, serves as the focal point for the Alliance's programs in medical education, continuing and inservice education and direct services. These services include a central EKG monitoring station linked to all the hospitals by telephone lines and a teleconference network, another telephone system that is the central tool in the educational programs.[1]

One of the largest hospital systems in the area is the huge 1,125-bed Baylor University Medical Center in Dallas, Texas. It includes five integrated hospitals linked together as an academic-service-research center for the

Southwest.   Another large Texas organization is the Baptist Memorial Hospital System in San Antonio. That three-unit system has 1,058 beds. But one of the most innovative hospital systems in the United States, an organization that made the satellite hospital idea come to life, is the Memorial Hospital System in Houston.

MEMORIAL HOSPITAL SYSTEM

The Memorial Hospital System, Houston, Texas, traces its roots to the Baptist General Convention of Texas, and 1907 when a 17-bed facility called Baptist Sanitarium was opened in the then small (population about 45,000) city of Houston.   The city has changed dramatically since those days. Houston has spread out into a creeping megalopolis of 1,999,316 persons, the nation's sixteenth largest standard metropolitan statistical area. Oil and petrochemicals have turned Houston into one of the most influential business and industrial city in the Southwest, a prototype of the "new money" areas and new power centers.

International events have contributed greatly to the growth of Houston and the Memorial Hospital System. After the Soviet Union rocketed its first Sputnik satellite into orbit around the earth in 1960, President John F. Kennedy committed the United States in the following year to landing men on the moon by the end of the decade and bringing them safely back to earth. Although the moon program spawned huge industrial and space complexes in Florida, Mississippi, Alabama and California, Lyndon B. Johnson, then Majority Leader of the U.S. Senate, secured the biggest space program plum of them all, the Manned Spacecraft Center, for Houston and his home state. The development of this center set off tremendous population and industrial growth in the Houston area.

In November 1961, W. Wilson Turner, now president of the system, completed a long-range development plan to point Memorial Baptist Hospital into the future. He said the hospital possessed a potential for future growth and development unequaled by any other hospital in our area. "We need only the wisdom and courage to launch out [Turner had mentioned the new "space laboratory"] and take advantage of its opportunities in order to further develop it into a truly great institution of healing." The city's estimated population at the time was 1.17 million; liberal projections said the city would grow to 1.78 million persons by 1970 and 2.85 million by 1980.

The development plan noted that Houston had 35 general hospitals either in operation or under construction, a total 6,498 short-term beds in 10 nonprofit facilities, 22 private hospitals, and 3 government hospitals. Turner, indicating that the city was developing a laced-doughnut configuration of

Figure 10:1

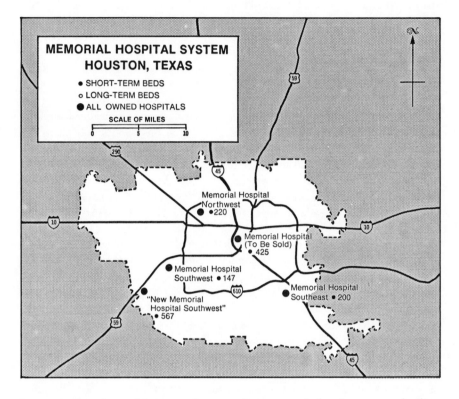

freeways that formed inner and outer rings around the downtown facility, said: "Memorial now draws most of its patients from the heavily populated area around the center of the city, with progressively fewer patients coming from the outlying areas. Practically all of the city's growth is in the suburban areas which are rapidly expanding while at the same time the central area is losing population or degenerating into sub-standard sections. While the development of the freeway system will make Memorial more accessible to all parts of the city and thereby enable it to continue to attract a high class clientele, we [Turner, the board of trustees and medical staff] feel that additional means should be found to protect its position of service to the community."

On the basis of this justification, Turner "recommended that Memorial Baptist Hospital develop itself into a hospital system, providing hospital beds in smaller branch institutions in the center of outlying suburban communities. The main, or central, hospital would provide special services to the smaller units, enabling them to upgrade patient care while at the same time, the smaller units would offer many advantages to both the main central institution and to the smaller branch units if the smaller units can be located on or near one of the feeder freeway streets." Facilities for inpatient care were proposed for the northeast, southeast, southwest, and west areas of Houston.

This plan would protect the main unit and preserve its role as a specialty referral center while creating strong satellite facilities that could draw on central medical and management expertise. Turner feels that the branch units would be an asset to the main unit in their capacity as feeder hospitals, referring to it patients. Another manner in which they would help the main unit would be in serving as proving grounds for key personnel, building up a reservoir of personnel from which to draw department heads." Turner listed twenty-five advantages to the systems concept. Memorial would be recognized as "pioneering a new concept of patient care."[2] The plan would protect Memorial's leadership position in the highly competitive Houston area. Hospital beds would be taken to the population centers. Centralization would result in greater economy and efficiency. Patient care standards would be raised. More and better personnel would be attracted to the system. Centralization of specialized and costly equipment would result in economy. Several of the prospective advantages were related to growth in services and programs at the main unit. Over-all, Turner said, the systems concept would be more attractive to everyone—the public, donors, doctors, nurses, patients and managers.

Turner's long-range plan, a detailed statement tracing population growth and the need for health care facilities is now being used in urban areas. That project rocketed Memorial Baptist Hospital into the future. By December 1964, three of the four satellites were open for business and renovation and upgrading of the main unit was well under way. The fourth satellite, Northeast Unit, was not built because there was not enough demand for new beds.

In the system's fiscal year that ended June 20, 1975, the four hospital units had admitted 48,717 patients. They provided 292,812 days of inpatient care, and 89,208 outpatient and emergency visits. A total of 1,032 beds were in service and the occupancy rate was 73.5 percent. Memorial had a medical staff of 585 active physicians, 311 courtesy members and 95 consultants. The full-time equivalent employees numbered 2,826. System assets were listed as $86.9 million. Expenses were $33.9 million including $18.5 million for payroll.

With high-speed freeways ringing the downtown unit, each of the three branches is only about a twenty minute drive from the main unit. The idea of satellite hospitals as "receiving stations," handling only the most routine cases, however, didn't work out.

In October 1965, two months before the Northwest Unit opened, the president of Memorial's medical staff said: "The satellites have grown in stature to where they need specialized equipment. The satellites can now handle most major cases. They have blood banks, recovery rooms, instruments and doctors. Selfishly, this is different than we wanted, but it is good. The satellites were originally like receiving stations with the major cases transported to the central unit. This has been changed because of the satellites' growth."[3] He then explained that the emergency rooms in the satellites were being used like a doctor's office, as a convenience.

In that early report on the system it was clear, however, that the satellite-main unit concept offered economy of scale in purchasing and shared services and valuable backup services in clinical medicine and management. There was also another manpower advantage: women out of nursing who didn't want to work in the city of Houston came back to their profession and took jobs in the convenient satellite facilities.

Memorial Hospital System made its next major move just a decade after Turner's long-range plan was put on paper; for as the satellites bloomed, the main unit floundered. Referrals went down as did the average occupancy rate.

Houston is like many other cities, but atypical in some ways. It is a bustling environment during the day as people work in air-conditioned comfort. At night, however, the people abandon their workplaces for homes in the suburbs. Unlike New York City or Chicago, Houston has very little "close in" living—high rise apartments, condominiums, public housing and ethnic neighborhoods of brownstones and row houses.

As the suburbs continued to grow, so did the three satellites. Each began as a 180-bed facility; by 1971 there were 200 beds at the Southeast Unit, 147 at the Southwest Unit, and 220 at the Northwest Unit. Houston's southwest area, in fact, was the metropolitan area's major growth area. As Turner said: "Detailed analysis of population and available health facilities selected the southwest sector and adjacent counties as the service area for a new hospital and projected a 450-bed to 500-bed hospital. Because no comparable facility existed or was being planned, the board voted to build a facility to replace the existing southwest unit and to convert that unit for extended care. A site was selected on a major freeway artery about 12 miles from downtown Houston."[4]

Memorial's links to the Baptist church were strong in the beginning, but only tenuous by the late 1960s. Direct financial support from the Baptist General Convention in 1971 was $168,059—0.62 percent of the gross total income. Other than Medicare/Medicaid reimbursement funds for patient care, the church had never allowed the hospital system to accept federal grants such as those available under Hill-Burton. The need for a new

Southwest Unit forced the issue. The trustees "requested the Baptist General Convention of Texas to release the hospital from its control in order to permit the hospital to reorganize as a non-profit community hospital in which non-Baptists could be elected to its board and all sources of financing be made available."[5] The church agreed in 1971 and the word "Baptist" was dropped from the system name.

By 1973, the area's bed needs had changed. The board, realizing that the community could best be served by relocating the system's beds rather than by adding beds, applied for and received a certificate of need for the new hospital as a replacement facility for the central and southwest hospitals, reducing the system's total number of beds by twenty-two.

Turner said, was that "patients were moving further and further away. It was becoming more and more difficult to attract the younger doctors to the downtown unit—they want to be close to their patients. And the average age of our medical staff members was increasing. Also, we suffered a decline in our census and you can't operate a system without a strong, main hospital." "At one time," Turner explained, "the downtown unit had 600 beds in operation and an occupancy rate in the mid-80s; in late 1975 only 425 beds were in service and the average occupancy rate had taken a nose dive to 70 percent."[6]

"By the mid-1960s," Turner said, "the system realized that simply continuing to add and expand services was no longer feasible. Methods for greater efficiency and economy of operation needed to be explored. A coordinated system for all levels of care was considered, to be blended with existing hospital services. Primary, secondary, and tertiary levels of care could be provided by altering services within Memorial Hospital System. These alterations would incorporate economies and help contain costs for patients."[7] When the new hospital was announced in 1971, Turner said: "Since the Hill-Burton Program began in 1946, developments in services and the growth of technology have increased requirements for support service four-fold. Today they occupy two-thirds of the total space in a teaching hospital."

The new $65 million total health care complex, being built in the southwest section of Houston on the campus of Texas Baptist University, will replace two facilities: the downtown Main Unit which includes three major buildings (600 bed hospital, school of nursing residence, and large professional building), and the "old" (circa 1962) Southwest Unit. The downtown buildings in Houston's business and financial center occupy valuable building sites and will be sold. The older hospital in the southwest area will be converted to office space and long-term care.

An immediate effect of this strategic change will be to: (1) move the base hospital to the southwest area and create a new tertiary care center there, (2) launch the system into long-term care and (3) reduce the number of acute care facilities from four to three and the number of authorized beds from 1,090 to 1,050. The long-term effect will be one of sifting out and altering the system's approach to care. The three acute care hospitals will become referral centers for their areas although they will retain centralized management and clinical services and refer very complex, high-technology need cases to such university complexes as the Texas Medical Center.

Eventually each of the acute care facilities will approach health care delivery at three levels. Primary services will be emphasized by working closely with "care as it is organized and provided in the physician's office. . . ." The objectives are to save physicians' time and provide new services such as outpatient multiphasic screening and "a family/community service center for coordinating social services and referrals to existing community agencies."

Care programs at the so-called "secondary level" will be available at the hospitals and open to patients of any physician and any hospital, not just those of Memorial Hospital System and its doctors. At the new Southwest hospital, this level of care will be coordinated through an outpatient/emergency center. "Services will include day surgery, ambulatory and extended care, rehabilitation, patient education, home care, and some psychiatric care.

"Tertiary care will be acute [care] based on existing hospital services. It will include comprehensive specialty procedures but will not overlap long-term research procedures available elsewhere in the city," Turner said, such as heart and kidney transplants.

The rationale of the three-level system was explained this way: "This approach not only will increase available patient services but also will allow Memorial Hospital System to integrate its services with those provided by other hospitals and community agencies. It also will allow patients to move easily between levels of care as needed, and will provide greater economy of operation through sharing of equipment and personnel between levels of care and through incorporating automation and support technology to reduce the ratio of employees to patients. . . . The strength of the plan lies in the fact that it addresses cost and service needs simultaneously."

In a period of two years, Memorial sold three offerings of taxable bonds worth a total $45 million without any trouble at all, which is the bulk of the capital needed for the new $64 million Memorial Hospital Southwest. This hospital will be the lead institution to establish the validity of the three-level approach. This complex is an integrated, thirty-acre campus of four buildings: (1) a so-called "technological base" for diagnostic, surgical, obstetric, emergency and outpatient facilities, and a 567-bed ten-story snowflake-shaped, patient tower rising from the base and connected by a vertical transportation system; (2) an Energy and Dispatch Building linked to the hospital by an underground transportation system; (3) a professional building joined to the hospital by walkways to each floor in the patient tower; and (4) an education building for seventeen programs.

This will be a technologically-oriented hospital, including such features as "elaborate computer and communications systems; all acute care beds in octagonal-shaped rooms equipped with oxygen, suction, and biomedical transmission capability; team nursing units; automated materials handling systems, and a central dietary department featuring ready frozen foods and microwave cooking."

The twenty-one-member Board of Trustees of the system includes attorneys, bank and oil company executives, three members of the Protestant clergy and one physician. The executive officers include Turner, a senior vice-president and secretary, five other vice-presidents and a controller. Each hospital unit is run by a vice-president.

Memorial Hospital System has had more than a decade of experience in shared services between a base hospital and its satellites. These services are categorized as: *contractual,* where nonmedical departments are responsible to each "client" hospital; *referral,* in the case of medical departments, and *cooperative* in instances involving highly specialized procedures and equipment. Turner explained that "the branch and the base departments for each service function as a unit, with a system coordinator. Advantages include medical direction for all departments, shared programs of continuing education, high levels of skill among employees, and the availability of backup personnel and equipment." System hospitals share about fifty services.

Greater economy can be gained by a high degree of sharing. The new complex under construction will use what Turner calls "high utilization methodology" in patient care and support areas to bring about further economies. The high capacity of the new hospital "opens the possibility for sharing services with small outlying hospitals to expand their capabilities, because the equipment and the personnel in the new health care complex will be able to provide some services in volumes greater than needed by Memorial Hospital System."

When compared to national ratios, Memorial's patient ratio of 2.4:1 is below the national average. After initial adjustments, and even if shared services are provided to outlying institutions, Turner predicts that the employee to patient ratio will decrease to 1.8:1, which "will have a terrific impact—reducing costs about $13 a patient day." This will come about by increasing the efficiency of technical and nursing personnel, and by reducing the workforce of housekeeping, dietary, and other support personnel, he explained.

In terms of outreach programs, an experimental program with 106–bed

Polly Ryan Memorial Hospital in nearby Richmond, Texas, was begun in late 1975. This institution is now tied in to Memorial's computer for patient accounts and general accounting. Turner said, "We know we can pretty well double their cash flow—of course, that's not saying too much for they are in poor shape. But we are using this as an experiment to see what we can do. We could provide this service to other smaller hospitals. This would help us too by increasing our volume and lowering per unit cost."[8]

NOTES

1. "An Alliance for Sharing," *Hospitals* (December 16, 1973), pp. 51-53.
2. "Long Range Development Plan, Memorial Baptist Hospital," Houston, Texas, November 1, 1961.
3. W.W. Turner, "Tri-Unit Complex Effects Economy," *Hospitals* (Sept. 1, 1975), pp. 49-52.
4. Ibid.
5. "Long-Range Development Plan," op. cit., note 2.
6. Telephone interview with W. Wilson Turner, January 6, 1976.
7. W.W. Turner, op. cit., note 3. All subsequent quotations from this article until otherwise noted.
8. W.W. Turner, op. cit., note 6.

Chapter 11
Mountain States

Large land areas, low population density, immense mineral resources and places for the U.S. population to expand—these are the characteristics of the eight Mountain States: Arizona, Colorado, Idaho, Montana, Nevada, New Mexico, Utah and Wyoming. Between the 1960 and 1970 censuses, this region grew from 6.8 million people to 8.2 million, more than a 20 percent gain. Montana is the nation's fourth largest state in land area; Wyoming is the second lowest in population density.

Possibly some of the best indications of hospital systems activity in the United States are contained in these states. There are 392 nonfederal hospitals and 43,865 beds in the eight states. The 1975 study of systems activity by the American Hospital Association and the Health Services Research Center of Northwestern University showed 126 nonfederal institutions and 19,762 beds as parts of hospital systems. Stated another way, at least 31 percent of the hospitals and 22 percent of the beds can be counted within systems.

Three major systems within the Mountain States are discussed here: Intermountain Health Care, with offices in Salt Lake City, Utah, has 15 hospitals and 2,101 beds in three states. The Presbyterian Hospital Center, Albuquerque, New Mexico, operates seven hospitals and have 834 beds. The Samaritan Health Service, Phoenix, Arizona, is a well-known system of seven hospitals and 1,256 beds.

INTERMOUNTAIN HEALTH CARE, INC.

Intermountain Health Care, Inc. (IHC), Salt Lake City, Utah, a newly named and reorganized hospital system with a rich history and an unlimited potential, was formed in September 1974, when The Church of Jesus Christ of Latter-day Saints (Mormons) decided to divest itself of fifteen hospitals in Utah, Idaho and Wyoming.[1]

197

The region is characterized by a rural-urban mix. While viable hospitals in the small communities that dot intermountain America are necessary for sustained economic growth, Utah's Wasatch Front, a geographical area stretching about eighty miles from Ogden to Provo, including the capital of Salt Lake City, is a rapidly growing urban area.

The Mormon church hospital system began to develop after the Mormons settled in the Great Salt Lake Basin in 1847. A 12-bed hospital, opened in an abandoned barn in Salt Lake City in 1882, was expanded to 50 beds but then closed in 1870 due to a lack of patients.

James A. Hamilton, a noted hospital consultant, explained the next development of the Mormon hospitals: "In 1895 Dr. William H. Groves, a dentist, provided $50,000 in his will for the express purpose of building a hospital for the church in Salt Lake City. The church contributed the rest of the necessary funds and, at a cost of $180,000, a 50 bed general hospital was opened in 1905. . . . The Thomas D. Dee Memorial Hospital in Ogden, Utah, was turned over to the church in 1912, and the hospital in Logan, Utah, opened in 1914. Three hospitals were added in the 1920s and the remainder have been established since 1939."[2]

At the time of Hamilton's report (based on 1956 data), the 12 hospitals (10 general, 1 maternity, and 1 pediatric) had a total 1,110 beds and an additional 307 beds were under construction. When the Mormon Church turned over its facilities to Intermountain Health Care, a nonchurch, nonprofit corporation, in 1974, there were 15 hospitals with a total 2,101 beds (see Figure 11:1). These hospitals employ 6,748 persons and have 1,100 physicians on their medical staff. They service areas with an estimated 1.5 million people. The hospitals have a physical facility replacement value of more than $107 million.

The Mormon Church is a growing religion. There are an estimated 3.3 million members worldwide, including 2,073,146 members and 4,828 churches in the United States. The church is experiencing very rapid growth in other countries, particularly in Central and South America and the Pacific Islands.

Why did the church get out of the business of health care? The First Presidency, the governing body and highest authority of the Mormon Church, consists of the President, Spencer W. Kimball, and two counselors. The September 1974 statement said: "After a thorough study and consideration, the Council of the First Presidency and Quorum of the Twelve Apostles has decided to divert the full efforts of the Health Services of the Church to the health needs of the *worldwide* Church membership. As a result of that decision and because the operation of hospitals is not central to the mission of the Church, the Church has also decided to divest itself of its extensive

Figure 11:1

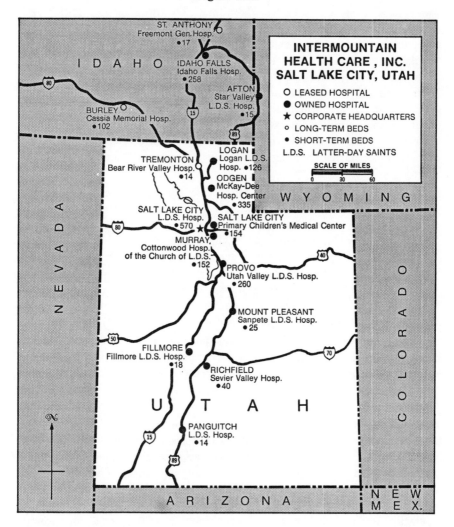

hospital holdings ... the growing worldwide responsibility of the Church makes it difficult to justify provision of curative services in a single, affluent, geographical locality."[3]

The Mormon Church entered the hospital field to serve its members and because of the need to provide community facilities and services where none existed. Other religious organizations, communities and governments also have built health care facilities in the same areas of Utah, Idaho and Wyoming. All these hospitals are used by Mormons and non-Mormons alike.

The church has had a long-standing policy against accepting government grants and contracts such as those available through the Hill-Burton program. It has, however, allowed its patients to pay for care through such mechanisms as Medicare and Medicaid. But the incongruity of federal regulations and programs with the church's philosophy seemed to be a motivating force in the church divesting itself of the fifteen hospitals.

In looking at the construction, renovation and service needs of the fifteen hospitals on a long-term basis, the capital requirements that would have fallen on the church were extensive. This financial commitment was not seen as germane to the church's worldwide health services orientation of medical missionaries stressing preventive medicine and public health programs.

The church had operated its hospitals in a quiet and efficient manner for many years. In 1970 the fifteen relatively autonomous hospitals were brought together into a centralized, multiple-unit system under the church-owned "Health Services Corporation" (HSC) headquartered in Salt Lake City. At the head of the organization was a ten-member board of trustees that met monthly. The board set policy that was carried out through an HSC Commissioner, Dr. James O. Mason, who functioned as the Commissioner of Health Services for the church, and an Associate Commissioner, Kenneth E. Knapp, who assumed operational responsibility for the hospital system.

The organization chart showed major positions in planning and management systems, finance, nursing and education, personnel and management engineering. Line management of the hospitals was vested in Knapp who was assisted by two field directors. Each hospital retained its governing board that directed the activities of an administrator.

Long before the divestiture decision was announced in the fall of 1974, the church employed Cresap, McCormick and Paget to do a major study of the effectiveness of its Health Services Corporation and to make recommendations on a future organizational and governing structure. The management consultants said formation of the HSC "was in accordance with trends under way in the health field to achieve economies of scale, as well as improved operations and a higher level of quality through enabling a group of hospitals to work together rather than on an individual basis." The consultants added, "Several distinct advantages have accrued to the individual hospitals and their communities as a result of the HSC's formation."

The consultants saw in addition to these advantages that the hospitals had become self-sustaining: "Cash management has been improved through the pooling of operating and capital resources to bring a higher return on monies invested and provide greater flexibility for the individual institutions beyond what they could achieve unilaterally. The increased return has generated additional interest income that more than pays for the total operating expenses of the corporate office."

Listing other pluses for the HSC, the consultants said personnel policies had been standardized, a program was under way to eliminate underwriting deficits in the uneconomic hospital operations, and management engineering programs had allowed the fifteen hospitals to evaluate the economic self-sufficiency of their operations by department service. In addition, the systems approach had enabled the reversing of accounts receivable trends, and there was a new emphasis on quality of care that "resulted in the development of corporatewide nursing standards, patient care audits, programs of continuing education, and access to a central pool of sophisticated equipment."[4]

On the other hand, the report said that HSC could not achieve its full potential because of a lack of consensus on why the Mormon Church was in the business of owning and operating hospitals.

After the consultants suggested several alternatives in August 1974, one was chosen and announced two months later to create the nonchurch nonprofit corporation to operate the hospitals. William N. Jones, a prominent Utah businessman, chairman of the board of Electro Controls Corporation, was named chairman of a fifteen-member, self-perpetuating board that includes ten members of the Mormon Church.

It should be pointed out, however, that while ten of the twelve positions on the HSC board were held by General Authorities of the church, none of the members of the new IHC Board of Trustees are Church General Authorities. The religious balance of the new IHC board is the same as that of the communities it serves, according to Jones.[5]

A search was soon under way for the president and chief operating officer of the new corporation, a position filled in April 1975 by Scott S. Parker, former administrator of 472-bed Hoag Memorial Hospital-Presbyterian, Newport Beach, California. After being on the job for only a few months, Parker talked about the outlook for IHC in an interview with the authors.[6]

To the question "Have you made any assessment of the management capabilities within the Intermountain Health Care hospitals?" he replied:

> A first review of the management structure reveals some positive news. We have a strong core of hospital administrators. I don't see any serious problems in the day-to-day management of the hospitals. Our focus has been on the overall organization of our central office, how that office will relate to the local hospitals, and how the central board will relate to the local hospitals' boards. We've come to some basic conclusions. Our central management will have three vice-presidents with functional responsibilities as follows: one will be responsible for finance, one will be responsible for the functions

that we do centrally for all hospitals—the traditional functions of purchasing, fund-raising, public relations, management engineering, and education. And we will have a vice-president for hospital operations to whom the administrators will report. Those three vice-presidents, in addition to myself, will make up the management team of the corporation. The vice-president for operations position was filled in 1975 with the appointment of David Jeppson, former director of hospitals at the University of Colorado Medical Center, Denver. Kenneth E. Knapp, formerly Associate Commissioner of Health Services for the LDS Church and who had operational responsibility for the system prior to its divestiture by the Church was appointed vice-president for central services.

We have a corporate board of trustees and, following the holding company pattern, we continue to have local hospital boards. The decision was a very simple one, recognizing that it's impossible, from a pragmatic point of view, to make policy decisions on a month-to-month basis for every hospital, and impossible to make management decisions on a day-to-day basis for every local operation. We want to have as much local initiative and responsibility as we possibly can and still maintain a system. We have expanded the hospitals' boards from a corps of LDS Church leadership, which was the basis before IHC, to a broader base of community involvement that is reflective of the composition of each community. Another reason for local involvement is that we have high capital needs. We need to develop strong fund-raising locally as well as centrally because we don't have the church to turn to for capital any more. It's impossible to raise money locally if the community does not identify with the local hospital. This happens if you don't have strong ties with the community leadership. We'd like that leadership on our boards both for the good of the communities and the hospitals.

Asked how the local board structure would work, he said:

The local board will deal 100 percent with local medical staffs in terms of applications to the medical staff, approval of membership, and the appeals process on credentials. We hope to keep local problems at the local level. The administrator in this functional organizational scheme reports to two people: his local board chairman and IHC's vice-president for hospital operations. In the traditional organizational sense, that will be a problem. I think it will be less of a problem if we go into it recognizing that we have to minimize the problem. I'd use this corollary. Maybe it's too simplistic, but it can be compared to a softball park with two contiguous diamonds. You have a line between that is the common boundary for the two diamonds; one diamond belongs to the local board and the local administrator, and the other diamond belongs to the central board and the central management. Once in a while we're going to hit a ball into each other's playing field. We will just try to minimize those foul balls and realize that it is going to happen occasionally. We will solve the problems as they come and learn from the process.

To the question "What are some of the central services that the corporate level management team will provide for all the hospitals?" Parker said some functions will fall primarily into the category of consulting while others could involve total functional responsibility. Public relations and fund raising, for example, are seen as consulting services to be provided the administrator, his board, and on-site specialists if they are available. Simultaneously those functions become operational as they relate to central functions. "Local hospitals need help in public relations. We basically are going incognito as a system right now, and as local hospitals."

Management engineering services also will be approached from a combined consulting and direct service approach, but in a different context by performing actual services in hospitals under certain circumstances. As he said, "Management engineering will provide a central corps that the smaller hospitals can call on for help if they cannot support or justify a full-time engineering person or team. For a larger facility, like our Salt Lake City hospital which is 500 plus beds, that hospital can justify and needs a full-time management engineering staff. In such cases the service of the central staff is consultative."

The central purchasing staff will be kept to a minimum, Parker said, but as he explained "of a quality so that the central offices can negotiate long-term contracts for selected items that will reflect significant savings. We will not totally centralize that function, recognizing that each hospital will have some routine needs that must be filled locally."

Another central function that will be developed is construction management. Parker said, "We do not have a high level of sophistication with either our administrators or our corporate experience in construction. We will be involved in quite a bit of remodeling and other major capital projects. I would like to give our administrators some assistance. And I would like to have the peace of mind that the construction programs we get involved in have a good degree of control. I have a keen appreciation of construction management within a system. Steve Morris [president of Samaritan Health Services] recruited a highly capable, former Navy captain with construction and engineering experience. This person served an excellent function —minimizing cost over-runs and getting quality construction for the dollar."

Educational functions within the Mormon system had concentrated on nursing and middle management, and Parker said, "We will continue with those programs, but I feel a need to expand this program to include education programs for our physicians, in the rural hospitals. We have an obvious need to assist them. We want to make it profitable for them to participate in educational functions. We want them to lead their communities and we plan to provide them some backup so that they can. The other motivation for a strong physician education program is to maintain and improve a referral system into our large regional centers and the system's principal teaching hospital in Salt Lake.

Parker, asked about the existing strengths of the Intermountain Health Care system, said "Tradition is one. This system has been operating for many years. There is built-in loyalty to the system. The hospital administrators have been with the system a long time, and they understand the need for central authority.

We have reasonable financial strength. As we inherited the balance sheet of the former church corporation, we inherited some liabilities to be sure. But we also were left with some reserves that we can use as the financial core to build upon. This will be very helpful. We should be able to negotiate good long-term interest and borrowing rates." Parker emphasized that the system's policy of central cash management would be continued in order to create financial leverage and make money with money through investments.

Several capital needs were evident, Parker said. "Our immediate capital needs are to build expansion wings at the Hospitals in Murray and Provo, Utah. [Murray, a suburb of Salt Lake City, is] a classic kind of suburban hospital that has been over-run with the population (running a 98 percent census) and needs to expand. We'll be doubling the size of that hospital and that will require roughly $10 million. We have seen the same kind of population expansion in Provo, forty miles south of Salt Lake and the home of Brigham Young University. There is only one hospital in the community—the one we own and operate. It needs an addition and that will probably cost approximately $15 million. That total $25 million will have to be borrowed and for the first time this organization will go into the market place for money." Parker also said that among other future needs would be the probable replacement of the 260-bed hospital in Logan, Utah, another one-hospital city.

As to future expansion, Parker said:

It's inevitable that we'll be faced with questions of acquisitions. We've already (after only three months) been approached by several communities in Utah and Idaho that have hospitals belonging to county governments. Many county governments are frustrated with the operation of their hospitals. They are confused by all of the regulations they are suddenly facing. They are having problems with recruiting and maintaining their medical staffs. They have all the classic rural hospital problems and are looking to us, exploring the possibility of generating our interest in acquiring or operating their hospitals.

If there was a situation where we really were interested and there was no other acceptable way to do it, it is feasible that we could either use reserves or borrow money to acquire the units. Leasing or contract management are desirable approaches under certain conditions and will be employed when such is the case. We have fifteen hospitals, eight of which we own and seven of which are on either a lease or a management contract. The majority of the seven are on management contracts. And, we have agreed to build a new hospital at some future date on a site we recently acquired from Sandy City, Utah which is another fast-growing suburb of Salt Lake City.

Intermountain Health Care is not unhappy with its contract management arrangements because it protects its cash, he said—"In many instances, it is a way to bring a hospital into our system without eroding our cash reserves."

"The board chose the term Intermountain," Parker explained, "because it has some flexibility. In vernacular common to our area, Intermountain means the states of Utah, Colorado, Wyoming, Idaho and eastern Nevada. You could expand it to include Montana and Arizona as well. And, if you take an even broader interpretation, you could include New Mexico. But, it would not include California."

Parker was asked about competition in Intermountain's service area. In most of the smaller towns and cities, he said, there is no competition from another system and Intermountain Health Care manages the community's only hospital. For-profit chains are another matter. "Hospital Corporation of America is building two hospitals in Utah. I am sure they view Utah as we do—as having tremendous potential for growth."

Intermountain Health Care already has the power to ensure that duplication does not occur within its fifteen hospitals, because:

All of the construction programs and major capital expenditures come under central review before approval is granted. We really do have the ability to do some shaping and to try to avoid duplication. There is only one radiation therapy unit in the entire system, for example. I think we'll be able to hold the line on that for quite awhile. I think we'll be able to hold the line on the EMI-type scanners, too. We probably have as much ability as any system to organize the high capital equipment and minimize its proliferation until justified.

Intermountain will not expand just for the sake of adding numbers. We'll grow at a pace that is comfortable and beneficial to existing operations. If we make an error, we'll make it on the side of caution rather than premature rapid expansion. The board already has made a decision to be intensive to the Intermountain Region.

Parker agrees with the traditional argument for multiple-unit hospital systems—survival in the face of pressures coming from governments and reimbursement agencies. And he adds: "A small independent hospital will have little if any impact on most major outside policy decisions affecting it. The systems themselves have a difficult time, but at least they do have some telling impact." Unions present yet another challenge, because "most hospitals have been dealing with local unions that are not well-financed and relatively immature. But it is inevitable that in the hospital field there will be the development of national hospital chains and central unions that will have central strength. That leverage against a small hospital will be tremendous. It will be very difficult for them to survive on a one-to-one basis."

At the time of the interview, Parker said IMC was already organizing its local boards so that they could be marshalled for a political thrust: "In our region, the legislatures are influenced a great deal by the rural representatives. If we have our local boards dealing with the local legislators, we should be able to have a positive impact in the state legislatures." Intermountain was not considering taking an independent national posture in dealing with the U.S. Congress, he said, but preferred to work through state and national hospital associations. Parker agreed though that a coalition of systems involved in meeting both rural and urban health care needs might benefit by presenting a united front before the rural caucus in Congress.

Asked if the Intermountain concept would work, he said, "It will work. It has worked and is working better all the time. I think it is an application of proven experience—and it will grow. We're continually being approached by hospitals that want to join our system. Other systems are being approached, too. This is a demonstration that smaller, independent hospitals are recognizing that there is strength in numbers. I think it is just the beginning of multi-hospital systems development in our country."

Speaking of the need for strong management, Parker added: "I think the successes that we have seen in multiple hospital systems nationally really relate to the vision of some individual managers, and their ability to implement, to gain, and to bring along and maintain the support of their boards. I don't know of any multiple hospital system that was created because of board pressure to do so; hospital boards tend to be conservative and traditional." Systems have been created, he continued, "because of management determination, innovation and dedication to a goal."

SAMARITAN HEALTH SERVICE

Hospital systems often begin on the basis of a merger. In the summer of 1968, for example, Good Samaritan Hospital in Phoenix, Arizona, and Southside Hospital in nearby Mesa, merged both physically and philo-sophically. The assets and liabilities of both organizations "were scooped up into one corporate body to become Samaritan Health Service, [explained Stephen M. Morris, president of SHS.] "Quickly and effectively a realistic three-pronged goal was established with the following contents: (1) to contain costs of patient care; (2) to develop a system of patient care, making it available to people no matter what their economic status, or how remote from the service they might be geographically; and (3) to continually strive to expand and escalate patient care in all areas."[7]

That merger created one of the widely publicized hospital systems in the United States. The system grew to include eight hospitals in the greater Phoenix area and north and northeastern Arizona in 1973. But SHS has gone through something of a "shaking out period" in recent years, so that today SHS has six inpatient facilities, 1,233 beds, a clinic and a unique air ambulance-emergency medical care system called "Air Evac."[8]

The facilities in this eight-year-old system are shown in Figure 11:2, which includes the hospital system managed by Samaritan's next state neighbor to the east, the Presbyterian Hospital Center in Albuquerque, New Mexico.

In 1962 early in his career, Morris became active in national hospital affairs when he was named a member of the American Hospital Association's House of Delegates. He served in the House until 1968, the same year SHS was formed, when he was named a member of the AHA Board of Trustees. In 1971, he was chosen president-elect of the AHA, and he succeeded to the presidency the next year. A good friend of Edwin L. Crosby, M.D., the full-time top executive of AHA until his death in 1973, Morris and the Samaritan Health system have been placed in the national spotlight for several reasons. The national crescendo of demands to "do something about the health care

Figure 11:2

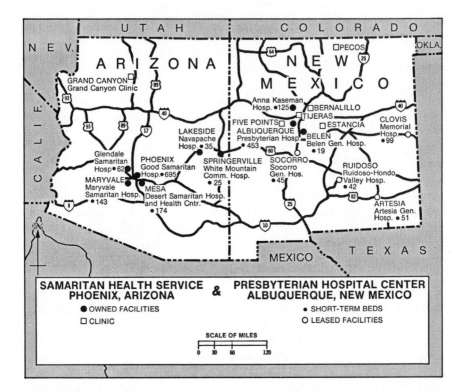

SAMARITAN HEALTH SERVICE
PHOENIX, ARIZONA
● OWNED FACILITIES
□ CLINIC

&

PRESBYTERIAN HOSPITAL CENTER
ALBUQUERQUE, NEW MEXICO
● SHORT-TERM BEDS
O LEASED FACILITIES

SCALE OF MILES
0   30   60   120

crisis" had risen to a high decible level in 1968. The Kaiser Health Plan stood out as an isolated example of how to do things—organize a system for care, stress preventive medicine, have committed doctor groups, and in these ways reduce the incidence of hospitalization and length of stay.

Around this same time, AHA had appointed its Special Committee on the Provision of Health Services headed by Earl Perloff, a trustee of Albert Einstein Medical Center, a two hospital system in Philadelphia, Pennsylvania. Morris was named a number of this committee that came up with the concept of Health Care Corporations, highly integrated hospital systems, that would be responsible to provide care in designated geographical areas of the United States. The HCC concept was later transformed into AHA's entry into the national health insurance sweepstakes, and packaged as Ameriplan.[9]

Still another related trend of the times turned nationwide attention on Samaritan Health Service and Morris. Around the end of the 1960s, Nixon Administration health policymakers had been sold on the idea of reorganizing the health care delivery system by putting major emphasis on the development of health maintenance organizations. Kaiser was often referred to as the prototype health maintenance organization. SHS became referred to as the same type of organization, but an example of a voluntary, not-for-profit initiative even more representative of what could be done nationally than the closed group practice approach that is the heart of the Kaiser System. At the time, Morris was a pioneer at the forefront of reorganizing the delivery system and an official with a high level position in AHA.

The same year that Morris was president-elect of AHA, SHS was only three years old and developing rapidly. That spring of 1971 Morris told a reporter for *Modern Hospital:* "If we are at fault, it was perhaps in developing too quickly. My only answer to that is the opportunities were there and if we didn't seize them they might not ever have come again." Morris, asked about SHS pioneering approach to urban and rural health care as a model for the nation, said, "We haven't really solved anything yet. But I think the general approach to comprehensive health care is in the right direction. The concept follows closely the proposals put forth by President Nixon's Health Maintenance Organizations and by AHA's Ameriplan. Our adaptation to an HMO could be made very easily." Later in the interview, Morris added: "I think we'll be in program development for about the next five years. We're through the formative stage. We've got the skeleton built, and now the model is ready to be fleshed out. We're entering the consolidation stage with stress on management, centralized services, and up-to-date program planning at each facility with emphasis on coordination between facilities." Another administrator in the system warned about being overly optimistic about cost savings in a system. "When you're talking about changing the whole structure from illness oriented to health oriented, it's going to cost a lot more money any way you cut it."[10]

Two years later, writing in *Hospital Administration,* Morris said SHS was aiming to do several things simultaneously—contain costs, increase accessibility, eliminate duplication and fragmentation, increase quality and emphasize prevention through treating vertical instead of horizontal patients. "If solutions can be provided for these five areas of health concern, [he said,] Samaritan Health Service will be well on the way to developing a prototype that will be ready-made for duplication throughout the nation. Already it is being carefully studied by groups in Colorado, New York, South Carolina, Missouri, Oregon and many other states as well as governmental health officials in Washington, D.C. The Health Services Research Center was the recipient of a contract from the Department of HEW which is being used to conduct a detailed evaluation of the effectiveness of what is going on within the organization. This major contract will enable the health care world to know what SHS is all about."[11]

In the early 1970s, two researchers from the Health Services Research

Center at Northwestern began studying SHS in terms of the impact of the merger between Good Samaritan and Southside Hospital. Sam A. Edwards, director of the center, and Adrienne A. Astolfi, director of research and development, reported their two-year study of the system in an article for *Hospital Administration*. SHS had expanded to eight hospitals. Edwards and Astolfi concluded that the merger "has enabled the member facilities to improve and expand services without incurring additional costs and while establishing the system on a solid financial base. In addition, merger resulted in an increase in comprehensiveness of services and improvements in quality and availability of care. Although the system is not without criticism, the system has been accepted by its employees, its medical staffs, and the communities it serves."[12] The studies would continue, the authors said, whose work was supported by a half million dollars in federal contract money from the National Center for Health Services Research.

There were many older hospital systems then in existence in the United States, but SHS had attracted nationwide attention. It was then suggested that Samaritan be compared with some of the older, more mature systems to see how it would stack up. This suggestion led to another two-year study, this time comparing SHS to seven other not-for-profit hospital systems.

This new study was taken up by James P. Cooney, Jr., as principal investigator, and Thomas L. Alexander, project director. They produced 900 pages of reports in four volumes in 1975, almost two inches of reading material. The four volumes, *"Multihospital Systems: An Evaluation,"* were subtitled "Overview," "Organizational Studies," "Cost Studies," and "Related Studies." The general orientation of these studies was toward the impact on people—particularly the effects of merger and system-building on the managers, physicians and other employees at the large and prosperous base hospital in Phoenix. Cooney and Alexander said: "Perhaps one of the most profound, and yet simplest, conclusions derived through this study is that the internal trauma of organizational change brought on by the formation of a multihospital system is mediated by age. The older a system becomes, the more smoothly it operates."[13] This SHS study was also financed by a contract from the National Center for Health Services Research.

The hospitals that SHS brought together were generally in financial trouble. Bruce R. Neumann of the department of accountancy, University of Illinois-Urbana, did a study of the financial aspects of the system and noted that the formation of SHS could be "characterized as the merger of a large, financially strong hospital with smalller hospitals that were, for the most part, experiencing severe crises. Each of the smaller Samaritan Hospitals required some form of capital input in order to survive. . . . Other Samaritan hospitals needed working capital loans to meet current liabilities and to increase the services available." Looking at the system post-merger, Neumann said the synergism of the system had produced three results: "1) spreading the risk of financial bankruptcy over a larger asset base, 2) stabilizing the flow of funds from operations for the entire Samaritan system, and 3) providing additional external sources of capital funds to individual Samaritan hospitals."[14] Neumann had trouble documenting cost savings. He did feel, however, that SHS had increased services available to patients throughout the system—and, of course, there was the over-riding effect of keeping other hospitals alive.

There have also been informal studies of SHS. A number of Phoenix-area community organizations, led in their zeal and probing by an official of the Motorola Corporation, put a microscope to the cost aspects of care within SHS. Their campaign was also against local money subsidizing system operations in other places, such as the rural hospitals, and the expense of Air Evac.[15]

Under SHS management organization, Morris reports to a thirty-eight— member board of directors. The system is divided into four operations and three service divisions, each headed by a vice-president, with operating divisions for Good Samaritan, Desert Samaritan, and Maryvale Samaritan hospitals. The fourth vice-president is in charge of Glendale Samaritan and is also the regional hospitals coordinator. Each of these vice-presidents also holds the title of administrator. The three service divisions are financial, human resources and development, and systems and services.[16]

The system's administrative offices are located in a building separate from the Phoenix hospitals. Many operational functions are centralized and shared. These include financial services, housekeeping, food service, biomedical information, materials management, patient services, human resources and development, and public relations. The centralized patient services function is called a prototype program set up to deal with admissions, patient problems, billing, insurance, and bed allocation. Two SHS facilities are shared by other hospitals in the area: an automated laundry, built in 1973, and a print shop.

AHA data for 1974, based on 1,138 beds in Samaritan's six hospitals, show these totals: admissions, 47,047; average census, 896 patients; average daily occupancy rate, 64.2 percent; total expenses, $55.26 million, and total full-time employees, 3,299.

SHS has total assets of $63.9 million and in 1975 moved to strengthen its financial position by retiring some debts and refinancing other debts. This is being accomplished through revenue bonds issued·under the governmental authority of Maricopa County. There were two issuances of bonds in 1975: $36.6 million were sold in July, and $58.4 million were sold in the last quarter of the year. This financial package puts SHS into a new alliance with the county for gross revenues are pledged against payment of the bonds into the next century. The bond issue also will provide capital for improvements and renovations in several facilities and allow SHS to build a new 256-bed Maryvale Samaritan.[17]

The 695-bed Good Samaritan Hospital is one of the best-known medical complexes in the Southwest. Founded in 1911 as the Arizona Deaconess Hospital and Home and renamed Good Samaritan in 1928, this full-service facility has all inpatient services, six outpatient clinics, twenty-eight sub-clinics and an around-the-clock emergency service. Specialized services and units include kidney transplantation and dialysis, and institutes for cardiovascular diseases, gastroenterology and rehabilitative medicine. There is a spinal cord injury center, mental health program and a radiation oncology center. There are educational programs at the graduate level, nine residency and five fellowship programs. There are also paramedical paraprofessional training programs in four fields. About 2,150 persons are employed at this facility and there are 750 members of the medical staff. Good Sam, as it is often referred to, occupies four city blocks and an eight-acre site. The main hospital has six, six-story wings. The Institute of Rehabilitation Medicine occupies a separate, five-story building.[18]

The old Mesa facility, called Southside, was replaced in 1973 by the 273-bed Desert Samaritan Hospital and Health Center. This modern, attractive hospital can be expanded to 1,100 beds. The system also includes two other hospitals in the Phoenix area: 147-bed Maryvale Samaritan that serves west Phoenix, purchased in 1969 at a bankruptcy sale, and the 62-bed Glendale Samaritan in the northwest part of the city. Glendale merged with SHS in 1969.

There are three rural-based system facilities. The 35-bed Navapache District Hospital at Lakeside, 189 miles east of Phoenix, is operated under a long-term management contract lease. The 25-bed White Mountain Communities Hospital, located 224 miles east at Springerville, is operated under the same arrangement as Navapache. SHS staffs and manages the Grand Canyon Clinic under a cost-reimbursement management contract with the U.S. Park Service. This institution, located 276 miles north of Phoenix, was built in 1968 as a 22-bed hospital to serve tourists visiting the Grand Canyon but was converted to a clinic operation in 1973. It has four employees and a medical staff of one. SHS operated the 23-bed Holbrook Hospital until September 1974, when the lease was terminated by mutual agreement.

There are 17 competing hospitals in the greater Phoenix area. These include the 560-bed St. Joseph's Hospital and Medical Center, an institution sponsored by the Sisters of Mercy of Burlingame, California, and the 250-bed Mesa Lutheran Hospital. Mesa Lutheran had an 81.2 percent occupancy rate in 1974. It is one of the larger facilities owned by the Lutheran

Hospitals and Homes Society of America, a large, competing system with headquarters in Fargo, North Dakota.

Policymakers would consider the Phoenix area highly over-bedded; nine of the seventeen competitors to SHS had occupancy rates under 70 percent in 1974. The four SHS hospitals had an overall occupancy rate of 77.1 percent.

The official document describing the revenue bond issue was instructive in terms of the description of "possible regulatory and other changes affecting health care facilities." It noted that the future was uncertain and a number of factors might affect SHS's operations, in fact, all hospital systems. These factors were listed as the possibilities of: new wage and price controls, reductions in Medicare funding, changes in Medicare regulations, development of health maintenance organizations, efforts by insurers and governmental agencies to limit the cost of services, possible changes in reimbursement by Blue Cross and Blue Shield plans, the cost and availability of malpractice insurance, the implementation of Public Law 93-641, and a ruling before the U.S. Supreme Court on the status of tax-exempt charitable corporations.

PRESBYTERIAN HOSPITAL CENTER

Albuquerque, New Mexico, founded in 1706 and now a bustling city of more than 333,000 people, still maintains many old west and Spanish characteristics. The largest city in a state of only 1,016 million people, Albuquerque is also the health care center of Bernaillo County and New Mexico. It contains 11 of the state's hospitals and more than 2,300 of its beds. Beyond its warm, dry air, spectacular scenery and thriving industry, however, the state is in desperate need of solutions to rural health care problems that plague many of the Mountain States. New Mexico's needs are compounded by great distances, communications problems, and secondary roads that are either dry and dusty or muddy and impassable. Another problem hampers a good health care system for the state: language. Many of the older citizens who need medical attention speak only Spanish; they are not oriented to primary care and only seek medical attention when their problems have advanced to an acute stage.[19]

The medical care and health care needs of the state were recognized many years ago by religious groups. The Presbyterian Church, for instance, opened a hospital in Albuquerque in 1908. The Dominican Sisters, Congregation of Our Lady of the Sacred Heart, with generalate offices in Grand Rapids, Michigan, established the 92-bed Nazareth Hospital, a facility for psychiatric care. And the Sisters of Charity of Cincinnati, with the generalate located in St. Joseph, Ohio, developed the 349-bed St. Joseph Hospital, an acute care facility. Over the years nine other hospitals have been established in

Albuquerque, including a 413-bed VA Hospital, a 73-bed U.S. Public Health Service Indian Hospital, a 65-bed Atchison, Topeka & Sante Fe Memorial Hospital, and other facilities.

Some hospitals in the urban areas, such as the Presbyterian Hospital Center and St. Joseph's have recognized the statewide rural health care needs. And they are reaching out in new ways to help the rural population, a good percentage of which is poor and living on poverty level incomes.

The Presbyterian Hospital Center (PHC) is a system that now includes a network of seven hospitals with 834 beds (see Figure 11:2). Two of the hospitals are located in Albuquerque and the other five are in the small and medium-size cities of Artesia, Belen, Ruidso, Socorro and Clovis.[20]

PHC has also joined with St. Joseph, through unusual arrangements involving competitors and differing religious philosophies, to establish out-patient clinics and primary care treatment sites in four rural communities.

PHC is the largest private, not-for-profit hospital in New Mexico. Presbyterian Hospital provides almost all services that would be available in a large medical complex, including facilities for surgery in a laminar flow operating room, open heart procedures and various specialized intensive care units. PHC co-sponsors a fully-accredited school of practical nursing in conjunction with Albuquerque Technical -Vocational Institute. The center also operates two major medical office buildings and several smaller offices. Management consultations have been provided for several hospitals in the state, sometimes informally and sometimes on a contract basis.

The driving force behind PHC is its president, Ray Woodham. PHC backed into a systems configuration, he said. In the mid-1950s, Albuquerque had experienced quite a population growth, particularly in areas northeast of the city. "The situation was ripe for a proprietary hospital to enter the community. In fact, one did acquire an option on a site and began to court the local physicians with the usual campaign promises, i.e. better services and lower costs. It appeared that the proprietary operation was going to get off the ground, so we played a little poker. We acquired an option on a site across the street from the proposed proprietary and announced plans to build. Frankly, at that point, our plans extended only to the sign that we erected on the property. Without reciting the trials and tribulations of putting this together, I'll just say that a 172-bed hospital was built and the proprietary folded."[21]

The satellite facility, named Anna Kaseman Hospital, opened in September 1970. So, a desperation move to block the construction of a for-profit facility launched PHC as a system. And in the next five years, the system grew and grew. New facilities, services and programs have been added so rapidly that the management abilities of Woodham and his staff were stretched, particularly during the days of the Economic Stabilization Program.

Woodham told his Boston audience that the total area of the six New England states is only about one-half of the area of New Mexico, a state with a low population density and a low per capita income. He compared PHC to a "motherhouse" and described it as an "overgrown community hospital" with nearly 15 percent of the state's general acute beds. Woodham then explained how the PHC system developed after Anna Kaseman Hospital opened.

The first expansion came in 1971 when PHC purchased the 19-bed Belen General Hospital, located in a rapidly expanding service area of about 25,000 population some 34 miles south of Albuquerque. Woodham said: "We are now facing questions of expansion, recruitment of physicians, and replacement of the facility, which is marginal. The community is just large enough that it is going to present some difficult questions in planning for the future. The problem, of course, is to infuse medical care and develop a different facility."

The 50-bed Atresia Hospital was added in the spring of 1972. It is located in a community of about 12,000 persons and is some 239 miles from Albuquerque. Woodham described the operation as one in which local politics and pressures typically influenced it. He said that before the acquisition the administrator "thought that the ultimate survival of Artesia Hospital would probably depend on its removal from local politics" and the ability to draw on the resources of the large institution. "So they came to us to see if we would be interested in leasing Artesia. By that time, I guess we didn't know how to say no, so we leased it for $1 a year for 10 years, which is the kind of offer you can't refuse. If we had looked at it a little more closely, I'm not sure we might not have bargained them down to 50¢."

In the fall of 1972, PHC became a five-unit system through another decade-long, $1 lease of the 42–bed Ruidoso-Hondo Valley Hospital, a county facility 191 miles south of Albuquerque in a resort community. "We thought it would be our vacationland, which shows how little we knew," [Woodham said.] "Ruidoso has skiing in the winter and horse racing in the summer."

Speaking of the system brought together to that time, Woodham explained: "We do have full management authority. We have advisory boards appointed in all three communities. They are policy advisory boards, and they make recommendations to our board of directors and to our management. The boards are designed to retain community commitment and involvement in the hospitals, and it is certainly far too early to tell whether or not they will be an effective mechanism. We think it would be ineffective if we did not have them. The plan was not to co-mingle funds, and we don't. We just send funds; we haven't gotten much back to mingle yet. We do anticipate full recovery, however."

A sixth hospital was added to the system in 1975. This is the 99–bed Clovis Memorial Hospital, which is being operated on a lease basis until a wholly-owned replacement is constructed. The institution is in a city some 220 miles from Albuquerque. In February 1976, PHC picked up its seventh system member—the 45–bed Socorro General Hospital—through another 10-year lease. This community is 75 miles from Albuquerque.[22]

According to 1974 American Hospital Association statistics, the seven PHC hospitals had 834 available beds. They had 36,984 admissions and an average daily census of 562 patients. The average occupancy rate was under 60 percent. This overall figure was pulled down considerably by the five hospitals outside the urban area of Albuquerque. Occupancy at the base hospital and its satellite was 76.0 percent. The seven hospitals had expenses of $26.4 million, including payroll of $13.4 million for 1,988 full-time employees.

Woodham believes that there are many advantages to the rural hospitals that accrue through system membership. He refers to central management expertise, inservice education programs, the availability of backup personnel, purchasing power, equipment assistance and partial removal from local politics. Another advantage, he said, is "the pace of change. We have time, talent, and money that can be applied to the problems of the affiliates in a way that it had never been applied to those problems (management, education, purchasing, and so on) before. It quickens the decision-making process, it quickens the pace of change and implementation. You have an opportunity to make your mistakes quicker under our system than you did under the old one."

Woodham added, "Another advantage is better board understanding. Our board is a progressive board. It is used to making decisions. It receives recommendations, gives them a yes or no, and we move ahead. Our board knows hospital business better than many small town boards, and that is a major advantage."[23] He also spoke about the ability to rapidly develop new services in the hospitals and the ability to supply backup operating capital.

There are fifteen members of the governing board, who are appointed by the Synod of the Presbyterian Church. This relationship ties PHC more closely to the church than most Presbyterian hospitals in the United States. Woodham reports directly to the board. The administrators of Presbyterian Hospital and Anna Kaseman report directly to Woodham, and administrators in affiliated hospitals, to a regional administrator.[24]

"There are a few advantages for the base hospital but, frankly, very few,"[25] Woodham said. Referrals have gone up slightly but the big advantage is in terms of a social commitment. "We have the advantage, I think, that any organization has of new challenges and in the type of self-renewal and satisfaction you get from doing something new, and doing something in a situation where you are demonstratively reaching out with a helping hand. It sounds corny, but we are helping the hospitals in those communities. I have no doubt about that."

Placing himself in the shoes of the people who work in member hospitals outside of Albuquerque, Woodham said they probably wish they were back dealing with the local politicians. PHC has replaced some department heads, set new standards and required new procedures. The continuing problem, he said, is to raise standards of quality of care. At the same time, he said, a central authority can bring on the danger of a decrease in local commitment, an attitude of, "Well, the big city boys are operating us now, and we don't have to worry about our problems because they are going to take care of it."

And the biggest headache for Woodham back at the "motherhouse" in Albuquerque is that PHC management staff is spending a large percent of its time and effort on system hospitals that only comprise a small percent of the overall business. And in the early years, each of the units was consuming PHC capital as an advance. Finally, Woodham said, there is the problem of "our inability to withdraw. A serious question exists in my mind as to whether we are ever going to be able to get out of some of these situations if we determine that some of them should not exist and some should not survive." What this comes down to is the need for informed communities and rural hospitals that will pull their fair share of the load. This will be accomplished, he believes.

Closer to home, PHC has been able to accomplish a degree of sharing with a Catholic-sponsored hospital that is rare in the United States. St. Joseph's had replaced its hospital with a modern plant, just before PHC built its satellite north of town, a few blocks away. Any new facility in the area was a threat, and PHC was strong competition. Woodham explained that

> to attempt to heal the wounds, we made strong overtures to St. Joseph's to develop some kind of cooperative efforts.
>
> The cooperation began modestly—shared purchasing and exchange of information. Then the health maintenance organization program came along. An 80-doctor clinic organized around 250-bed Lovelace-Bataan Medical Center found the HMO program to be an opportunity to generate additional income and they proceeded to organize one and targeted the largest, highest salaried industrial operation in town—one having over 7,500 employees and a source of about five percent of our patient load. We [PHC and St. Joseph's] saw this as a threat, so for all the wrong reasons, we decided we had to have an HMO too. This brought us together faster than anything else could have....

This joint offensive move to be competitive with another hospital-based HMO and protect existing referral patterns, led St. Joseph's and PHC to organize a separate venture called Cooperative Health Services, which "was formed in 1971 to pursue solutions to the broad problem of cost and availability of health care in both urban and rural New Mexico through the application of resources from the private sector."[26] So far, the cooperative has launched into four major programs.

The HMO, called New Mexico Health Care Corporation, is an open panel arrangement that began operations in January 1973. This prepaid plan provides comprehensive services to more than 14,000 enrollees. The HMO brought together 230 physicians on the medical staffs of the two hospitals. The benefit package is called Mastercare.

Albuquerque Ambulance is a second venture of Cooperative Health Services. This not-for-profit company, the only certified emergency transport system in the area, operates eight vehicles and serves all hospitals.

A third program, Hospital Home Health Care, is Medicare certified and provides care to homebound patients within a forty-mile radius of the two hospitals.

A fourth venture, called Southwest Health Care Corporation, is a new delivery system model, a not-for-profit health care organization that manages five outreach clinics in medically underserved rural and urban communities (see Figure 11:2). Clinics at Tijeras and Estancia are staffed by family nurse practitioners and at Pecos, by a physician's assistant. Doctors provide care in the clinics at Bernalillo and Five Points, an area also designated as South Valley. Demographic descriptions of the five service areas are distressing. While there is beautiful scenery, the human, medical and health care needs are compounded by low educational levels, poverty-level incomes, high unemployment, high fertility rates, poor road systems, and language barriers.[27]

Woodham's board viewed this rapid development, within only five years, with mixed emotions. As he pointed out, the board asked: What are you really seeking to do? After a lot of soul-searching, he said, the board came up with a three-point policy: "1) there should be no action which would impair the ability of Presbyterian Hospital to improve and expand existing Albuquerque services; 2) Affiliations should be sought that will strengthen the PHC operation, and 3) PHC has a social obligation to assist other health programs in New Mexico, provided PHC can afford to help."[28]

By the time he spoke to the New England meeting, Woodham could point to other expansion possibilities appearing on the horizon. PHC was receiving requests for assistance from other hospitals that wanted to link into the expertise available at the big medical center. The center had a request to open a clinic in Ruidoso, where it already had a hospital, because another hospital in the community was about to close. In Albuquerque, PHC was under political pressure to open a clinic in a deprived area of the city. At the same time, there was the question of whether PHC and St. Joseph's could merge.

The cooperation with St. Joseph's extends to joint medical staff committees, joint purchasing, information exchange, some success in the agreement and nonduplication of services and the joint venture, Cooperative Health Services. Woodham said: "An informal study of our operating expenses between the two hospitals located a few blocks apart lead us to estimate approximately $2 million per year would result in savings if the two institutions were merged.... Our relations have improved to the point that we can sit down and discuss these things. The stumbling block seems to be based on the differences of the religious ownerships of the institutions." The owners of PHC, the Synod of the Presbyterian Church of Arizona and New Mexico, gave Woodham's board the authority to form a holding company that would remove the religious aspects of ownership, "and in that process we would offer board membership to other hospitals in the holding company. This has not been effected yet, nor has it been acceptable yet."[29]

In an article for the January 1973 issue of *Hospital Progress,* Sister Celestia, S.C., administrator of St. Joseph Hospital, explained the history of the development of the HMO with Presbyterian Hospital Center. Her paper dealt primarily with the details of that organization, but she concluded by saying:

> What benefits does a Catholic hospital derive from being involved in the development of a new type of health delivery system? Such involvement permits the Catholic health care facility to exert a broader leadership role than would otherwise be possible, since no single entity in the health delivery system today can be expected to meet increasing needs. The emphasis is placed on the Catholic hospital working with others in a geographic area who share common goals. Hopefully, this kind of involvement will have an effect on the way in which health care is delivered, the people to whom it is delivered, and the way in which the health care dollar can be best spent to deliver service....[30]

NOTES

1. Press release, September 6, 1974.
2. J.A. Hamilton, *Patterns of Hospital Ownership and Controls,* Minneapolis: University of Minnesota Press, 1961, p. 92.
3. Press release, op. cit., note 1
4. "A Study of the Presiding Bishopric's Office, Phase I: The Health Services Corporation," The Church of Jesus Christ of Latter-day Saints, August 1974.

5. Personal letter from Scott S. Parker, February 9, 1976.

6. Interview with Scott S. Parker, August 18, 1975, Chicago, Illinois. All subsequent quotations are from this interview until otherwise noted.

7. S.M. Morris, "An Emerging Health Care System," *Hospital Administration* (Spring 1973), pp. 76-85.

8. Samaritan Health Service, Phoenix, Arizona, an undated brochure containing 1974 statistics.

9. "Ameriplan Modified by House of Delegates, praised by H.E.W. Secretary Richardson," *Modern Hospital* (September, 1971), p. 35.

10. D. Maddox, "Arizona's Voluntary Chain may be Model for Future," *Modern Hospital* (June 1971), pp. 89-94.

11. S.M. Morris, op. cit., note 7.

12. S.A. Edwards and A.A. Astolfi, "Merger: Cause and Effect," *Hospital Administration* (Summer 1973), pp. 24-33.

13. J.P. Cooney, Jr. and T.L. Alexander, *Multihospital Systems* (four volumes), Health Services Research Center of the Hospital Research and Education Trust and Northwestern University, 1975.

14. B.R. Neumann "A Financial Analysis of a Hospital Merger: Samaritan Health Service," *Medical Care* (December 1974), pp. 983-988.

15. "Planning Agency Tries to Mediate Motorola-Hospital Controversy," *Modern Hospital* (July 1972), pp. 35-36; and "Motorola and Samaritan Health Services Renew Battle Over Costs," *Modern Hospital* (February 1973), p. 24.

16. This information is contained in a prospectus for a Maricopa County, Arizona, bond issue to finance Samaritan Health Service improvements, dated July 14, 1975.

17. Ibid.

18. Ibid.

19. The characteristics of the area are discussed in descriptive material about Cooperative Health Services, a joint venture by Presbyterian Hospital Center and St. Joseph Hospital, undated.

20. Personal letter from PHC.

21. R. Woodham, untitled address before the New England Hospital Assembly, March 1975. Until noted otherwise all subsequent quotations are from this address.

22. Telephone interview with Ray Woodham, January 8, 1976.

23. R. Woodham, op. cit., note 21.

24. Explained in a personal letter, January 14, 1976.

25. R. Woodham, op. cit., note 21. Until noted otherwise all subsequent quotations are from this address.

26. Op. cit., note 19.

27. Ibid.

28. R. Woodham, op. cit., note 21.

29. Ibid.

30. Sr. Celestia, "St Joseph Hospital, Albuquerque, and The New Mexico Health Care Corporation," *Hospital Progress* (January 1973), pp. 30-42.

Chapter 12
Pacific States

The Pacific census division shows the highest level of hospital system activity in the United States. This five-state area includes Alaska, California, Hawaii, Oregon and Washington. The 863 nonfederal hospitals in this division contain 141,887 beds. The 1975 study conducted by the Health Services Research Center (HSRC) of Northwestern University, in cooperation with the American Hospital Association affiliate organization, Hospital Research and Educational Trust, showed 344 hospitals and 77,479 beds in the states that were reported as members of systems.

Most system activity is in California. And there are several reasons why. (1) There are many Catholic-sponsored hospitals in California. The 1975 Catholic Hospital Association directory lists forty-one hospitals sponsored by twenty-four different religious groups. (2) The biggest multiple-unit system in the nation, the Kaiser Health Plan, is concentrated in California. Kaiser also accounts for many of the system hospitals in Oregon and Hawaii. (3) California is a furious center of activity for for-profit, investor-owned chains. Of the thirty-two major for-profit systems in the United States, fourteen have their headquarters in California, mostly southern California and the Los Angeles metropolitan area. The Federation of American Hospitals' accounting in 1975 showed that the fourteen California corporations own seventy-three hospitals in California. Those same chains manage other California hospitals through contracts.

There is still another reason for hospital system activity in the most populous state—19.9 million people, according to the 1970 census. The population density of California increased considerably during World War II. As the war began for the United States in the Pacific, the state's defense industries grew rapidly. Existing industries, such as Kaiser's ship-building plants, received a major economic boost, as did Kaiser's fledgling hospital system.

The population influx to California also offered opportunities for the growth of proprietary hospitals. Unlike well-established hospitals in the East, particularly the New England states, voluntary hospitals in California were not as well established. They couldn't respond with new buildings and new programs to meet the demands presented by rapid population growth. Chains of hospitals developed and expanded after Medicare and Medicaid placed higher standards on hospitals. The chains continued to grow after the war by purchasing many of the autonomous for-profit institutions that had been built to keep up with the need created during World War II.

The HSRC study is limited. It is not believed to include an accounting of all hospitals that are members of systems in this census division, or any other U.S. census division for that matter. However, the information about California is believed to be quite significant—that around half of the state's nonfederal hospitals and almost 70 percent of the beds can be counted within systems.

In this chapter, three organizations are discussed in summary form: the University of Washington Hospitals, Seattle; the Kaiser Health Plan; and Adventist Health Services, Glendale, California. A fourth system, the Lutheran Hospital Society of Southern California with offices in Los Angeles, is discussed in detail.

The Los Angeles region deserves special mention because it is saturated with competing hospital systems—the Adventists, the Lutheran Hospital Society of Southern California, Kaiser's southern California region and others, such as the giant Los Angeles County-University of Southern California Medical Center with its four hospitals and 2,105 beds, a public hospital system only slightly overshadowed in size and scope by the facilities of the New York City Health and Hospitals Corporation; the Cedars-Sinai Medical Center, a large private system operating two division 'and 733 beds; and the Memorial Hospital Medical Center of Long Beach, a two-unit system of 737 beds. Nearby in the same region, a system is developing around 472-bed Hoag Memorial Hospital-Presbyterian at Newport Beach.

Southern California is unusual in other ways. Orange County, part of the Los Angeles metropolitan area, is often referred to as one of the most over-bedded regions in the nation. The combined factors of over-bedding, existing systems, and systems now being built will probably present the federal Health Systems Agency in the area with the most formidable challenges available anywhere in the fifty states.

UNIVERSITY OF WASHINGTON HOSPITALS

The University of Washington Hospitals system includes two units of care in Seattle. An unusual organization because of the management structure and the primary orientation toward graduate medical education, University Hospital has 301 beds and serves as a referral center for the entire state. It is a state-supported facility that is ultimately controlled by the university's seven-member board of regents appointed by the governor. The other institution is the 245–bed Harborview Medical Center located five miles from the campus in another section of Seattle. It is owned and governed by King County. It receives direction from a six-member board of trustees appointed by the county executive. This board functions very much like a community hospital board.[1]

In 1974 these two hospitals had 16,896 admissions and an average daily census of 403 patients. The average occupancy rate was 74.0 percent and there were total expenses of $35.3 million, including $19.9 million for payroll to 2,319 full-time employees.

The two hospitals are linked under a central management organization headed by Roy S. Rambeck, executive director of hospitals. Referring to the two hospital system, specifically to Harborview, Rambeck explained: "This institution has served for more than 40 years as the 'public hospital' which has provided care for the poor of the county. The two hospitals together comprise the largest and most comprehensive health delivery system in the Northwest region of the country. Each has an outpatient volume of approximately 150,000 visits per year and each has many progressive units. Together they provide the University's health professional schools with the bulk of their clinical training facilities."

The university has schools of medicine, dentistry, nursing, public health, pharmacy and social work. The center has affiliations with three other hospitals. The Seattle system is of a special type—tied as it is to a university education center. Some individuals may argue with Rambeck's claim of being "the largest and most comprehensive" system in the Northwest. But, as Rambeck said, "Although the two hospitals are quite different in many ways [including ownership and control], they function as a highly integrated, single hospital system. Both hospitals are supported partially by the state legislature through an appropriation to the University of Washington so that they may be maintained as effective teaching resources for the health professional schools."

The state support literally saved Harborview Medical Center. In 1967 legislators authorized the university to contract to manage Harborview, then known as King County Hospital. "It was clear that the impact of Medicaid and Medicare, a major change in attitude of the county government, and other factors left everyone in doubt as to whether the hospital had any kind of future," Rambeck said. The management agreement with Harborview is likely to continue for a long time. Under the arrangement, there is a strong attempt to keep the county hospital free of political control.

Rambeck explained that "the county is required to provide a board of trustees to govern the institution so that local politicians will have no way to control or influence its policies, programs, or operations. The University provides all of the management direction including the provision of all medical services. All of the employees were transferred to university status so common personnel policies and personnel interchanges between the two hospitals can be facilitated. All of the members of the medical staff at Harborview ... are required to be members of the University of Washington medical school faculty."

Unlike many hospital systems, including many university-based systems, Rambeck explained, "There is no 'super board' to provide overall governance coordination of the two-hospital system. The primary mechanism for maintaining the two units as components of a single hospital system is provided through the administrative structures. All medical affairs and educational programs are coordinated within the structure of the medical school and the five other health professional schools of the university. For example, all of the clinical services in both hospitals are under the control of the chairmen of the medical school departments."

Rambeck continued: "Within the university's overall administrative structure, all deans of the health sciences and the executive director of hospitals are accountable to the vice-president for health affairs who brings about overall coordination of the general administration, medical care administration, and academic administration within the entire two-hospital system."

The University of Washington system is different from the Rush University System for Health, for example, where a Medical Center Cabinet is responsible for overall coordination. And it is different from the approach in Detroit whereby the Detroit Medical Center Corporation is an overall coordinating unit for six hospitals and the Wayne State University school of medicine's outpatient clinic.

Under the Rambeck approach, each of the two hospitals has an operating administrator. But Rambeck maintains system-wide directors for finance and systems services who answer directly to him. "These four key people and a personnel director make up my senior management staff," he said. Rambeck's senior managers have also helped bring about a sifting out of services between the two hospitals.

Harborview has all of the programs in community mental health, a trauma center, burn center, public health clinics, involuntary treatment programs, alcoholism and drug abuse programs and other services. University Hospital has the obstetrical services, radiation therapy, organ transplantation, renal service, laundry, perinatal center, heart surgery, neurosurgery and family medicine. Both hospital pharmacies have been consolidated under a single service. And Rambeck said the two hospital dietary departments would be merged in 1976.

Late in 1975, Rambeck said he felt a need for "some type of governance structure in the university which can focus exclusively on the University Hospital's matters and we expect to have a sub-board developed by mid-1976. In our special situation, it is unlikely that we will ever develop a third board to facilitate joint planning and make hospital-wide policy decisions."

As to future ventures, Rambeck said, "our management system is presently engaged in only the affairs of these two hospitals. As a system, we have developed many sharing arrangements with other hospitals and agencies in the area, but we do not offer direct management services outside the system. We are developing plans for a continuing care center and we may get into a health maintenance organization later which will expand our sphere of system activity, but I doubt that we will otherwise make any significant changes in the range of our management activities."

KAISER-PERMANENTE MEDICAL CARE PROGRAM

The entire content of this book could have been devoted to one hospital system—The Kaiser-Permanente Medical Care Program. As the most studied and best known of the U.S. systems, however, it seems only important at this time to briefly describe the Kaiser plan. This description may serve as a benchmark for comparison to the less mature, developing, and smaller hospital systems in other parts of the United States.

Studying Kaiser is a massive task. Greer Williams, while assistant professor of community health and social medicine at Tufts University, was commissioned by the chairman of the Kaiser Family Foundation to taken an outsider's look at the plan. Williams' report, published in a special issue of *Modern Hospital,* indicated that "health professionals seem to gaze upon the Kaiser health plan either with stars in their eyes or bile in their livers."[2] He conducted over 100 interviews and talked to everyone from corporate-level officials to doctors and nurses. "One of the most frequent comments [he] encountered was, 'This is not easy to do.' It was refreshing to find so much rationalism and so much good contact with reality in a program that has become high fashion among health care planners."

In his report, published in February 1971, Williams said: "The Kaiser Foundation Health Plan annually provides, in round numbers, 2,000,000 members with 7,600,000 doctor office visits and 1,000,000 days of hospitalization, plus a large volume of x-ray, laboratory, prescription drug, and other medical services, at an average cost of $150 a member or $450 a family.

This is a snapshot dated 1970. Every year all figures increase. In any year, seven or eight of every ten members use these services in California, Oregon, Washington, Hawaii, Colorado, and Ohio."

The Kaiser-Permanente Medical Care Program consists of three organizations set up in each of the six service regions to provide comprehensive health care to plan members. A fourth organization in each service region, called a Permanente Service Corporation, provides support services.

Kaiser Foundation Health Plan, Inc., is the central component of the program. This organization contracts with individuals and groups to arrange for a comprehensive package of benefits. In 1975 there were 2.7 million plan members. The health plan then contracts with Kaiser hospitals and the medical groups to provide coverage.

The 24 Kaiser Foundation Hospitals and 4,823 beds are organized as nonprofit, charitable corporations. They are also community hospitals and "staff privileges are available on the usual basis to qualified doctors in the community"[3], Williams reported.

Permanente Medical Groups assume the full responsibility to provide professional and related medical care to plan members in a specific region. "These physician groups are organized as partnerships or professional corporations, and each is responsible for its own physician recruitment, selection and staffing patterns. In some regions, this includes the employment of allied health professional and administrative personnel."[4]

The Permanente Service Organizations are six separate business corporations that provide certain support services to the plan, the hospitals and the medical groups in each region. These services include data processing, accounting, and purchasing. These corporations also operate prescription pharmacies at nonhospital locations in all regions.[5]

The Kaiser System provides proof for the proposition that systems have advantages in economy, accessibility, accountability, quality of care and power—when compared to autonomous units.

At the same time, Kaiser is atypical. The complete linking together of physician groups, prepayment plan and hospitals gives this system a measure of control not available in any other U.S. system. Still another feature makes Kaiser unique. This control occurs in a system that is not the creature of government.

While Kaiser is atypical, some U.S. systems are moving in this same direction. They control hospitals and are beginning to talk of prepayment plans. They may compromise on the medical staff organization, however, and maintain a willingness to work with physicians through various business arrangements. The Lutheran Hospital Society of Southern California, a system discussed later in this chapter, is taking on some characteristics of a Kaiser-like system.

SEVENTH-DAY ADVENTIST HEALTH SERVICES

There is a religious fervor that has marked the development of many hospital systems, such as the Catholic-sponsored systems, and the three major Lutheran systems based in North Dakota, Kansas and California. Perhaps the least-known of the religious-sponsored systems are those of the Seventh-day Adventist Church. The Adventist Church operates dozens of hospitals and thousands of beds in the United States and foreign countries. In Rio de Janerio, Brazil, an Adventist health care system is self-insured, a sort of South American "blue cross" plan.[6]

The Seventh-day Adventists are a minority religion—3,301 churches and 464,276 members in the United States—with a unique philosophy. Their church

> believes that man was made originally in the image of God. The entrance of sin into the world marred the image and resulted in a separation of man from his Maker to his detriment—physically, mentally, and spiritually. The church believes that the health ministry, in the relief of suffering and the treatment of disease, may contribute directly to the restoration of the whole man.
>
> The health ministry of the church—by education, by precept and example, and by making the laws of healthful living understood and accepted—can assist mankind in avoiding those illnesses caused by the violation of health principles. Thus, the health ministry may contribute to the avoidance of illness, to the restoration of health here on earth, and to the reconciliation of man to God, which is preparation of eternal life hereafter.[7]

Many leaders in public health advocate these very principles. These are strong beliefs; federal policymakers might reduce them to an argument for health maintenance organizations. More specifically, however, this philosophy says that the Seventh-day Adventists are in the business of health care and intend to stay. Faced with realities of the times, however, nationwide authorities of the church have directed each church-sponsored hospital to become a member of a hospital system—either an Adventist system or an organization with compatible philosophical beliefs.[8]

The objectives of Seventh-day Adventist hospitals (there are two other Adventist groups in the United States) are grounded in fundamental religious principles too. "To witness," an employee handbook says, "employees of Seventh-day Adventist medical institutions should think of themselves as 'ministers of Christ,' healing, comforting the sick, teaching and inspiring hope and courage. Their lives should be exemplary in word and deed." There is a second objective: "To relieve pain. Relieving pain and suffering and the treatment of the sick calls for love and compassion. Compassion and love are the very elements of the character of God. Enlightened scientific medical service is to be rendered with Christian compassion, reverence for God, and an abiding faith in the Great Physician."[9]

There are five formally-organized Seventh-day Adventist hospital systems in the United States. These corporations are members of the General Conference of the Seventh-day Adventists that has its world headquarters in Takoma Park, a suburban area of Washington, D.C. At the end of 1974, the systems had 51 hospitals, 7,533 beds, and a number of nursing homes and retirement centers. The church also has many hospitals located outside the continental United States. There is another church organization that also owns and manages hospitals in the United States—the Association of Privately-Owned Seventh-day Adventist Services and Industries.

The hospital systems formally organized under the General Conference are: the Central Union of Health and Hospital Services, Denver, Colorado; the Northwest Medical Foundation, Portland, Oregon; the Southern Adventist Health and Hospital System, Orlando, Florida; the newly formed Eastern States Adventist Health Services, Takoma Park, Maryland; and the Pacific Union Conference of the Seventh-day Adventist Health Services, Glendale, California.[10] The Glendale, California system and another hospital system in California, the Lutheran Hospital Society of Southern California are shown in Figure 12:1.

The Glendale-based system, whose president is Erwin J. Remboldt,[9] is the managing authority for 11 hospitals located in three states; 9 of the hospitals are in California. The facilities have 1,701 short-term beds and 131 long-term beds. American Hospital Association statistics are available on 10 of the hospitals. In 1974 these data showed that based on 1,601 short-term and 131 long-term beds, there were 52,516 admissions. The average census was 1,172 and the average occupancy rate was 78.2 percent. Total expenses were $72.2 million and there were 4,213 full-time employees. (These statistics do not include the 50-bed Hanford Community Hospital, Hanford, California.) System-wide statistics for 1975 showed that costs in the 11 hospitals came to a whopping $95.1 million. That same accounting listed 4,605 full-time equivalent employees.[11]

Each of the hospitals is in the full-service category and provides at least basic medical, surgical, and emergency care. Two of the institutions are quite sophisticated. The 452-bed Glendale Adventist Medical Center and the 362-bed White Memorial Medical Center, Los Angeles, are major teaching hospitals of the Loma Linda University school of medicine. Loma Linda, started by the Seventh-day Adventists, is a well-known school emphasizing primary care with over 500 medical students in training. Adventist Health

Services (AHS), therefore, is tied into a major manpower production center. As Remboldt said:

> The purpose of the multi-hospital system in these three states, as far as the ... church has been concerned, is that we have large hospitals in metropolitan areas, and we have small hospitals in rural areas. Some hospitals have as few as 49 beds, such as Port Hueneme Adventist Hospital in California, and, of course, we have one hospital with 452 beds. The feeling was there would be a need as we faced the health care problems in the future to provide additional expertise in areas of management, finance planning, purchasing, and so on.
>
> The organization is set up in such a way that the church body is the constituency for the health care corporation which is my office and staff. The board of trustees for AHS [16 members] is the constituency for the 11 member hospitals. This is the constituency that meets and appoints the local boards of trustees at the various hospitals. Under the articles of incorporation, I am designated as chairman of the board of all of these individual hospitals, which gives us in the health care corporation the necessary authority to direct these institutions in a unified way. Each individual hospital has a board of trustees made up of local people, but should that local board be unwilling to follow the overall directions or policies, we have the authority ... to remove that board ... and administration. To date, this has not been a real problem because on a cooperative effort, there is really no problem of exercising authority or direction—that becomes automatic.[12]

Although only a little more than two years old, AHS has moved rapidly to pull together a central management corps and central policies. A personnel commission composed of representatives from each of the eleven hospitals has come up with a uniform personnel and fringe benefit program. Centralization allowed the corporation to produce and buy employee handbooks on a volume basis, a seemingly small but nevertheless significant cash savings—50 percent on the printing, for example. This is a group purchasing program. And a materials management program "helps us keep control of the inventory and has cut down the inventory in each institution materially by proper management."

The church government is divided into ten areas in the United States, and there are health care corporations in each area. Only the West Coast (Glendale) corporation has a group purchasing program, but there is a plan to combine all of the North American Adventist groups into a unified, national purchasing plan.

Rightfully so, AHS has placed major emphasis on financial management. There is a vice-president for financial affairs who is chairman of the finance committee of each of the hospital boards. As Remboldt explained, "We have standardized our financial reports in the corporate area, making comparisons of the hospitals by size and reporting this back to the administration. This points out areas where they may have some problems either under revenue or in expenses that are in excess."

The central corporation has conducted workshops for the hospitals in budgeting, labor relations, medical staff relations and other areas. "The corporation is self-insured for unemployment compensation, workmen's compensation and malpractice, and they have established a uniform claims management service and engineering service for the prevention of malpractice problems [which] has tremendous potential for the future." Medical staff recruiting is also handled by the central staff. In early 1976, the system hired a planning director.

Remboldt is thinking of new programs, such as a health maintenance organization that may be organized at City of Industry, a growing community in east Los Angeles County. Remboldt said AHS had been approached to organize this program as part of the nationwide group practice project supported by The Robert Wood Johnson Foundation. The program is being coordinated by Donald Madison, M.D., of the University of North Carolina and a graduate of Loma Linda.

Speaking of the system approach, Remboldt said: "I am personally convinced that this has been a very positive affect on all of our hospitals. As we look to the future, we believe that this is the only way that some of the smaller hospitals, especially in more rural areas, can continue to have a viable, competitive program."[13]

The Adventists have worked quietly and effectively behind the scenes in Washington. In the 1974 amendments to Taft-Hartley that removed the exemption of not-for-profit hospitals, Adventists were successful in getting a conscious clause inserted in the final bill. That clause says health care employees who have a conscious feeling against unions don't have to join, even though the hospital is organized.[14]

In some ways, it may be thought that AHS is a closed, go-it-alone system. But this is not so. Remboldt is one of four systems managers who were brought together in 1975 by Ernst and Ernst, the accounting company, to consider pooling their resources to develop a large computer center to serve their combined hospitals. The other managers represented the Lutheran Hospital Society of Southern California, Intermountain Health Care, and Samaritan Health Service. "I hope that out of this we can get together on some other programs of mutual interest," Remboldt said, "such as purchasing and malpractice.[15]

LUTHERAN HOSPITAL SOCIETY OF SOUTHERN CALIFORNIA

Many American corporations have found that one way to survive is to diversify, and the familiar terms of "conglomerate" and "spin-off" have not been lost on some multiple unit hospital systems, such as the Lutheran Hospital Society of Southern California (LHS) and its president, Samuel J. Tibbitts.

In May 1975, LHS announced that it had formed a profit-making subsidiary called Western Health Management Services, Inc.[16] Tibbitts explained: "This organization evolved over three or four years, mainly in my own mind, as to what the Society should be doing. We had several difficulties in growing, particularly in California because proprietary strength represents about 50 percent of the hospitals. The provinciality of non-profit hospitals and our name inhibited our growth too. The boards of hospitals we really wanted would finally decide against us because of our Lutheran image. They felt they were community hospitals and not lined up with any particular religious sect. And, of course, Catholic hospitals wouldn't even look at us."[17]

A reason to grow, Tibbitts said, was that "we were continually being asked to do consulting work and helping people out, which we were happy to do. But you know you can only do so much of that and do it for free. We began to see that the proprietary, investor-owned chains were making quite a bit of money through management services, and this sort of thing. Over the years we had developed the expertise to do as well as they could, possibly even better."[18]

The most rapid period of LHS growth began in 1966 when the society began to fully develop central management techniques. At that time, a full time executive staff was created at the corporate level.

LHS was founded in 1920 by "a group of Lutheran laymen who believed that it was God's will to provide services for the sick and injured."[19] The health care program remained small for twenty years, until 1940, when a second hospital was acquired. As a system, LHS is thirty-five years old. Today, the Society owns two hospitals, manages five others on a lease basis, and has strong shared service and management ties to an eighth hospital (see Figure 12:1). Considering all eight facilities together for statistical purposes, there were 1,479 beds and 62,594 admissions in 1974. The average daily census was 1,825 and the overall occupancy rate was on the low side at 71 percent. The eight hospitals had $67.7 million in expenses, including $33 million for payroll to 3,899 employees.

Figure 12:1

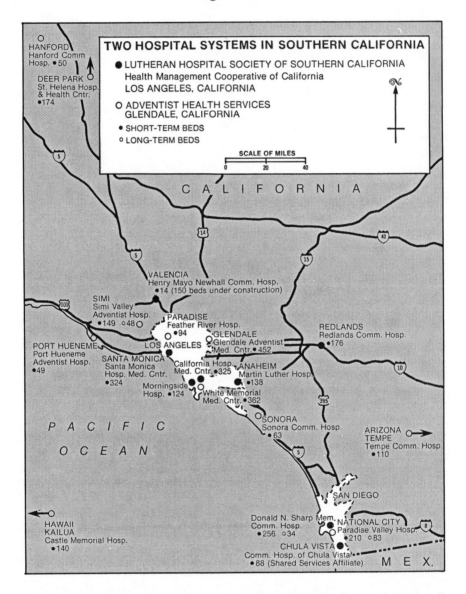

TWO HOSPITAL SYSTEMS IN SOUTHERN CALIFORNIA

● LUTHERAN HOSPITAL SOCIETY OF SOUTHERN CALIFORNIA
   Health Management Cooperative of California
   LOS ANGELES, CALIFORNIA

O ADVENTIST HEALTH SERVICES
   GLENDALE, CALIFORNIA

● SHORT-TERM BEDS
o LONG-TERM BEDS

Western Health Management Services has 500,000 shares of stock, all owned by the Lutheran Hospital Society of Southern California. The corporation's central service functions were shifted into this profit-making organization, including purchasing, accounting, data processing, construction and design, management engineering, health planning, fund raising, public relations, printing and electronic equipment maintenance and engineering.[20]

When Western Health Management Services was formed, the society also took another significant step. All of the hospital operations and management relationships were spun off into a nonprofit, 503(c) corporation called Health Management Cooperative of California. The president of this organization is Frank R. McDougall. There are boards of directors for both the management company and the cooperative. Those boards report to the Society's board, a widely-representative group of community citizens although the membership is at least 51 percent Lutheran.

There are two classes of membership in the cooperative. Tibbitts explained: "Seven founder members are the hospitals either owned or managed by the cooperative. These institutions have agreed to take the full services available from Western Health Management Services. They also receive the benefit of Western in that all profits . . . go back to the board of LHS and that board then decides what to do with the profits. And it will undoubtedly use them to benefit the founding members."

The other class of members is "participating hospitals." The only other LHS facility, Community Hospital of Chula Vista, falls into this category. "A participating member only has to take certain services of Western," Tibbitts explained, "and it is not really under full management—it is under sort of a shared services arrangement."

The objective in establishing the two new corporations was to try and get the best of all worlds by maintaining the benefits inherent in a community hospital and the philosophy of LHS, and still compete with other management and shared service corporations by turning a profit. Government controls and regulations are forcing hospitals "to go out and develop some other revenue basis."

The society has proven the concept of centralized expertise and economy of scale. According to Tibbitts, "Now, we want to develop more volume. We want to get into consulting. When we started this thing, we really didn't think about industrial concerns being clients. Right now they are some of our biggest clients." These firms have included Southern California Edison, Union Oil and Farmer's Insurance. There is growth potential in services to private industry, Tibbitts agreed, particularly in industrial and environmental health programs.

But the most immediate target for expansion is hospitals. The marketing strategy is designed to convince potential systems hospitals that the cooperative [and Western Health Management Services] can save them money through shared services and by the ability they will have to tap the available management expertise. Tibbitts hopes eventually "to get them [hospitals] into the cooperative—as participating members, and then somewhere along the line they may become founder members. In the meantime, we can make a little profit. But we would rather have 100 hospitals over here [in the cooperative] than make any profit over here [in Western]."

Another route to expansion could be the acquisition of investor-owned hospitals in the southern California area. Tibbitts said they had "been offered two or three in the past month (July, 1975). We are taking a serious look at one." Asked if he were strong enough to wait, he replied, "Yes. Our approach has always been conservative. I am going to go 'gung ho' on consulting and any management contract where we have no risk. That is hot. But as far as buying hospitals, we will be very cautious."

The two new corporations would be launching an organized marketing effort in southern California and the western states. Tibbitts also thought that there was a good possibility LHS would tie in for shared service programs with Intermountain Health Care (Salt Lake City, Utah), Adventist Health Services (Glendale, California), Samaritan Health Service (Phoenix, Arizona), and the Lutheran Hospital and Home Society of America (Fargo, North Dakota). He said, "This could be in purchasing, could be in data processing, management training—again getting the volume and power. We have talked about it, but there is nothing firm in it." By December 1975, these organizations had hired Ernst and Ernst to do a major feasibility study on a combined EDP network. Tibbitts also said there is a possibility that these same multiple-unit systems could go together in capital formation, because "if you could get all of those groups together, God you could form your own underwriting firm ... sell your own bonds."

To the question "Would this be made possible because the systems would know their exact volume?" he said: "That is right. This is very possible. I am a firm believer in finding other ways to generate revenue for hospitals because I think we are going to have to. The curve organizations, the non-profit ones, can form new profit-making subsidiaries. We could give McDonnell-Douglas a run for their money ... very easily." McDonnell-Douglas Automation Company has a widely used shared computer system called MCAUTO.

Tibbitts, interviewed by the authors the same day that the American Hospital Association's hearing committee had met in Chicago, was asked: Why is there so much current interest in multiple unit systems? He replied:

> I have preached this sort of thing for years, saying, "This is the only way to go." But people don't want to change until they have to. And I think they find out now that they're going to have to change ... with all the problems ... all the government controls.
>
> Some people wondered this morning why the review committee only lasted 20 minutes. One guy got up and asked a question about

a typographical error in the report. That was all that was said. Period, end of meeting. Now that says something doesn't it? It says that there are so damn many problems facing hospitals that people don't know where to start to talk about them. I think that is what is going on. I think administrators are scared to death. I think boards are getting scared. And there is some security in a system.

There are many arguments for systems, Tibbitts said, beginning with the political one: "I think we have got quite a bit of clout in California. That is part of the reason for a system. You start developing your relationships, not only with state government but on the local level with the county board, the supervisors, city councils, and mayors. That is part of the organizational plan so that when something does occur you have got all those units out there that are ready to respond because they have been trained to respond. And they are used to being in the political arena."

Another source of systems strength, he believes, is an alliance with physicians: "I think it is obvious that doctors are becoming more closely associated with hospitals. Not that they are all going to work for hospitals on salary." But a close association does benefit doctors, he said, predicting a tremendous growth in hospital-based primary care physician groups. The development of this pattern of practice is receiving a push through grants from The Robert Wood Johnson Foundation.

LHS has two primary groups going and is developing others. "They are operating out of the emergency room and the clinics. That is the way it starts, and you move it from there to a health maintenance organization. It is surprising—the medical staff members don't mind that too much." Tibbitts said this degree of acceptance may be because primary groups feed referral patients to the specialists, "any hospital that doesn't have its own physician population group is going to be in trouble." Group practice is no longer such an emotional subject among specialists in southern California. Indicative of this, he said, is that "thirteen specialty groups have joined together and formed an Independent Practice Association—and they are ready to go on an H.M.O."

This type of organizational arrangement may also allow LHS to try rural health care delivery efforts. Tibbitts said, "I do see us going into rural areas. I do see us putting small hospitals together with larger hospitals and feeding the rural hospitals out of the primary-based groups. I see contract groups of doctors becoming a very fertile field, particularly in California. There is one physician [in our area] who serves as manager of 43 emergency rooms. He currently has 150 doctors in his group. He is a very smart guy. He treats doctors fairly and is strong on continuing education and quality of care. He is also the guy we are contracting with for our primary based groups. So, he sees the picture coming. And that sort of scares you. If a guy can get that many hospitals and doctors contracted with him, he has got a lot of power. So you have to watch that because he can have a pretty strong union."

As for cost containment, Tibbitts referred to the three traditional means of saving money: group purchasing that creates economies of scale; nonduplication of facilities, such as electronic data processing; and the greater expertise available that can show a manager in need how to save money. Placing a new and important twist on how to figure cost savings, Tibbitts said in 1971 that there had been $1.1 million dollars in annual savings to the LHS hospitals. This was the estimated cost to duplicate services in the individual hospitals that were already being provided by the central organization. Other savings were projected on the basis of size and volume. "The studies we have done, and they have been done by our staff so nobody has certified them, show that we are saving about $5.50 a patient day in our hospitals."

In terms of the federal/state stance on the cost issue, Tibbitts believes it is a problem of taking "the least of two evils. It is either arbitrary controls on the part of individuals within government or taking your chance with independent state commissions that will control beds, rates, and so forth. I would rather throw my lot with an independent commission. It is still a state commission, but with some reasonable people on it, you hope."

Financial control and reimbursement are areas of LHS management that have received plenty of emphasis. A vice-president of finance handles capital financing and overall supervision of the following: a controller (general accounting and accounts payable), a financial analysis group (budgeting and cost benefit analysis) and a government reimbursement group that is continuously reviewing regulations and trying to get the maximum amount of money from third-party agencies.

LHS is self-insured for unemployment compensation, life insurance, long-term disability and Workman's Compensation. On October 1, 1975, the society took a giant step into another self-insurance program called the Pacific Western Employees Health Plan.

An estimated 3,000 LHS employees and their families (about 7,000 persons in all) were covered as the plan went into action. The Society has been insured through Blue Cross but was facing a 60 percent premium hike. Tibbitts explained: "We wanted to improve the benefits because our employees had griped about certain things, particularly accessibility to doctors. We have improved the benefits. Through self-insurance and using our own utilization review control system, we think we can get by with a 10 percent increase in premiums while at the same time increasing benefits."

Under the Pacific Western Employees Health Plan, the Society's employees who use the eight systems hospitals are covered 100 percent for hospital care. They are covered 80 percent in other hospitals. Blue Cross remains as the claims processor and the provider of stop-loss insurance. Employees also are issued a Blue Cross card.

NOTES

1. Personal letter from Roy S. Rambeck, December 31, 1975. Until otherwise noted all subsequent quotations are from this letter.
2. G. Williams, "Kaiser: What is It? How Does it Work? Why Does it Work?" *Modern Hospital* (February 1971), p. 67.
3. Ibid.
4. Kaiser Permanente Medical Care Program, *Facts 1975.*
5. Ibid.
6. Interview with Erwin J. Remboldt, Atlanta, Georgia, November 20, 1975.
7. Adventist Health Services Employee Handbook, updated.
8. E.J. Remboldt, op. cit., note 6.
9. Employee Handbook op. cit., note 7.
10. Adventist Health Care Systems, undated list furnished the authors by the national headquarters.
11. American Hospital Association Guide to the Health Care Field, 1975 edition (Chicago: American Hospital Association).
12. Personal letter from E.J. Remboldt, January 9, 1976. All subsequent quotations are from the letter until otherwise noted.
13. E.J. Remboldt, op. cit., note 6.
14. E.J. Remboldt, op. cit., note 12.
15. Ibid.
16. Press release, undated but received by the news media in May 1975.
17. Taped interview with Samuel J. Tibbitts, Chicago, Illinois, August 18, 1975.
18. Ibid.
19. S.J. Tibbitts, "Multiple Hospital Systems," *Hospital Administration* (Spring 1973), pp. 10-20.
20. S.J. Tibbitts, op. cit., note 17. All subsequent quotations were taken from this interview.

Chapter 13
Catholic-Sponsored Systems

Catholic-sponsored hospital systems deserve a special chapter in this book for several reasons: (1) there are many of them, although they don't always fit neatly into defined geographical categories; (2) they have always been guided by a unique strategy—that of espousing and promoting a religious mission through the delivery of medical and health care, and (3) they have an almost unlimited potential, if congregations decide to work as systems bound together by needs and realities of the Twentieth Century, rather than continuing to operate as autonomous institutions held together only by the common bond of a sisterhood.

Government regulation, rising costs, competition from other hospitals, moral, legal and ethical issues—all of these problems are forcing Catholic-sponsored hospital systems to think in new terms. The leaders and representatives of the Catholic hospital systems are beginning to respond forcefully as they sense challenges coming from the environment.

Several years ago, Sister William Joseph, R.S.M., administrator of Mercy Hospital, Scranton, Pennsylvania, and a former president of the Catholic Hospital Association, told the Catholic Health Services Leadership Program conferences: "That our destiny among American hospitals should be that of a 'sub-system' is an historical accident, not necessarily a devine plan. Categories rise out of philosophical origin, not out of the incidence of reality. Sub-systems like ours can be the leaven of a society and can, if guided rightly, work toward the changing of the whole structure. And this is where our opportunity for leadership lies."[1]

Sister Mary Maurita, R.S.M., executive director of the Catholic Hospital Association, had explained at the time that the primary thrust of the conference "is to develop the relationships and maximize the potential strength and resources of our Catholic sponsoring groups and their various multi-faceted health care facilities. We believe that this is a timely step and an exercise of leadership at a time when the total health care system is on the verge of being restructured." She predicted that the Catholic subsystem would evolve into new forms and "eventually become molded through legislation which brings the voluntary and governmental segments together in a more formalized approach."[2]

Catholic hospitals have always been a tremendous force in the United States. James A. Hamilton said, "There were more than 300 Roman Catholic religious orders in the U.S. in 1956, and approximately 180 of these orders owned and/or operated hospitals. Of the latter group, all but three were sisterhoods. Many sisterhoods control just one hospital while others own and/or operate a large number of such institutions." In 1956, the 180 or so sisterhoods operated 874 hospitals (137,628 beds) in the continental United States. This was more than two-thirds of the church-sponsored total. Discussing the philosophical orientation of the Roman Catholic Religious orders at that time, Hamilton said they are "communities of men or women bound together within the Church by the vows of poverty, chastity, and obedience. Most religious orders are expected to be self-sufficient and are relatively independent of each other and of other Roman Catholic organizations; however, *all* orders must abide by the canon laws of the Church."[3]

The world has turned precipitously since that statement was made. Fewer candidates are entering religious life thus reducing the number of religious personnel in hospitals. The Catholic Hospital Association's annual report for 1973-1974 listed the number of religious (persons who had taken formal vows) working in health care institutions as 8,978. But comparative data are not available either for previous years or more recent years.[4]

Economic pressures have caused some Catholic organizations to do one of several things: close their hospitals, sell to a community group, sell to a for-profit organization, lease the facility, merge with another institution, or consolidate with another institution.

The Catholic Church and Catholic hospitals have been fighting on other fronts too. State abortion-on-demand laws, a liberal interpretation of sterilization laws, and U.S. Supreme Court decisions upholding the legality of those laws, have prompted tremendous moral, legal and ethical debates all across the country. The Catholic Church and its hospitals have stood firm in their "right to life" orientation.

In 1972 Paul R. Donnelly, director of the Catholic Hospital Association's department of hospital administration and now a vice-president of the association, said

> the full potential for achieving a strong integrated subsystem within the larger health system context has not been realized.
> There are 1,270 individual inpatient health care institutions

identified as "Catholic" in the United States. They are sponsored by 296 different religious congregations and 20 dioceses. These 1,270 institutions exist in varying states of relationship to their sponsoring group and to each other. The expected unity or integration does not always exist even though the framework comes close to existing through past congregation ties and identification with the organized Church. In short, there has not always been a unified approach by and between those "Catholic" facilities. Furthermore such unity of effort has not always existed even between health facilities sponsored by the same religious congregation—even, I might add, when two hospitals operated by the same religious congregation are located in the same city or are in close geographic proximity.

In short, although we have an identifiable subset of health care facilities which exist as "Catholic," we do not have a Catholic health care "system" which is coordinated and directed toward pervasive mutually-agreed-upon goals.[5]

In 1974, the 669 institutional members of the Catholic Hospital Association included 647 short-term general hospitals, 9 rehabilitation, 7 psychiatric, 5 maternity and pediatric, and one cancer hospital. The 161,448 beds were divided into 156,001 short-term and 5,447 long-term. Catholic facilities recorded 5,670,075 admissions, 45,554,614 patient days of care, and have an average occupancy of 77 percent. The average length of stay in short-term institutions was 7.7 days and the average number of beds per hospital was 241.[6]

The Catholic Hospital Association's Project 1980 Committee has studied the implications of the times and their potential impact on the viability of Catholic-sponsored health care institutions. Sister Grace Marie Hiltz, S.C., administrator of Good Samaritan Hospital, Cincinnati, Ohio, was the 1974-1975 chairman of the CHA. In her incoming address to the association, as reported in *Hospital Progress,* she identified four issues that surfaced as a result of Project 1980 deliberations: "The issues are pluralism, continued freedom to practice religion, the need for the Church to serve the sick, and religious congregations' viability." The report also said: "The Church will continue to serve the sick through institutions, she stated, but many tensions and pressures threaten the vitality and survival of all the Catholic health apostolate. The future role of health care facilities under Catholic auspices in the United States is directly related to and dependent upon the commitment of religious congregations to sponsor and directly influence such facilities. Sr. Grace Marie thus asked: Are many congregations, by turning their hospitals over to profit management firms, accepting short-term responses to long-term problems and rationalizing the consequences? Why are religious congregations reluctant to cooperate, to share information with each other about any plans to dissociate themselves from a health facility?"[7]

A year later, the Project 1980 Committee reported:

> Between 1970 and the present [June 1975], the number of institutional members of CHA has declined from 796 to 669. The committee projected that by 1980 the CHA will have between 650 and 625 members, excluding long-term care facilities. However, these hospitals will increase in average size from approximately 241 beds today to 270 beds by 1980, the average hospital admitting about 7,900 patients per year. The average census of this hospital will decrease from 77 percent today to between 65 and 75 percent, depending upon the impact of PSRO and other constraining forces.
>
> Today 202 religious congregations sponsor health care facilities. In the past six years, seven congregations have withdrawn totally from the health apostolate. However, the committee projected that, although fewer [congregations] will be sponsors in the 1980s, the number of disengagements will not exceed more than five congregations.
>
> Continuing an established trend, fewer religious will staff Catholic-sponsored hospitals in the future. Presently, 251 Catholic hospitals have lay chief executive officers. By the 1980s, the number of lay administrators will increase to about 300, making about half of the institutions sponsored by religious congregations under the direct management of lay personnel. In addition, most will have boards of trustees with civic community representation.[8]

In summary, between 1956 and 1970, the number of Catholic-sponsored hospitals decreased from 874 to 796. And in just five more years, 1970 to 1975, the number of Catholic hospitals decreased from 796 to 669, a loss of 127 hospitals. Some members of CHA considered the Project 1980 Committee report overly pessimistic. It is clear, however, that Catholic hospitals are undergoing serious self-reappraisal in an effort to cope with economic, social and political forces of the times.

In her paper on "The Catholic Sub-System—An Opportunity for Leadership" (October 1971) Sister William Joseph, R.S.M., commented: "The basic structure to achieve a broad influence is already established in an existing network of health facilities." She then asked a question that was fundamental to all Catholic hospitals: "Can we capture the system's benefits so that they accrue to local hospitals?"

Sister William Joseph interpreted the decline in the total number of

Catholic hospitals as "reflecting the reality of changing needs and of religious congregations facing the fact that a given institution may need to be closed in the interest of serving the greater needs of a community." At the same time, she said, hospital beds under Catholic auspices had grown in recent years by 4,000 beds. This to her illustrates two things: "1. The Catholic health system is responding in an orderly way to changing needs and conditions, and 2. We are a viable and growing system in terms of services offered to the communities we serve. But how do you read statistics like these? It is possible to read them mournfully, if we take the dangerous view of quantitative thinking."[9]

More recently, Donnelly commented in a personal letter:

> I would say that since the initial undertaking of the Catholic Health Services Leadership Program there has been a continual assumption on the part of staff and Board [of Trustees] alike that the strengthening of the multi-hospital arrangements, which have been traditional with Catholic hospitals, would be of prime importance to the Association. The assumption being that faced with external pressures, greater strength can be achieved through a unification of effort, rather than considering each hospital as an individual autonomous unit.
>
> At the present time [December 1975], under the general thrust of Project 1980, we are looking at various alternatives to multi-hospital arrangements that would maintain strength within the Catholic system even though in certain situations the traditional relationship between a religious congregation and a given hospital may be altered. Donnelly added that the CHA would be holding a conference "to identify the issues that will be involved in any modification of the present arrangements into a pattern that resembles more a geographical thrust than a purely religious congregation thrust which is often not geographical and quite widespread in terms of the location of its hospitals."[10]

While Catholic hospitals represent a strong systems trend in many ways, in many other ways they are *not* strong multiple unit systems. Control tends to be highly decentralized so that while a hospital identifies with a religious order, it does not always identify with a strong central management system. Donnelly gave an example:

> There are 30 religious congregations who operate four or less health care facilities in the New England area plus New York. All but four of the total health care institutions which these 30

congregations sponsor are in this same geographical region. There is a total of 56 health care facilities in this category in this region and they account for 10,886 beds. Fourteen of these 30 religious congregations operate one hospital. This information illustrates that there is a definable population which may have a quite different set of issues to face than those religious congregations who sponsor a larger number of hospitals. There may be a great deal of potential benefit to be derived from these religious congregations getting together to begin dialogue to explore how cooperative efforts between congregations may be worthwhile—and begin the process of intercongregation cooperation.[11]

Similar comments could be made about Pennsylvania, Ohio and other states.

THE CATHOLIC MEDICAL CENTER
OF BROOKLYN AND QUEENS

The New York area does contain a good example of a highly advanced multiple-unit Catholic hospital system, The Catholic Medical Center of Brooklyn and Queens, (CMC), Jamaica, New York. The center represents a voluntary commitment to two boroughs of New York by five institutions: the 236–bed St. Mary's Hospital that serves the Bedford-Stuyvesant area of Brooklyn; the 93–bed Hospital of the Holy Family that serves downtown Brooklyn; and three member hospitals in Queens: the 273–bed Mary Immaculate Hospital serving the central area; the 308–bed St. John's Queens Hospital serving the northern area, and St. Joseph's Hospital serving the southern area of the borough. These hospitals provide care for patients from diverse ethnic and religious backgrounds, including non-Catholic black communities and Jewish communities.[12]

"At present, the CMC has a complement of almost 1,200 beds, affords privileges to over 900 physicians on its staff, annually provides some 360,000 patient days with over 88,000 outpatient visits, more than 115,000 emergency clinic visits, and almost 38,000 ambulance calls, and thereby effectively serves a large number of the city's communities," according to a statement explaining the concept of the center. The consolidation of the five hospitals "under one central management provides an unusual opportunity to provide premium health care with the accomplishment of totally interrelated working arrangements between these five hospitals of the CMC and to establish an important regional medical program."

All of the hospitals retain separate boards although they are linked by their regional concept through a central office and management team headed by

Alvin J. Conway, executive vice-president. In the systems concept, Mary Immaculate Hospital has been designated as the "hub" institution of this vertically and horizontally integrated hospital system. Highly specialized programs (heart surgery, burn center, radiotherapy, pediatric I.C.U., and transplatation and dialysis) are centered there.

A strong argument for CMC and its regional system is the need for physicians in inner-city areas. "This shortage is most apparent in the unavailability of care to the poor, to the isolated in city ghetto areas, and to the members of minority groups. Private physicians are as hard to find in some neighborhoods of New York City as in backward rural counties of the South," the report said.

Conway believes CMC is "well advanced and far ahead" of many other developing multiple systems in the United States. "I'm getting a query every two weeks or so about our system, mostly from Catholic hospitals," he told a reporter.[13]

SISTERS OF THE SORROWFUL MOTHER

Sister M. Regina Bruen, S.S.M., provincial of the Sisters of the Sorrowful Mother, Milwaukee (Wisconsin) Province, explained how her order has met the technological challenges of the times facing thirteen sponsored hospitals: "We have established management services at a central level, as a separate corporation with an executive director, in order to provide member hospitals with a valuable new resource. As a result, we are able to assist each hospital in administering its finances, in developing progressive business practices and methods, and in adapting the latest medical and scientific techniques to its specific needs. In addition, we have established a centralized computer system and hired data processing experts to manage it."

Sister M. Regina added: "With our hospitals ranging in size from 100 beds to 850 beds and located in an area stretching from Rhinelander, Wisconsin, to Roswell, New Mexico, serving the needs of rural areas, urban centers, the poor, the middle class, the affluent, whites, blacks, Chicanos, Indians, the young and the aging, we are faced with dichotomy. On the one hand, we derive strength through totality; yet, on the other hand, there is a natural tendency for our individual communities to draw apart from one another. Then, too, as we devote more and more of our time to becoming proficient in the field of health care, it becomes all too easy to lose sight of our over-all purpose."[14]

Geographical dispersion, then, is a problem faced by many Catholic hospitals along with these questions: How can inter- and intra-congregational cooperative efforts, i.e. systems concepts, be brought about when sponsorship is so diverse and authority so decentralized? If the bonds of the Roman Catholic Church are not sufficiently strong to bring diverse (in terms of congregational sponsorship) Catholic hospitals together into systems, what will bring them together? Government regulation? Fiscal problems? Moral, legal, and ethical issues? Health Systems Agencies?

While the leadership of the Catholic Hospital Association has been wrestling with these issues, through such programs as its Catholic Health Services Leadership Program and Project 1980 Committee, a few of the orders have also examined the issues in some detail.

CONGREGATION OF
THE SISTERS OF THE HOLY CROSS

The Congregation of the Sisters of the Holy Cross, Notre Dame, Indiana, operates nine hospitals in six states, a system stretching from Maryland to California.[15]

These facilities are: 72-bed Holy Cross Hospital, San Fernando, California; 230-bed Saint Agnes Hospital and Medical Center, Fresno; 338-bed Holy Cross Hospital, Salt Lake City, Utah; 227-bed Saint Alphonsus Hospital, Boise, Idaho; 338-bed Saint Joseph's Hospital, South Bend, Indiana; 344-bed Holy Cross Hospital, Silver Spring, Maryland; 333-bed Saint John's Hickey Memorial Hospital, Anderson, Indiana; 504-bed Mount Carmel Medical Center, Columbus, Ohio; and 194-bed Mount Carmel East Hospital also in Columbus. According to 1974 statistics, these nine hospitals had 2,580 short-term beds and recorded 107,367 admissions. The average census was 2,150 and average occupancy rate was 82.9 percent. Expenses were $101.9 million, including payroll of $51.7 million for 6,392 full-time employees.

Sister Geraldine M. Hoyler, C.S.C., while a student at the University of Denver, examined the issues of the times in some detail and proposed that the order establish a multiple unit hospital system. She explained, "Originally a community devoted solely to the educational apostolate, the Sisters of the Holy Cross entered the nursing field at the time of the Civil War staffing hospital boats on the Ohio and Mississippi Rivers, as well as hospitals at Mound City and Cairo, Illinois and Memphis, Tennessee. As a result of this experience the sisters entered into the operation of hospitals across the United States."[16]

Each of the nine hospitals is a separate corporate entity with nine members. All members of the so-called "motherhouse corporation" are Sisters of the Holy Cross. Each hospital also has a board of trustees with a general membership ratio of 50 percent sisters and 50 percent non-sisters. A third level of management is that of the administrator and her assistants in each hospital. There is also a consulting arm known as Central Administrative Services (CAS) with headquarters in South Bend. A creature of the congregation, CAS is charged to assist the corporations, boards of trustees, and individual administrators. Sister Geraldine explained, "This staff arm currently consists of two CPAs, an industrial engineer, a personnel expert, and a purchasing and procurement expert. Besides functioning in a consultative role, they also are responsible for group purchasing including such items as liability insurance. In this light it is important to note that they are employed by the Congregation, not any hospital corporation, or even the group of hospital corporations."

The one thing that links together the nine hospitals is the "sponsoring tie" back to the Sisters of the Holy Cross. The "motherhouse corporation" has retained many of the real powers—establishing objectives, selection of executives, disposition of profits and assets and the determination of mergers and acquisitions. But when local boards of trustees were implemented in 1968, the balance of power between the corporation, boards, and administrators became confused. In an effort to repair this situation, the congregation created a position of director of hospitals in mid-1975 to bring about "the preservation and development of . . . values in a corporate Holy Cross health care system." But, as Sister Geraldine explained, the role of the director has been largely that of consultant and advisor with no direct authority over Central Administrative Services. This management structure could create conflicts, but she said "the results should not be regarded as negative, however, for it cannot be stressed too strongly that here, at least, is a first step toward the creation of a better way, an affirmation that a system is desirable."

Sister Geraldine briefly discussed, but then turned away from presystem and systems concepts such as merger, management contracts, joint ventures and investor-owned hospital chain techniques. She prefers an application of the bank holding company concept as the organizational form for the Sisters of the Holy Cross to consider.

Two conditions would be assumed in the implementation of a multiple-unit system for the Sisters of the Holy Cross, Sister Geraldine said: "(1) The legal structure of the organization will not change, and (2) The role and functions of the director of hospitals are open to potential expansion of both authority and power." Acknowledging that change is never easy, she said the sisters would have to consider the following if they wanted to develop a system: "(1) definition of the multi-hospital system as envisioned for those hospitals operated under the auspices of the Congregation of the Sisters of the Holy Cross; (2) development of a structure to implement the system concept: (3) definition of function, authority and responsibility and inter-relationships at: (a) the corporate level, (b) the board level, and (c) the administrative level; (4) development of tools to measure success of the new structure; (5) development of formal and informal methods of education for each level in the new structure, and (6) development of communication channels in the new structure."

The most difficult problem the present system faced, Sister Geraldine said, was one of role perception at all three levels of governance: corporate membership, board of trustees, and administration. "What was needed," she said, "was a new psychological contract between the corporate and administrative levels."

"As long as the present situation exists," Sister Geraldine said in July 1975, "the central staff will continue to be merely consultative, lacking any authority to effect change and caught in the resultant binds. A hospital system implies that the Congregation acknowledge that sponsorship includes control."

SISTERS OF MERCY OF THE UNION

The Sisters of Mercy of the Union (R.S.M.), founded in 1831 in Ireland, has eight provinces with its generalate located in Bethesda, Maryland. These Sisters of Mercy operate eighty-four medical and health care units, making this order the largest of all the Catholic-sponsored multiple-unit systems (see Figure 13:1). The eighty-four units include fifteen long-term care facilities that are identified either as homes, villas, nursing homes or continuing care centers. The other sixty-nine facilities are identified as hospitals. Mercy province headquarters are located in: Baltimore; Chicago; Cincinnati; Dobbs Ferry, New York; Omaha; Farmington, Michigan; St. Louis; and Dallas, Pennsylvania. There are Sisters of Mercy facilities in twenty-four states.[17]

Although the Catholic Hospital Association's *1975 Guidebook* lists 84 health and medical care facilities owned and operated by the Sisters of Mercy of the Union, including 69 hospitals, statistical data available through the American Hospital Association's 1974 survey of hospitals identifies only 65 institutions. The summary data for 65 hospitals in the eight provinces show:

Beds—16,724
Admissions—603,386
Total inpatient days—4,870,518
Occupancy rate—79.8 per cent
Average daily census—13,344
Average length of stay—8.1 days[18]

The Sisters of Mercy "sponsors the largest number of hospitals in the United States,"[19] according to Sister Elizabeth Mary Burns, R.S.M., director of the health services board in the provincilate at Farmington Hills,

Figure 13:1

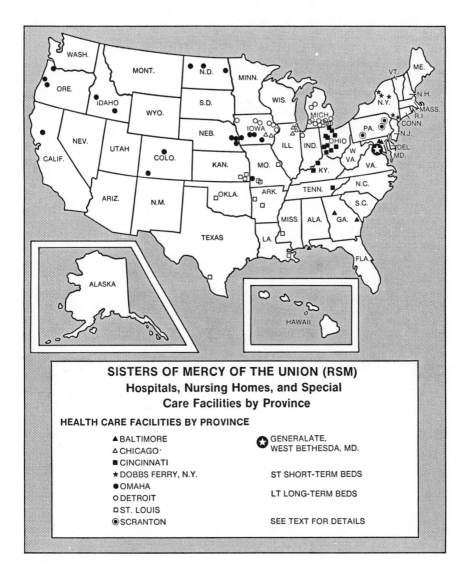

SISTERS OF MERCY OF THE UNION (RSM)
Hospitals, Nursing Homes, and Special
Care Facilities by Province

HEALTH CARE FACILITIES BY PROVINCE

▲ BALTIMORE
△ CHICAGO·
■ CINCINNATI
★ DOBBS FERRY, N.Y.
● OMAHA
○ DETROIT
□ ST. LOUIS
◉ SCRANTON

✪ GENERALATE,
WEST BETHESDA, MD.

ST SHORT-TERM BEDS

LT LONG-TERM BEDS

SEE TEXT FOR DETAILS

Institution and Location	ST	LT
PROVINCE OF BALTIMORE		
Villa Mercy, Daphne, Alabama		45
St. Joseph's Infirmary, Atlanta, Ga.	280	
St. Joseph's Hospital, Savannah	273	

Institution and Location	ST	LT
Mercy Hospital, Baltimore	364	
Stella Maris Hospital, Baltimore		355
PROVINCE OF CHICAGO		
Mercy Center for Health Care Services, Aurora, Ill.	328	
Mercy Hospital and Medical Center, Chicago	517	
Mercy Manor (residence), Chicago		100
Misericordia Home (handicapped children), Chicago ...		136
Mercy Hospital, Davenport, Iowa	298	
Mercy Hospital, Iowa City, Iowa	248	
PROVINCE OF CINCINNATI		
Sacred Heart Home (ambulatory care for aged), Louis- ville, Ky.		64
Our Lady of Mercy Hospital, Owensboro, Ky.	130	
Clermont County Hospital, Batavia, Ohio	63	
Our Lady of Mercy Hospital, Cincinnati	152	
Siena Home for the Aged, Dayton		98
Mercy Hospital, Hamilton, Ohio	306	
St. Rita's Hospital, Lima, Ohio	426	
Mercy Medical Center, Springfield, Ohio	331	
Mercy Hospital, Tiffin, Ohio	115	
Mercy Hospital, Toledo	350	
St. Charles Hospital, Toledo	260	
Mercy Memorial Hospital, Urbana, Ohio	86	
St. Mary's Memorial Hospital, Knoxville, Tenn.	525	
PROVINCE OF NEW YORK		
McAuley Centre (infirmary care for aged Sisters), Dobbs Ferry		26
Uihlein Mercy Center, Lake Placid, N.Y.	96	
St. Francis Hospital, Port Jervis, N.Y.	108	
Mercy General Hospital, Tupper Lake, N.Y.	56	
Mercy Hospital of Watertown and Madonna Home, Watertown, N.Y.	400	120
PROVINCE OF OMAHA		
St. Elizabeth Community Hospital, Red Bluff, Calif.	75	
Mercy Hospital, Denver	370	
Mercy Hospital, Durango, Colo.	105	
Mercy Medical Center, Nampa, Idaho	144	
St. Anthony Community Hospital, Pocatello, Idaho	127	
St. Joseph Mercy Hospital, Centerville, Iowa	77	
Mercy Hospital, Council Bluffs, Iowa	330	
Bishop Drumm Home for the Aged, Des Moines		147
Mercy Hospital, Des Moines	366	
St. John's Medical Center, Joplin, Missouri	367	
Archbishop Bergan Mercy Hospital, Omaha	455	
St. Catherine's Hospital Center for Continuing Care, Omaha		260
St. Vincent's Home for the Aged, Omaha		300
Mercy Hospital, Devils Lake, N.D.	110	

Institution and Location	ST	LT
Mercy Hospital, Valley City, N.D.	75	
Mercy Hospital, Williston, N.D.	96	
St. Catherine's Residence and Nursing Center, Portland, Oregon		109
Mt. St. Joseph's Residence and Extended Care Center, Portland, Oregon		316
Mercy Medical Center, Roseburg, Oregon	106	
PROVINCE OF DETROIT		
Our Lady of Mercy Hospital, Dyer, Ind.	275	
St. Joseph Mercy Hospital, Clinton, Iowa	146	
McAuley, Center, Dubuque, Iowa		32
Mercy Medical Center, Dubuque	376	
St. Joseph Mercy Hospital, Sioux City, Iowa	340	
St. Joseph Mercy Hospital, Mason City, Iowa	312	
St. Joseph Mercy Hospital, Waverly, Iowa	45	
Mercywood Hospital (psychiatric), Ann Arbor, Michigan		125
St. Joseph Mercy Hospital, Ann Arbor	558	
Leila Y. Post Montgomery Hospital, Battle Creek, Mich.	228	
Mercy Hospital, Cadillac, Mich.	185	
Mt. Carmel Mercy Hospital, Detroit	557	
St. Joseph Mercy Hospital, Detroit	269	
St. Mary's Hospital, Grand Rapids	370	
Mercy Hospital, Grayling, Mich.	66	
Mercy Hospital, Jackson, Mich.	201	
St. Lawrence Hospital, Lansing, Mich.	306	
Mercy Hospital, Muskegon, Mich.	238	
St. Joseph Mercy Hospital, Pontiac, Mich.	471	
Mercy Hospital, Port Huron, Mich.	119	
PROVINCE OF ST. LOUIS		
St. Edward Mercy Hospital, Fort Smith, Ark.	227	
St. Joseph's Hospital, Hot Springs, Ark.	249	
Mercy Hospital, Fort Scott, Kans.	163	
St. Margaret's Mercy Hospital, Fredonia, Kans.	42	
Mercy Hospital, Independence, Kans.	85	
Mercy Hospital, New Orleans, La.	216	
Mercy Regional Medical Center, Vicksburg, Miss.	200	
St. John's Mercy Medical Center, St. Louis	607	
Mercy Villa, Springfield, Mo.		134
St. John's Hospital, Springfield, Mo.	550	
Mercy Health Center, Oklahoma City, Okla.	400	
Mercy Hospital of Laredo, Texas	234	
PROVINCE OF SCRANTON		
Mercy Hospital of Johnstown, Penna.	202	
Mercy Hospital, Scranton	316	
Mercy Hospital, Wilkes Barre, Penna.	330	
TOTALS	17,398	2,367

Michigan, headquarters for the Mercy Province of Detroit. While the Sisters of Mercy of the Union is the largest sponsoring group, she said, "there are a number of smaller congregations of Sisters of Mercy. . . . Altogether, there are between 125 and 140 hospitals in the United States sponsored by the Sisters of Mercy, whether they are united under one religious government plan or have remained independent."

An estimated one-fourth of all U.S. hospitals are Catholic facilities and about 90 percent are sponsored by religious communities. Organizations such as the Sisters of Mercy of the Union are taking steps to bring these vast resources together in some new ways and turning to lay experts for help. In late 1975, for example, the Generalate at West Bethesda hired H. Joseph Curl, former director of Georgetown University Hospital, Washington, D.C., as a health care and financial advisor. In 1974 the Detroit Province hired Edward J. Connors, the former director of the University of Michigan Hospital, Ann Arbor, as a staff consultant.

Sister Elizabeth Mary, looking at the issues of the day facing Catholic hospitals, specifically those institutions in the Detroit Province, recalled that as early as 1965 the province had begun to study its future. In the next five years, the sisters had before them consulting reports that recommended more of a local focus for the hospitals. And there were many indications of change: the number of Catholic-sponsored hospitals in the province had decreased from 25 to 20; the religious management group decreased from 143 to 83, and the average age of sisters in the health care mission was going up.

A consultants group recommended in 1968, Sister Elizabeth Mary said, "that we 'tap local communities for equal or greater amounts of citizen talents and interest and for equal or greater amounts of financial support. . . .' " The consultants also recommended "that there be an effort 'to differentiate and clarify the total top management responsibility; to equitably, fairly and uniformly separate the policy making, appraisal and control functions from the executive management functions.' This recommendation . . . seems to be more important as time proves its wisdom," Sister Elizabeth Mary told Duke University's Tenth National Forum on Health and Hospital Affairs.

The result of these recommendations was that the Sisters of Mercy developed a decentralized management approach, creating five small hospital systems that "developed their own policies and long-range planning with limited aid and coordination from the Provincialate." But external forces led the order to believe that there were larger issues to consider. A thirteen-member Perspectives Committee was created to look at the issues in detail, including a reorganization of the system. Connors became a consultant to this group. Outside advice was sought from several experts. The sisters made site visits to a number of the better-known hospital systems in the United States, including two for-profit chains.

A canonical consultant advised the Sisters that in any reorganization they should reserve certain rights. These were the rights to articulate the philosophy and theology of the hospitals, sell and lease real property, veto operating and capital budgets, appoint trustees and administrators, amend articles of incorporation and bylaws, and "enter into any agreements of merger or consolidations with other health care facilities."[20]

Financial consultants urged the Sisters of Mercy-Detroit to consider an overriding fact: efficient Catholic-sponsored hospital systems, like other systems, could generate financial resources to enhance the mission of the corporation and the sponsoring body. The financial group said the sisters should consider one of two courses: either give the autonomous hospitals legal and fiscal responsibility or place those functions under a central management staff.

"The present corporate structure lends itself to cost savings through centralized management, but with few exceptions are these advantages being utilized,"[21] the consultants said. There is a scarcity of sisters trained to manage hospitals, the report pointed out, and one way to create leverage for those scarce managers would be to restructure the system into an overall corporate structure rather than retain the seventeen autonomous management structures. The consultants favored the formation of a corporate holding company.

If the sisters were going to stay in the business of running community hospitals, the consultant recommended, "then it is in your best interest to run them as aggressively and business-like as possible—this includes the necessity of maximizing profits for equity growth which will provide for future growth, replacement, and continuity of operation." The report added that this money-making stance "is not necessarily contrary to serving the public; for you are depleting your future capacity by operating with losses or not making maximum use of your resources."

The consultants recommended a reorganization based on service area concepts and less attention to geography. Three corporations were suggested: one for the four Iowa hospitals, a second for the eight urban, Detroit-area hospitals, and a third organization called Suburban Community Hospital Corporation that would consolidate the management strengths of six facilities located in areas outside of the Detroit region (see Figure 7:2).

The third consulting company, a law firm, recommended that the sisters adopt a "parent-subsidiary concept" of governance. This would not require the participation of a large number of sisters, the attorneys said. "Yet, it puts Policy Control where it belongs—vested in the Sisters of Mercy. Further, it puts Operating Control in the local health care institutions—where it belongs." The "parents" would be the three holding companies (Iowa, suburban and urban) who relate back to the province in Detroit. Each hospital would form a subsidiary operating company relating to its appropriate holding company.

The corporate reorganization studies began in early 1974. In May 1975, Sister Elizabeth Mary prepared a document "to provide the basis for consideration of corporate reorganization of the hospitals operated by the Sisters of Mercy, Province of Detroit."[22] That document reaffirms the basic philosophy and mission of the Sisters of Mercy, and the need to maintain compliance with canonical and legal requirements.

Her analysis of the issues facing the Sisters of Mercy continued with an observation that management roles were not well-defined and staff resources were not available in the current organization. "With the exception of a few selected functions," Sister Elizabeth Mary said, "the hospitals have not taken advantage of the strengths inherent in a 'system' of hospitals. Shared services among members, multiple assignments of scarce human resources, uniform corporate policies, mobility of key personnel, clear delegation of authority are examples of 'system' characteristics that have not been optimized to date."

Taking a hard look into the future, she said: "It would be unwise to reduce the number of health facilities sponsored by the Sisters of Mercy primarily on the basis of a reduced number of Sisters. The scope of management influence for the Sisters can be expanded in a new corporate structure through such approaches as satellites, management 'division,' and corporate staffing. While a new corporate structure should evolve with a commitment to the utilization and development of the skills and abilities of the Sisters of Mercy, further consideration should be given to the question of whether a Catholic health facility, supportive of the basic philosophy and mission statement of the Sisters of Mercy, could exist under a new corporate structure with no Sisters of Mercy serving within the institution."

There is little question that the Sisters of Mercy feel that their mission is unique and that it sets apart Catholic hospitals from other hospitals. Sister Elizabeth Mary said: "In an age pressured by dehumanization and technology, our health care facilities should assume a leadership role in preserving reverence for the human person by: a. providing excellence of health care in a personal, compassionate, and humanistic manner, and b. safeguarding and witnessing to the right to life for all persons."

Sister Elizabeth Mary also quoted this statement from a sister in the health ministry who said that health care " 'really is big business, yet more than ever, we are convinced that to withdraw from this service at this time in history when national health insurance and health maintenance organizations are so close upon us, bringing within their structures cold, heavy bureaucracy, we would not be living up to our goals. Also, we feel that the dignity of personhood could be lost in that dimension.' "

Early in 1976, Connors said the sisters were working effectively to take the corporation toward consolidation of its five corporate units into one centrally-oriented hospital system. The sisters proposed that each corporation, its trustees and sponsoring organizations approve the plan, Connors said. He said the reorganization should bring more efficiency into the governance and management of the institutions while also reaffirming the sisters' commitment to the hospitals and health services.[23]

By October 1975, the Sisters of Mercy had come up with two working documents that form the basis for organizing a closely integrated hospital system. "Guidelines and Planning Assumptions for Corporate Reorganization" states much of the realism and philosophy contained in papers by Sister Elizabeth Mary, along with pertinent information from the consultants' reports. A second document, "Study of the Corporate Organization, Governance & Management of the Health Care Institutions Sponsored by the Sisters of Mercy, Province of Detroit," spells out detailed plans and recommendations as the twenty hospitals consider reorganization.[24]

This is the summary of conclusions that the Perspectives Committee listed in its document:

1. The impact of the *Church's ministry* will be strengthened by the extent to which we maximize our opportunity to enhance our province ministry in the healing mission of the Church.

2. Sponsorship of health care institutions provides tangible evidence and public witness to the vital role of the Catholic Church in serving the health needs of people and is a valid and an appropriate expression of the philosophy and mission of the Sisters of Mercy.

3. Reaffirmation by the Sisters of Mercy of the commitment to sponsor health care institutions, is desirable in order to provide a renewed sense of direction for the health services ministry of the Province.

4. The strengths of our present operation are a solid foundation on which to build competent and responsive service. This foundation includes: (a) a history of competence in health care; (b) dedicated and well-prepared Sisters; (c) lay staff, doctors and community persons desirous of working with us; (d) significant corporate improvement since the 1969 restructuring, (e) fiscal soundness and good physical resources.

5. Change in our present corporate and management structure is required in light of internal difficulties and because of the increasing external changes and pressures of the future.

6. Weaknesses exist in the present operation which can be overcome. The proposed system will enhance our capability to: (a) be on the cutting edge of responsiveness and innovativeness in meeting the needs of the people; (b) address the gospel witness of the institution; (c) address the spiritual development and spiritual input of Sisters and staff; (d) attract

candidates to this ministry and to this religious community; (e) obtain greater participation of laity in governance and management than the present structure allows.

7. In our present service, we are significantly involved in serving a broad population spectrum of our country, (rural-urban, affluent-poor) and in touching the lives of many in their hour of suffering and need.

8. There is a level of need, an opportunity to serve and a justification for the existence of our hospitals that is broader than the internal problems of the Detroit Sisters of Mercy.

9. It is essential to maintain a voluntary non-profit health system within the U.S. as a responsive and innovative alternative to the government and for-profit systems. Within that voluntary system, the delivery of health care will be significantly enhanced by the health-care efforts of religious.

10. Nationally, multi-hospital units are replacing the traditional pattern of single hospital units. The Detroit Sisters of Mercy have talents and resources which makes it appropriate for them to assume leadership in structuring and maintaining a health care system.

11. Our number of established institutions represents a potent resource envied by other hospitals. This very strength can be a force for good. The dimension of our existing operation gives us a unique opportunity for competent and responsive service in the civic community and within the Catholic Church.

12. The Detroit province should not continue with the current scope of health service without more extensive and effective use of lay persons in governance and management.

13. There is a definite urgency to the need for the Sisters of Mercy to change the governance and management structure of their hospitals. There is a readiness for change within the Province, and enthusiasm and support for the bold and imaginative changes that are recommended.

14. The scope of these recommendations will require carefully-timed phasing. The changes recommended are within the manpower and financial capabilities of the Detroit Sisters of Mercy and their lay colleagues.

The Perspectives Committee also listed this summary of recommendations:

1. Establish an integrated system for the governance and management of our health institutions and health services that is a careful blend of local responsibility, Province-wide integration, improved management capability and enhancement of R.S.M.'s in both governance and management. The key elements of the system include:

　　a. creation of a Subsidiary Board of Trustees at each local level with carefully delegated authority.

　　b. creation of a single corporation (Mercy Health Corporation) responsible for the governance and management of all hospitals and health services.

    c.   provision for the Provincial Administrative Team to be the members of the Mercy Health Corporation with appropriate reserved powers.

    d.   provision for the Trustees of Mercy Health Corporation to be charged with broad responsibilities for governance and management.

    e. appointment of four Trustee Officers of Mercy Health Corporation on a full-time basis to provide defined lines of accountability for the Chief Executive Officers for the individual institutions.

    f. appointment of a corporate management staff to provide the skills and support necessary to the Trustees and the local institutions.

    g. development of a Mercy Health Advisory Council to act as an advisory body to the Mercy Health Corporation.

    h.   enhancement of the opportunity for all R.S.M's to carry their responsibilities as owners-sponsors, both individually and corporately.

2.   Maximize the influence of Sisters by placing selected Sisters in positions to which they can have significant influence on several or all institutions.

3. Utilize qualified lay persons for corporate management functions and positions as institutional CEO's corporate management staff and corporate executives.

4. Finance the cost of the system through revenue generated by member hospitals based on an approved annual budget. This financing will replace the current central management fee, the current corporation costs, and other current shared program costs.

5. Evaluate the system on a scheduled basis and report the results of the evaluation to the entire religious community.

6. Develop and implement the system in a manner that is flexible for future change and sensitive to the unique requirements of a religiously sponsored service.

7. Institute a process of review, decision-making and implementation that balances the urgent need for action with the requirement of understanding and support of the sponsoring group and the current corporation.

8. Conduct the activities of the new structure in a manner and style that will enhance the ministry of Church in healing and serving the needy.

Through the statements, the Sisters of Mercy, Detroit Province, have carved out a new future and a new systems configuration. Although major changes such as these will not occur overnight, the Detroit-based organization is well on its way to becoming the first multiple-state Catholic organization to form a highly integrated hospital system.

NOTES

1. Sr. W. Joseph, "The Catholic Sub-System—An Opportunity for Leadership," *Hospital Progress* (October 1971), pp. 64-69.

2. Sr. M. Maurita, Introduction to the Catholic Health Services Leadership Program, 1971.

3. J.A. Hamilton, *Patterns of Hospital Ownership and Control,* Minneapolis: University of Minnesota Press, 1961, p. 92.

4. CHA 1973-1974 Annual Report, p. 36.

5. P.R. Donnelly, "A Progress Report on Phase II of the Catholic Health Services Leadership Program," *Hospital Progress* (September 1972), pp. 75-79.

6. The Catholic Hospital Association 1974-1975 Annual Report.

7. Sr. G.M. Hiltz, "Developing Community Requires Sound Management Plan," *Hospital Progress* (December 1974), pp. 59-61.

8. "Issues Raised Challenging Questions But No Pat Answers—Sr. Grace Marie," *Hospital Progress* (July 1974), pp. 38,39.

9. Sr. W. Joseph, op. cit., note 1. All subsequent quotations are from this interview until otherwise noted.

10. Personal letter from P.R. Donnelly, December 19, 1975.

11. Ibid.

12. "Comprehensive Health Services for Five Hospitals and Their Communities by Regional Cooperative Arrangements—The Concept of the Catholic Medical Center of Brooklyn and Queens, Inc.," undated and unpublished. All subsequent quotations until otherwise noted are from this citation.

13. Telephone interview with Alvin J. Conway, November 13, 1975.

14. Sr. M.R. Bruen, "Challenges Facing Sponsoring Groups," *Hospital Progress* (March 1973), pp. 61-63, 78.

15. The Catholic Hospital Association 1975 Guidebook.

16. Sr. G.M. Hoyler, "A Proposal for a Multi-Hospital System, Congregation of the Sisters of the Holy Cross," unpublished May, 1975. Until otherwise noted all subsequent quotations are from this proposal.

17. The Catholic Hospital Association 1975 Guidebook.

18. Personal communication from H. Joseph Curl, February 13, 1976.

19. Sr. E.M. Burns, "Changes in Church Operated-Systems," Tenth Annual National Forum on Hospital Affairs, Duke University, May, 1975. Until otherwise noted all subsequent quotations are taken from this citation.

20. Rev. A.J. Maida, "Canonical Analysis of the Hospital Care Facilities Owned and Sponsored by the Sisters of Mercy Province of Detroit," September 18, 1974.

21. Third Working Draft, "Study of the Corporate Organization, Governance and Management of the Health Care Institution sponsored by the Sisters of Mercy, Province of Detroit," submitted by the Perspective Committee of Health Services Board of the Province of Detroit, October 1975. Until otherwise noted subsequent footnotes are taken from this draft.

22. Sr. E.M. Burns, "Supplement to a Paper 'Changes in Church Operated Systems' " unpublished, May 24, 1975. Until otherwise noted all footnotes were taken from this cite.

23. Telephone interview with Edward J. Connors, January 19, 1976.

24. Third Working Draft, op. cit., note 21.

Chapter 14
Performance and Power

The arguments stated in Chapter 2 evolve around this premise: A central corps of managers created by a hospital system has certain advantages over the small group of managers of an autonomous hospital.

Individual hospitals rarely have the bed size and volume of care to afford the specialists they need. Individual hospitals don't present continuous opportunities for specialists to develop and use their skills to highest capacity. It appears that the voluntary, nonprofit, free-standing autonomous community hospital may simply be too small to make effective use of all the talents it needs. No matter what its size, every hospital must have experts in management, technical and legal fields if it is to operate effectively and be able to cope with the government bureaucracy. The single hospital can neither react quickly nor effectively to poorly conceived regulations. It can't afford to operate at a deficit, knowing that it may not be able to meet its financial commitments. A single hospital may not either effectively change its services to meet new needs or alter its environment, if it is no longer able to survive in one location. The autonomous hospital is a captive of its environment. It has little flexibility to plan and exercise control over its own destiny. Its strategies are limited.

Within a system, the managers would include individuals with specialized skills and knowledge in quality patient care assurance, human resource development, labor relations, capital financing, reimbursement, financial controls, planning, building, data systems, technology, insurance and risk management, purchasing, materials control, public relations and legislative affairs.

The central corps of managers in a system can assist in the design, development and implementation of appropriate standards and systems for the individual units of care. The managers provide a monitoring capability to ensure that individual units are performing at capacity and within limits.

259

And the central management corps provides a perspective to ensure a systems-wide breadth of vision that goes far beyond the bricks and mortar orientation of a single institutional location.

Samuel Tibbitts suggests another important dimension of the quality of management issue for large and small hospitals, "Obviously, seven heads are better than one, and this is not only true on the top management level—it is carried throughout the organization to the departmental level. . . . Also, peer group review of operations is definitely helpful."[1]

The advantages of hospitals systems are sometimes inherent in the giant industrial corporations that operate on a national and international basis. But the concept of such advantages in the highly complex service field of hospital care is new and still not fully proven. It is fair to say, however, that hospital systems emerging across the United States do have certain advantages over autonomous institutions in terms of economy, quality of patient care, accessibility, and power. Systems have more strategy alternatives.

ECONOMY

Systems and autonomous institutions alike face severe problems in cost containment. Health and medical care now absorb 8.3 percent of the Gross National Product. Hospital care is rising about 20 percent a year on the Consumer Price Index.[2] There is every possibility of wage and price controls again, either through federal or state governmental actions. If price increases are beyond the control of the individual hospital, and the multiple system hospital, this fact must be explained to Congress, governments, consumers, members of the press and third parties. Some states have already responded to skyrocketing costs with rate-setting and denials of insurance company and Blue Cross requests for rate increases. These reactions will surely intensify and probably accelerate in the remaining years of the 1970s. The federal government could put a limit on the amount of the GNP available for medical and health care.

Economy is a critical argument that is difficult to prove. There are several reasons for this difficulty: (1) there have been very few long-term studies of the ability of hospital systems to either contain or reduce costs, and (2) many savings occur in terms of programs not attempted, beds not built, and equipment and new technology not purchased, rather than through increases in productivity. The health care field is just now trying to apply this proven industrial concept within its highly personalized service environment.

Tibbitts reported in 1973 that the Lutheran Hospital Society of Southern California was saving patients $5.50 a day. This figure was computed from an annual savings of $1.158 million to $1.820 million that the society estimated it was saving its member hospitals because those system hospitals did not have to duplicate equipment and services available on a central basis.[3]

Several researchers seem to confirm the claims of the managers of investor-owned, for-profit chains. These claims are that proprietary systems can accumulate savings in initial construction costs, volume purchasing, judicious use of special personnel, standardization of procedures and systems, strict controls on manpower and the ability to attract capital at favorable interest rates.

For-profit chains have shown the way to effect economies through rigid controls on staffing, the most variable and expensive management cost. The first place a for-profit management contracting arm looks to save money, and turn a failing hospital around, for example, is in employee to patient ratios. The next place it usually concentrates its efforts is in cash flow and optimizing reimbursement. One chain gave an example of a radiologist who bragged about having all results back to doctors by noon on the day the test was initiated. The for-profit manager's answer to economy was to cut the radiologist's staff in half and get all work back by the end of the day.

Sam A. Edwards and Adrienne A. Astolfi directed the first major study that evaluated the development of a not-for-profit hospital system through merger, the Samaritan Health Service of Arizona. During the early stages of the systems development, they reported, there were benefits in cost effectiveness, comprehensiveness of care, availability of care, organization and management, and community acceptance of the system.[4]

The most extensive study of economy in hospital systems, published in 1975, was completed by James P. Cooney, Jr. and Thomas L. Alexander of the Health Services Research Center of Northwestern University in cooperation with the Hospital Research & Education Trust, an affiliate of the American Hospital Association.

Cooney and Alexander studied eight systems and compared each to a control group. The systems were not identified by name. The researchers concluded that seven of the systems experienced a slower growth in per case cost, a lower level of average case cost, a lower price level, a lower rate of growth in prices, a higher output, a level of service comparable to other hospitals, a lower average length of stay, a higher wage rate without higher labor costs and a slower rate of growth in manhours provided per case. They also argued that these savings were passed on to the community through lower costs and charges. However, none of the systems studied were for-profit. The for-profit systems usually charge prevailing rates and profits are returned to stockholders or reinvested.

In the Cooney-Alexander study, only one system failed to perform in a more cost effective manner than its control group. This system was apparently carrying a heavy medical education load and had higher administrative overhead costs. Cooney and Alexander speculated that the lower length of stay and the more intensive use of resources might be due to stronger managers in the systems who could persuade physicians to modify their practice styles in order to achieve high usage patterns.[5]

Every system discussed in the previous nine chapters seems to be saving money for its hospitals and in many cases affiliated institutions too through the economies of scale created by the system.

But some of the potentially large savings in systems are difficult to measure, such as beds taken out of service and closed, potentially duplicate equipment not purchased, and employees not replaced or hired because centralization of services eliminated the need for additional technical and support personnel. Memorial Hospital System in Houston, Texas, believes it can contain its future costs by using labor-saving devices that reduce employee to patient ratios.

The impact of utilization of beds and services on economy has yet to be measured within systems to any great degree. Nationally, the potential for saving money is overwhelming.   Bernard R. Tresnowski, senior vice-president, federal programs, for the Blue Cross Association, has noted: "The American Hospital Association's annual statistical survey for 1974 shows that 25 percent of the nation's 903,000 short-term hospital beds are empty on any given day."[6]

Available beds and services tend to be used because they are available. This is what Milton I. Roemer found in his study of bed distribution and occupancy rates many years ago.[7] This indictment is still true today. And it is a major reason for Public Law 93-641.

"Of equal importance are the inappropriate decisions associated with the scope of services," Tresnowski said.   "In a report from the President's Commission on Heart Disease, Cancer and Stroke it was demonstrated that 11 percent of the hospitals equipped with open-heart surgery units did not perform a single operation during the year."

Tresnowski also said: "A personal experience illustrates the problem of demonstrating positive net present value. I was recently invited to speak in Oakland County, Michigan, an area where I served as a hospital adminis-trator for six years.   A friend—the clinical pathologist at the hospi-tal—invited me to examine his clinical laboratory covering an area of approximately 10,000 square feet and equipped with all of the latest technology in automated and computer-related laboratory equipment.   I estimated the economy of scale for this institution as being four times its current usage.   I am also aware that other institutions serving Oakland County were similarly equipped resulting in no real opportunity to achieve economy of scale, unless a considerable amount of inappropriate laboratory examinations are provided."[8]

Tresnowski brought up three economy of scale issues: overbedding, underused open and closed-heart facilities, and duplicate clinical laboratories. Duplicate and underused clinical services, such as cobalt therapy units, present yet other examples.

In Detroit and Minneapolis, systems integration will lead to a net loss of available beds. But the bed issue is nowhere near resolution because fundamental questions have not been answered, such as: What is an acceptable occupancy rate in an urban institution? What is an acceptable rate in a suburban institution? An acceptable rate in a rural hospital? When will surgeons and hospitals agree routinely to waiting lists for elective surgery?

Will patients go along with this approach for the national economic good? How many hospitals are willing to "bank" beds or put them in "mothballs" in order to drastically reduce the costs of unoccupied beds? How many hospitals are willing to convert beds to other uses, such as long-term care or hotel-type accommodations for senior citizens? In at least one instance, systems seem to do a good job. The Lutheran Hospitals & Homes Society of America frequently converts short-term beds to long-term bed use in order to achieve overall higher rates of occupancy.

An idle open-heart or closed-heart surgery unit is a tremendous drag on the nation's economy too because of the investment in space, equipment and personnel—factors that apply to any underused clinical facility. Systems are in a much better position to control these costs because of central decision making. The Rush-Presbyterian-St. Luke's Medical Center in Chicago does about 750 heart operations a year, about half of the total performed in Illinois.

The criticism of underused clinical laboratory facilities is a problem that occurs all over the United States, most usually in highly competitive urban and suburban areas. This problem is continuing to accelerate because of malpractice claims and the practice of defensive medicine. It is further complicated by the fact that the laboratory is usually a profit center. With the pinch on other sources of revenue, most administrators won't want to tamper with this money-making department and face a confrontation with pathologists.

Within a system, the consolidation of facilities such as the clinical laboratory need not necessarily be a major problem, because the revenue involved is retained under common ownership although costs may be reduced, quality enhanced and services added. One of the early systems, the Youngstown (Ohio) Hospital Association, has a centralized laboratory serving three physically separate facilities. The Northwestern University-McGaw Medical Center, a Chicago system tied to a consortium of institutions, came into being partially because pathologists at two hospitals wanted to consolidate the clinical laboratory. There are several examples within hospital systems where the marketing of laboratory services to smaller, rural hospitals is providing much needed expertise while also helping to increase utilization of equipment.

Integrated hospitals should be able to standardize a basic battery of clinical laboratory tests and through high volume usage keep those costs low. If systems can break down the barriers of transfer between units of care and institute a common medical record system, this procedure should eliminate the need for duplicate laboratory tests and reduce the cost of care.

Integrated systems of care can contain costs, perhaps even reduce the cost of care, because they create economies of scale through shared services and central management. They offer the opportunity to control duplication in services, equipment and personnel. Through a strict control of the utilization of beds, clinic space and services—systems should be able to increase productivity and ensure less idle capacity. Savings that could be realized through bulk purchasing, inventory and warehousing control, and material and systems management should develop as systems grow in size and efficiency. Standardized and tested construction and renovation methods should be more economical within systems.

The central element in bringing about economy is the element of control. Who decides which institutions should provide which services? The answer to that question has always been controversial, but less so where systems are in operation. Final decisions about services can be made by governing boards after an appropriate assessment of the system's financial ability and the medical demand for the service. This decision-making process can significantly reduce the expense of interhospital bargaining, conflicts and competition.

Systems control is usually vested in a governing board but delegated to a central corps of experts and advisors. In effect, the central corps of managers perform in somewhat the same capacity as a management contracting company. Under a management contract, one survey shows that a managed hospital may have available as many as thirty-five different services. These services range from help with admitting practices and labor relations to systems analysis and physician recruiting.[9]

Once a core of management experts become available in a system, their knowledge and service can be sold either to wholly-owned institutions or hospitals owned by other corporate entities.

The managers of multiple-unit hospital operations, both for-profit and not-for-profit, have learned that advantages can accrue to them through large-scale organizations, if the facilities are properly used. They quickly learned that a profit can be realized from almost any operation within a hospital because their organizations have advantages of scale over businesses with smaller volumes of service.

The soundly planned hospital is almost recession-proof. The real estate around the hospital affords the owner an advantageous investment opportunity. The spreading of combined debt guarantees over many hospitals significantly reduces the lender's risks. More and more systems are buying larger parcels of land around their new hospitals and developing a range of community services and related business enterprises as a way to make money. Fairview Community Hospitals in Minneapolis provides a good example in its socio-medical campus.

There's always been profit in the health care system—doctors have always worked that way. Institutions organized "not-for-the-purposes-of-profit" differ from for-profit institutions in their philosophical orientation. For-profits have to keep one eye on their stockholders and the stock market. Nonprofits have to worry about board members, community needs and frequently a religious mission too. They must ensure that they have enough income beyond expenses to accumulate capital for modernization and growth.

Systems can use money more efficiently. Central cash management makes it possible to increase earnings on short-term investments. Intermountain Health Care, LHHSA, Hospital Corp. of America, Peoples Community Hospital Authority, and others mention this advantage. In addition, the consolidation of assets and guaranteeing of a loan across the system make it easier to gain access to the capital markets and get more favorable interest rates. The Sisters of Mercy, Henry Ford Hospital, LHHSA, and other systems mention this advantage.

Systems also place more stringent controls on new capital investments. Any unit that wishes to invest new capital must provide a strong justification for that investment. The Capital Area Health Consortium puts a $25,000 limit on expenditures that must be approved centrally. In any central organization the rules are quite clear: individual operating units have financial autonomy, but only up to a point.

In effect, systems are creating a regional resource allocation decision model to help ensure that depreciation of other sources of capital will be put to the most effective use. While one unit within a system may generate more dollars than another, that money-making unit will not necessarily be allowed to use those dollars at its specific site, unless the investment is cost beneficial to the whole system.

Systems automatically have some basis of comparing the operations and aspirations of any one unit with another. This knowledge provides valuable information for a decision process. The administrator in a system hospital has other administrators and specialists to back up his recommendations. And his recommendations are based more often on hard data and careful studies.

The administrator may routinely use experts to conduct feasibility studies. This means that the manager will not have to go to his operating board without facts to buttress his concerns. Physicians and other health professionals are no longer dealing with an administrator whose expert backup must come from a limited staff, if one exists at all, and a manager whose expertise and personal prestige is limited.

Systems have the advantage of internalizing the resource allocation process making it more difficult for one hospital or one medical staff to successfully argue for the duplication of high cost facilities and services. If third-party reimbursement schemes are modified to promote efficiency and if systems are allowed to share in the economy, the financial rewards could be passed back to consumers as reduced charges.

QUALITY OF CARE

There are no known studies to support a conclusion that systems either provide better or worse patient care. However, many of the procedures and programs observed in the hospital systems described in previous chapters seem destined to improve the quality and comprehensiveness of medical care. This conclusion is not meant to avoid the issue, but it is fair to point out that there is no general agreement on the definition of quality care. Most policymakers say that quality must be based on outcome review. The development of such concepts is now the province of the various specialty boards and specialty societies that are working to set up standards for Professional Standards Review Organizations.

Across a hospital system, there is an opportunity to consolidate strong services and phase out weak services. There is the advantage of higher use of specialized facilities, such as open-heart surgery suites, that should help keep the surgical-technician-nurse team effective through the frequent use of their special skills. Systems also create an ongoing peer review situation, both in hospital administration and medical practice, so that managers and doctors have to justify the appropriateness of their decisions.

Duplication of services and programs is costly, both in terms of economy and quality. It seems rational to argue that duplication can lead to low use and thereby low performance which can affect quality. Systems managers, operating as a central corps of experts, should be able to centralize highly specialized services and demand quality.

The Capital Area Health Consortium, for example, is deeply involved in a sorting out of roles among hospitals in the Greater Hartford, Connecticut, area. This internal examination is designed to ensure that the institution with the greatest capability for mounting a cost-effective and high quality program will be assigned that effort. This should reduce the potential for duplication so often associated with underutilization and the attendant low quality. A similar sifting out of roles has occurred within the Detroit Medical Center, the Greenville Hospital System, the Memorial Hospital System in Houston, and others.

At the same time, these hospital systems are ensuring that physicians practicing within their systems will have direct access for their clients to these quality services. Such systems more readily promote the admission of patients directly to those institutions having the specialized programs. In addition, personnel practicing and working within specialized programs and departments of hospitals are more likely to have developed the skills needed for their jobs and to maintain those skills through frequent use. While the obvious example is an open-heart surgery team there are other examples as well: critical care nurses, radiological technicians, medical technologists, physical therapists and admitting clerks.

All of the systems are promoting continuing education and are supplying a wide range of educational programs to ensure that physicians and other health personnel utilize effectively the most up-to-date knowledge available. Many of the systems are directly connected or strongly affiliated with educational institutions which supply these educational services. If this new knowledge is put into practice, it should contribute to an improvement in quality of patient care.

Several systems are being developed with close ties to manpower production centers. These include the Capital Area Health Consortium in Connecticut, the Wilmington Medical Center in Delaware, the Detroit Medical Center Corporation, the Rush University System for Health in Illinois, and the Adventist Health Services in Glendale, California. Still other systems, such as those in Charlotte, North Carolina and Greenville, South Carolina, have close ties to educational centers through Area Health Education Center programs. In those cases where systems are not closely tied to the education of doctors, such as Appalachian Regional Hospitals, this factor often holds back the development of new services.

ACCESSIBILITY

Systems of hospitals under single management can improve access to medical and health care in several ways: (1) by ensuring that existing, needed facilities do not abandon the service area, (2) by retaining physicians where they are needed, (3) by experimenting with new forms of care, and (4) by offering the possibilities of integrating all levels of service together so that patients receive care on a graduated and planned scale of need.

Many of the reasons that systems developed in the first place are directly related to problems of access to care. Religious orders, such as the Catholic-sponsored hospitals, and the Lutherans are prime examples of organizations that are providing care where it is needed, particularly in rural areas. In response to population growth and population shifts to the suburbs and new town areas, hospital systems have developed satellites, branch hospitals and outpatient facilities. The contract management of hospitals by systems is a direct response to a community's inability to keep services accessible without help from a stronger management group. Several systems have developed ambulatory care programs and outreach efforts to develop easier access to general care services and to meet specific problems, such as chemical dependency, mental illness, problems of the aging and home-bound patients.

In Detroit, the Henry Ford Hospital has made a conscious effort to establish low-cost, high-need services in low income and ghetto areas. The Abbott-Northwestern Hospital has done much the same in Minneapolis and provides services for one of the nation's outstanding programs for the aged—the Minneapolis Age and Opportunity Center.

Other systems have abandoned the inner city, such as the Evangelical Hospital Association which first opened for business in a rough neighborhood on Chicago's South Side but followed its doctors and patients to the affluent suburbs west and north of Chicago in 1972. The Memorial Hospital System is leaving Houston's inner city. And the Wilmington Medical Center is moving its base hospital to the suburbs.

The ability of systems to secure capital has made it possible for them to generate programs in geographical areas that would have had difficulty obtaining such services without the systems-wide approach. Some specific examples include the Rush network's health maintenance organization called ANCHOR, the Lutheran Hospital Society of California's prepaid health plan for its employees and the various outreach facilities and programs established in rural areas by Appalachian Regional Hospitals and the Presbyterian Hospital Center in Albuquerque, New Mexico.

Some of the hospital systems have met the rural health care problem head on. The Lutheran Hospitals and Homes Society of America was born in rural American hard times and continues to provide the margin of efficiency necessary to keep small and isolated community institutions in operation. While long-term subsidy is not possible, short-term assistance probably makes the difference between staying open and failing. For the people in the areas served, this difference is critical. Great Plains Lutheran Hospitals has a similar story to tell. Primary, secondary and long-term care are accessible to people in the communities served by these systems.

In the Carolinas, a not-for-profit shared service organization, Carolinas Hospital and Health Services, is managing five rural hospitals. A circuit riding, highly experienced rural hospital administrator provides backup to on-site administrators. Such help was absolutely essential for the rural hospitals to survive. Some of these rural and very small (twenty-five to fifty beds) institutions may eventually become ambulatory care sites with long-term beds as well. Whatever they become, it is essential for these hospitals to have the kind of talent for planning and transition which is rarely if ever available in communities where health systems are failing. Rural areas face continuing health care crises. Some areas have found that giving up some autonomy is a small price to pay for the kind of help available to them by systems integration.

Systems can help solve the problems of accessibility. This can be accomplished when smaller institutions are tied into multiple-unit systems that have greater management expertise and more sophisticated technology. The movement of patients to services and the movement of services to remote locations should be more easily accomplished in a system. Patients can be moved within the system as necessary and doctors can follow their patients without costly new admissions testing and processing. Those systems that have established satellite and branch hospitals, for example, appear to have made care more accessible to shifting populations. Scaling up or scaling down services to meet more precisely local needs is easier when an entire organization isn't dependent on one operating site.

By creating capital and economies of scale, systems are in a better position to experiment with new health care delivery forms, such as neighborhood health centers, health maintenance organizations, mobile clinics, first aid stations, links with elderly housing and cooperative plans with other institutions.

Systems provide opportunities to bring all types of institutions together into an integrated and coordinated system of care. Competition for available resources, such as health professionals and paraprofessionals and other support personnel, does not just occur between community hospitals located in overlapping service areas. It spreads to special purpose institutions in the areas too—whether it be a Veterans Administration hospital, a state mental hospital, a county general hospital, a prison hospital, a Public Health Service hospital, a military hospital, a long-term care unit, a nursing home or a home health agency.

Hospital systems can help eliminate duplication between community hospitals. They also offer governmental agencies new options, if they want a system to manage a county general hospital, for example, or a prison hospital on a contract basis. Again, the system can draw on its experts in management and the clinical sciences. Systems and the new Health Systems Agencies have the potential to bring together all types of health care delivery units, perhaps even orienting the Veterans Administration and military hospitals toward their communities. And perhaps even opening up state mental hospitals to public scrutiny.

Systems can help attract, retain and more effectively use physicians. Integrated care units offer doctors financial stability, a wide range of services and equipment and valuable colleague relationships not always found in solo, small institutions. Systems provide physicians with educational opportunities and educational resources. They create something of a buffer zone between the physician, Blue Cross and Blue Shield plans, and governmental agencies and entities such as PSROs and Health Systems Agencies. By bringing a number of facilities together in a system, there is an opportunity to bring doctors together too. A central management that can prove its effectiveness should be able to create respect within the medical staffs of the various facilities. The Lutheran Hospital Society of California is willing to work with doctors under a variety of arrangements—group practice, solo, fee-for-service and contract arrangements.

The system should also be able to create respect within the communities it serves. If a system has a monopoly in an area, there is no guarantee that that monopoly will be efficient just as there is no guarantee that a utility will be efficient. But as the system becomes more visible, consumers can relate to one large organization instead of several smaller ones. All hospitals will have to depend on public philanthropy and tax-exempt bonds for capital in the future. Once consumers realize this, hospitals will have to become more accountable if they want to survive. And accountability may be forced on hospitals through state public disclosure laws.

Hospitals traditionally have drawn support and guidance from local leadership. Public hospital authority systems depend heavily on consumer support in order to get bond issues passed for capital expansion. Most nongovernmental multiple-unit systems are operating with links to the local power structure and are increasingly dependent on local support for capital.

Public-based systems, such as those in Charlotte, North Carolina, Greenville, South Carolina, Fort Lauderdale, Florida, and Wayne, Michigan, have to be responsive to community demands. Without community support for bond issues, these systems have no means of capital expansion. In other cases, such as Appalachian Regional Hospitals and the Memorial Hospital System, managers have had to assume a new community focus in order to keep the system alive. The ARH had been dominated by coal interests and coal unions; now they are trying to assume an overall community focus. The MHS in Texas was once closely tied to the Baptist Church. Intermountain Health Care was once controlled by the Mormon Church. The church organizations didn't fight a severing of ties to the systems hospitals because medical care facilities were draining away scarce economic resources. These resources must now be generated in communities.

In terms of understanding the cost of care and quality of care, systems offer consumers certain advantages. Managers should be in a position to account for local accomplishments and give economic perspective to consumers by providing comparable data in understandable form. Systems provide a larger liability target than single hospitals, but a more centralized organization should be able to ensure more quality of care procedures and continuous peer review.

POWER

What are the problems facing hospitals? There are massive government programs that bring with them new laws and regulations. There are efforts on the part of the purchasers of services, including government as the largest buyer, to reduce the cost of care. Major advances in medical technology are leading to demands for higher priced equipment that requires more highly educated support and backup personnel. Higher standards are being demanded of institutions through laws such as the Occupational Safety and Health Act. These are capital demands, and coupled with workers' demands for higher pay, they have created high capital requirements at the same time federal grant programs have either dwindled or disappeared and reimbursement formulas have not matched costs. How are hospitals to cope with these forces? Do hospital systems make a difference?

All of the previous arguments for systems come down to the accumulation of power as the central advantage. The administrator increases his visibility and his relative power, compared to the governing board and the medical staff, for example, because he is the spokesman and top manager for an organization that inherently has more power. There are more beds, more physicians, more employees and more dollars to manage and spend. The larger numbers create clout, to use the political Chicago term, for dealing with other power structures operating within the hospital's internal and external environments.

In a historical case study of a single hospital, Charles Perrow identified three major periods in the history of a community hospital that reflected the more critical problems facing the institution. In the early stage, trustees were the controlling influence because of the need to acquire capital and gain community acceptance. In the second stage, physicians dominated the hospital because of the increasing complexity of medical practice and the importance of their professional skills. In the final stage, the administrator gained the most influence because of an increasingly complex environment that required the manager to coordinate and interact with outside agencies. This was the power distribution over time in a single hospital and before the days of Medicare, Medicaid, comprehensive health planning and regional medical programs. The single hospital did not face the complexities added through operating multiple units at multiple sites.[10]

Many of these same power forces were examined in a historical case study of the Greenville Hospital System in South Carolina and its relationship to a planning and development agency. Like the study by Perrow, the power trends were occurring long before the major events of the mid-and late-1960s began to unfold, the new medical care public policy initiatives exerted by the Congress and the administrations of Presidents Lyndon B. Johnson, John F. Kennedy, and Richard M. Nixon. As these initiatives unfolded, the power of the administrators within the hospital system began to grow.

A major source of this power flowed to the chief executive officer because he had to take on the new role of securing capital from outside sources. He had to operate an efficient hospital in order to generate operating revenue. Physicians benefitted from an institution in the black and an institution that had the money to buy new equipment. In the process, doctors accepted a greater rationality in the allocation of resources and power within the hospital system.

As more powerful external forces were brought to bear on the institution, the administrators had to focus their attention on the decision processes within those agencies. What those agencies said or did not say was becoming critical to the question of which hospital systems programs would receive capital financing.

In the Greenville study, as the new planning agency developed its expertise, other related health and welfare agencies were involved in the planning process. The administrators found additional opportunities to broaden the interest of their hospital system into such areas as primary care, preventive care programs with the health department and other health-enhancing efforts. As the system's spokesmen, the administrators gained new power.

As the external agencies became more visible, more physicians became involved as well to protect and enhance their interests. The pulling and tugging of balancing forces created something of a tug-of-war in the short run. Eventually, however, all of the participants in the power struggle seemed to have broadened their perspective. The administrators solidified their position because they demonstrated a new expertise within the organization. They were dedicated to ensuring proper care for patients in a cost-effective manner. Their position was greatly enhanced by public policy. The administrators represented the needs and aspirations of both the medical staff and the community within the decision arenas of government and planning agencies.[11]

In the long run, competing interests must be balanced. Power must be balanced between administrators, medical staffs, communitites, consumers, governments, third-party agencies, Blue Cross and Blue Shield plans, insurance companies, labor unions, industries, trade associations and others.

Hospital systems represent a major step toward effective economies, ensuring quality of care, providing access to medical and health care and striking a balance of power between competing groups and forces. There is no magic in systems. Hospital systems are not a total answer. Greater pressures for public accountability and the regionalization and integration of health care systems must still be grounded in public forums, such as the Health Systems Agencies, and in professional and public bodies.

The struggle for power and the debate will be concentrated, one hopes, at the community level where the problems of medical and health care must be solved. The issues of overriding importance to the medical and health care systems include answers to these questions: Even as we use scarce economic and human resources for medical and health care, is the quality of life enhanced: Is mortality reduced? Is life lengthened? Even if the answers to these questions are "yes," is the expense of 8.3 percent of the GNP justified? Or, should more money be spent on better education, better housing, income maintenance and nutritious food?

Autonomous hospitals and hospital systems must now sift out beds, services and programs, and relate them to need, demand and economy. If providers do not perform these tasks voluntarily, this will be accomplished eventually by others. Hospitals also face a second task and an opportunity. They may have to close some beds and services, but they can become community centers of preventive medicine, health education, and health maintenance for their service areas.

Anne R. Somers, associate professor in the department of community medicine, College of Medicine and Dentistry of New Jersey, Rutgers Medical School, has proposed that hospitals coordinate all the health services in their communities. She said, "The one institution capable of assimilating and directing the new medical technology is the hospital."[12] Perhaps it is the time to say, paraphrasing her article's headline, "Only the hospital system can do it all—now."

NOTES

1. S.J. Tibbitts, "Multiple Hospital Systems," *Hospital Administration* (Spring 1973), pp. 10-20.

2. C.W. Weinberger, "A View of the Federal Government" an address before the Commonwealth Club of San Francisco, San Francisco, California, July 21, 1975.

3. S.J. Tibbitts, op. cit., note 1.

4. S.A. Edwards and A.A. Astolfi, "Merger: Cause and Effect," *Hospital Administration* (Summer 1973), pp. 24-33.

5. J.P. Cooney, Jr. and T.L. Alexander, *Multi-Hospital Systems,* four volumes, Health Services Research Center of the Hospital Research and Education Trust and Northwestern University, 1975.

6. B.R. Tresnowski, "National Health Planning and Resources Development Act of 1974, Its Meaning and Implications," a speech before the American Society of Internal Medicine, Portland, Oregon, October 3, 1975.

7. H.L. Lewis, "Hot Words Over Empty Beds," *Modern Healthcare* (April 1975), pp. 51-54.

8. B.R. Tresnowski, op. cit., note 6.

9. M. Brown, "Contract Management: Latest Development in The Trend Toward Regionalization of Hospital and Health Services," *Hospital & Health Services Administration* (Winter 1976), pp. 52-53.

10.   M. Brown, "The Impact of Changing Inter-Organizational Relations on the Policy Structure of a Hospital: An Historical Case Study of a Health Planning Organization in the Hospital System," a dissertation for the Dr. P. H. degree granted by the University of North Carolina, 1972.

11. Ibid.

12. A.R. Somers, "Only the Hospital Can Do it All-Now," *Modern Hospital* (July 1972), pp. 95-100.

Chapter 15
Outlook

If present trends continue, what will hospitals systems of the future look like? What does the future hold for administrators and managers, small autonomous hospitals and large tertiary care centers, such as medical school-teaching hospital complexes? What are the implications for local, state and national hospital associations? What are the general national implications of hospital systems for third-party agencies and government regulatory agencies?

National, multistate and regional hospitals systems will continue to emerge across the United States. The Kaiser Foundation Medical Care Program, the Lutheran Hospitals and Homes Society of America and many of the Catholic-sponsored systems are already multistate in nature. Their service programs and economic power are already spread through more than one census region.

LHHSA is a primary candidate that could develop as a nationwide hospital and nursing home system for rural areas because of its solid reputation and rural experience. It may truly become "of America" as its corporate name implies. In early 1976, the Society had management control over ninety institutions. At the same time, the Society's managers had nine acquisitions under active consideration. The requests for help had been sifted out from over eighty formal invitations to come into communities in several states.[1]

The survival and growth outlook for LHHSA is excellent. Harry Malm's philosophy of self-help in each of the communities, but with central banking and cash management in Fargo, North Dakota, could be applied to any size system. This system might buy its own bank for the convenience of money operations. This system will grow thoughout the United States, perhaps into the Appalachian states because of the tremendous rural health care need in those areas. A group in Silver Spring, Maryland, wants the Society to build a nursing home. Such an expansion could attract the attention of troubled hospitals in the area and present other opportunities for growth.

There are also opportunities for the Society to grow within its current areas of service interest, because of the search for and development of new sources of energy and the increasing emphasis being placed on the importance of farm and dairy products to the nation's survival and growth. These factors have underlined the importance of meeting the social needs of rural America. Malm and the Society have a tremendous amount of political clout that could be exercised within the Rural Caucus of the Congress. In 1975 the Society's annual meeting brought about 600 people together at Hayward, Wisconsin. One can imagine the LHHSA meeting some day in Washington, D.C., and delegates from more than 100 hospitals arriving by train from the west, and being met on the platform by 28 senators and over 100 representatives who had come to greet their constituents.

There also seems to be a possibility that LHHSA will link up with other multiple hospital systems. Some of the merger candidates would seem to be: the Good Samaritan nursing home system in Sioux Falls, South Dakota, the Great Plains Lutheran Hospitals, Inc., Phillipsburg, Kansas, and the Lutheran Hospital Society of Southern California. The three major Lutheran systems could join together into a formal alliance, perhaps even a consolidation, and create a vast network of hospitals and nursing homes stretching from the West Coast through the Great Plains, and expanding eastward.

The outlook for Great Plains Lutheran Hospital appears bright. Federal programs continue to push the need for strong, rural health care systems of the Great Plains-type. Wheat has become almost as precious as gold or crude oil. The United States will be forced to maintain critically-needed institutions in rural areas, such as hospitals, if it wants to continue to depend on a productive agricultural system to help maintain the international balance of payments and feed a hungry world. The Phillipsburg region would appear to be a prime location for an Area Health Education Center run by a university school of medicine. Such a center could help provide critically-needed manpower in the area. It also might form the basis for an expanded hospital system.

The Lutheran Hospital Society in southern California is a strong system that is developing its financial base. LHS's management services group provides a strong underpinning for a corporate capability that could parallel and compete with Hospital Corporation of America, Hospital Affiliates, and other national systems, perhaps even Kaiser. This financial capability is further strengthened by Sam Tibbitt's willingness to work with physicians on most any practice basis. Tibbitts' personal leadership and political skill has attracted widespread attention among administrators, who frequently refer to him as the logical chairman of the board of the American Hospital Association. Should this occur, the industry's major trade association would undoubtedly turn more toward a posture of supporting hospital systems.

Truly nationally integrated Catholic-sponsored hospital systems would seem to be a natural evolution too. The Catholic orders must either move soon to gain the advantages of systems or find their influence on the wane. They will lose out to regional systems, such as the Lutherans and for-profit chains, if they remain restricted by the local nature of their boards. The Sisters of Mercy of the Union (R.S.M.), and the Daughters of Charity of St. Vincent DePaul (D.C.) are primary candidates as national Catholic systems.

These two organizations each have assets approaching $1 billion, as large as many successful business corporations. They may move to integrate their hospitals into systems when it becomes clear that a new strategy is necessary to survive, to keep local units from folding, and that such an organization can be put together without either sacrificing the autonomy of the local administrator or diffusing the principles of the Religious.

The future of the Catholic-sponsored systems will depend on the interaction of two sets of forces: those forces working inside the Church structure of generalates, provinces and individual hospitals, and those forces working outside the church.

Within the church, the idea of systems configurations would seem to require a great deal of selling and persuasion; efforts to that end have begun in earnest, but there is a long way to go.

Health Systems Agencies are working outside the Catholic church. They have the job of sifting out all of the resources in a defined geographical area in order to come up with an integrated system of care. This could mean that pressure will be put on some Catholic hospitals to either go out of business, expand their services, or merge with another institution. The issue here may come down to a Constitutional one—separation of church and state —particularly if Catholic hospitals strengthen their apostolic orientation based on canon law.

Just how far the separation arguments will go may depend on the ability of individual hospitals to reorganize into strong systems configurations whereby religious managers trained in hospital and health care administration interpret and make policy in accordance with directives that come from generalates and the Catholic Church in the United States. The constitutional issue may also be drawn on such issues as abortion, sterilization, extraordinary extension of life, genetic engineering and control, and other moral, legal and ethical issues—particularly when Catholic hospitals and their physicians approach the issues from a different standpoint than other hospitals.

The argument that Catholic hospitals deliver more humanistic medical care needs to be proven and demonstrated. If this argument can be sustained, it could provide Catholic hospitals with a distinction that would set them apart from many other hospitals. This humanistic characteristic is not necessarily something that could be "marketed" with Health Systems

Agencies, governmental regulatory agencies and third-party payment plans. But it is a characteristic that might be sold to consumer groups and patients who are the constituents of those who make the laws and regulations.

The uniqueness of Catholic hospitals, particularly those of a few decades ago, was that patients were admitted to an institution that was also a home for Religious. There are still Catholic hospitals where nonmedical people, young and old alike, live in the hospital. There's a Catholic hospital in Minnesota, for example, that is also the home of a freelance artist. The "home" atmosphere of Catholic hospitals of the future could integrate sick and well people of all ages into a community of understanding and compassion, an opportunity open to any hospital. Catholic hospitals also have another opportunity. They could create groups of semi-Religious of both sexes by offering a new type of dedication and formal allegiance to the church and its medical care and health care principles, without requiring the total vows traditionally required of the Religious.

As systems grow larger through mergers, consolidations and the linking together of hospitals with common philosophical and geographical interests, what are the implications for nonsystem hospitals?

The path ahead for small hospitals is clear. Whether they are in urban, suburban or rural areas, small hospitals will have to become parts of systems if they want to survive. They need access to top management. Population shifts, a change in a road and highway system, the loss of a doctor or two, a bad year with reimbursement formulas and a competing hospital down the street or in the next town—all of these forces can place the small hospital in an untenable position. Small hospitals need access to the top management available within a system.

Any large hospital of 400 or more beds is a potential site for the nucleus of a hospital system. And the development of large regional and multistate systems has particular implications for medical school teaching hospitals and the VA system.

As not-for-profit hospital systems without close ties to VA, public and university hospitals grow in size and influence, they will begin to compete head on with medical schools. They will be able to sell the concept of systems-wide integration of services and it won't be long until policymakers will ask: Should the medical schools abandon their go-it-alone, we-want-one-of-everything approach? Private, competent hospitals within systems will begin to skim the cream of referrals and take more paying patients away from medical school hospitals. Even if medical schools strike close alliances with public and VA hospitals, they may take on the image of hospitals for the indigent. As the Congress goes along its piecemeal route toward national health insurance, new groups of Americans will be picked up for coverage.

They will then have a choice of where they seek care—perhaps near home, and perhaps in a systems hospital.

Medical schools have alternative strategies, however. First, they should link into a system, preferably one with urban, suburban and rural components. This would link the university teaching commitment to a variety of roles and problems and should enhance its public image and support. Some newer medical schools have no teaching hospital at all or at least a small one. With long delays in getting new capital, they find it easier to make direct links with community hospitals from the beginning. Systems offer this continuing opportunity and could be the sites of the new medical schools—perhaps in Central Appalachia and the Dakotas.

There are still other strategies for medical schools. Where they have flexibility to operate within an academic environment, often controlled by politically-appointed regents, medical schools might take on a new role. They could build a system through purchase, lease and contract arrangements. This is the Rush University System for Health approach and it seems to be working. Medical schools might also consider the same approach to mental health—stringing together a group of state -owned mental hospitals with clinics located at systems hospitals. This also could be done through contract, lease and purchase arrangements. It would be the ultimate in an outreach effort.

In order to survive, medical schools will have to take a cue from the not-for-profit hospital systems. Many systems managers frankly admit that the reason they are helping small hospitals in rural and urban areas is to ensure the survival of their base hospital. They need referral patients in order to survive. And so do medical school teaching hospitals.

The kind of specialization once reserved almost exclusively for the medical school hospital can now be developed in a variety of systems. Systems are going out and doing the tough work of building rural resources, often saving failing hospitals. In the long-term, these systems are developing control over future cities. And they will get the attention of state and federal legislators whose constituents are served by the systems hospitals. Eventually, they will compete with medical schools for leadership in a specialty of rural medical practice.

Medical schools which have paid little attention to serving the needs of suburban and rural areas, for example, helping them to recruit doctors and furnishing continuing education programs, can hardly expect more than token assistance in the future, and possibly hostility, if they are competing with a system hospital that has helped out in time of need. And in urban areas, if the medical schools inherit the VA and public hospitals, they will end up with high-rise facilities in densely developed areas that are not accessible to patients.

What medical schools have to do is be willing to surrender some of their autonomy and to reach out to existing systems or form their own systems. Will this happen? A nationally known hospital executive commented: "The deans just aren't ready to face up to the fact of systems development. It's too threatening."[2] Some deans have, however, and medical schools have before them a new opportunity.

Major medical schools and teaching systems, alone or in combination with neighbors in adjoining regions and states, will soon realize that they must either build a hospital-education system or lose their freedom to preserve their primary mission. Medical schools already possess an adequate power base—programs in education, research and service. They also have political power and prestige. What they need now is a new community focus. This new focus is already developing in some regions through the eleven Area Health Education Centers programs and the efforts of several schools to decentralize medical education to off-campus branches and divisions. The University of Illinois medical school has four branches located in four cities, for example, and West Virginia University has one geographically dispersed division and is developing two others.

AHECs represent a major opportunity to tie the medical research and development, health manpower production and continuing education capabilities of universities to emerging hospital systems. Other related approaches to linking educational capabilities to hospital systems include the Rush University System for Health in Chicago, the University Health Center of Pittsburgh, and the University of Washington Hospitals in Seattle.

VA SYSTEMS

The VA System is highly dispersed throughout the United States but about 95 percent of its facilities are affiliated with medical schools. The linking of medical schools with public and VA hospitals is a natural way for the large teaching centers to build a system, increase utilization and cut down on duplication of services and programs. It is also a way for universities and hospitals to relate more specifically to geographical areas. The VA System is not growing at the inpatient bed rate that it experienced in past years, but it is adding new outpatient facilities. The potential links between public hospitals, VA hospitals and university hospitals is a natural one: the training of medical students and the need for teaching patients.

The VA is trying to make more formal links with medical schools and is even developing its own schools. The VA Department of Medicine and Surgery provides the bulk of its services to veterans in its own referral hospitals. The department could make a major contribution to the strengthening of health services in smaller, more rural areas by buying services locally near the veteran's home. This approach would have the twin advantages of providing a stronger revenue base for local services and avoiding the necessity of separating the veteran from his home and family. This would also save the VA (and the nation's taxpayers) money required to transport the veteran to distant medical complexes. It would allow the VA to make a more judicious use of its own beds, perhaps even closing some beds. This service approach would also help local hospitals develop their capabilities in early diagnostic work and follow-up care after the veteran returns to his home from the specialized treatment centers. In early 1976, these kinds of questions were being examined in a major study by the National Academy of Sciences, which is designed to ask an appropriate question: Where does the VA System fit into the overall U.S. health care delivery system?[3]

CITY HOSPITAL SYSTEMS

Just such questions are being asked in the Chicago metropolitan area. The Northwestern University-McGaw Medical Center, for example, is geographically isolated in a crowded area of Chicago near Lake Michigan. A change in referral patterns would seriously affect this great center. In order to obtain patients, the center will have to innovate.

One of the tallest buildings in the world, the 100-story John Hancock Center that includes several floors of condominiums, is located a few blocks from Northwestern-McGaw. A few years ago, Northwestern University students did a marketing study of permanent residents of the skyscraper to find out where they obtained medical care. The idea was that the medical center might organize a primary group practice located in the building. Northwestern-McGaw did not organize the practice.

What would happen to referral patterns if the Rush-Presbyterian-St. Luke's Medical Center decided that a group practice at John Hancock Center was a good idea? This idea is not new; a hospital in Canada runs a clinic in a shopping center area with a daytime population of about 40,000 persons.

Clinics need not even have doctors on the premises. They could be linked to the hospital by closed circuit television. Such a telemedicine system was established by Massachusetts General Hospital several years ago—tying MGH to a first aid station at Boston's Logan Airport that serves travelers who are between flights. MGH also does consultations with a VA hospital in the Boston area via a telemedicine hookup.

The Rush University System for Health in Chicago recognized the necessity to link up with a network of community hospitals in the early 1970s and is a prototype for others to consider. It seems likely that Rush will extend its efforts in contract management to more hospitals in the metropolitan Chicago area. These moves may pre-empt some markets long taken for granted by other hospitals. Logical places for Rush to expand include the Gold Coast area of north Chicago and high-rise building sites where clinics could be established. A program marketing preventive medicine, diet plans and treatment for alcoholism would seem a natural in these areas of affluence and sometimes negative life styles. To take care of its share of poor in Chicago, Rush will also have to secure a share of the most affluent, paying market.

Chicago systems are in a stage of transition. In response to such moves by Rush, it would seem logical for other medical complexes and autonomous hospitals to tie in more closely with their medical staffs and patient markets. This is what is happening in other cities and metropolitan areas. It only takes one move by a strong, fully integrated service institution to force others to consider a strategy to protect its own position in the market.

There are other possibilities of change in the Chicago area. Catholic-sponsored hospitals might form consortia that cut across the lines of sponsoring religious orders. Northwestern-McGaw Medical Center, specifically Northwestern Memorial Hospital, will very likely look for ways to make strong ties to suburban markets. The University of Chicago owns its own hospitals but may find itself isolated and competing for referrals. One of the center's major teaching affiliates, the Michael Reese Hospital and Medical Center, has wanted a medical school of its own. Eventually this institution may become a de facto extension of the university. If that is not palatable, Michael Reese could negotiate a strong teaching role with either the Rush System or Northwestern-McGaw.

A primary expansion target for several medical schools in the Chicago area is the Christ Hospital of the Evangelical Hospital Association. This hospital is now affiliated with Rush. As a system within a system, the outlook for EHA is good because of the location of its hospitals in growing suburban areas near primary care doctors and paying patients. The association's nursing school helps provide the personnel needed to deliver care. EHA is strong as a stand-alone system. An Evangelical-Rush system might be even more powerful. Will the two ever get together through a merger or consolidation arrangement? "I don't think so," Paul Umbeck said. "We might start doing some things together, such as contract management. They would like to be able to absorb us or take us over. They are short on primary care; they needed those branch hospitals."[4]

In other areas of the United States, there are other systems integration possibilities.

In Utah, Intermountain Health Care could form a system with a manpower production center by joining forces with its strong competitor, the University of Utah. In the Los Angeles area, the Lutheran Hospital Society and Adventist Health Services are geographically near each other and are planning some joint ventures with other systems in the West. An LHS-Adventist System also would give all the hospitals access to the medical school at Loma Linda, California. Other western linkups might see these two organizations joining forces with Samaritan Health Services, Intermountain, and the Presbyterian Hospital Center in Albuquerque that may merge with a Catholic hospital, St. Joseph.

The nationwide Adventist goal of having all of its hospitals as members of systems is an idea that will likely catch on with other religious-sponsored systems. The Adventists strongly advocate keeping religious and moral values as fully a part of the health care mission. There seems to be an important point to be made—religious systems have a strong base of common understanding and mission. These facts should make it easier for church organizations to link their hospitals to others with a common understanding. This is the very reason that Catholic Systems, or Ecumenical Systems could develop.

How will the hospital systems in the Minneapolis-St. Paul area shake out in the years to come? They are characterized by competitiveness and oriented toward growth, expansion and survival.

The University of Minnesota Hospitals and Health Science Center is not a system in itself. But it is a powerful referral center for the Twin Cities and Upper Midwest with a strong voice in medical education. Carl N. Platou, president of Fairview Community Hospitals, said in late November 1975, that "the three other systems are out competing too." What about the University of Minnesota? "They are not a system, but they are a little concerned about what we [Fairview] are doing. We are seen as an intrusion into their backyard."[5] There is competition of another sort, he said, for the ear of state legislators. As private systems reach out to community and rural hospitals, the legislators might want the university to do the same thing.

Abbott-Northwestern Hospital Corporation (and the Minneapolis Medical Center, Inc.) are committed to building a strong medical center in downtown Minneapolis. But this system also wants to grow and its managers see the Services To Other Institutions program as the mechanism for growth. The management contracting arm of STOI has had problems in the early stages, but this concept would still seem to be a good one offering potential for growth.

United Hospitals of St. Paul has all of the opportunities for growth that are available to any system. It appears ready to challenge Fairview and Health Central in the same areas of Minnesota.

Will Fairview Community Hospitals and Health Central merge? Without considering any of the affiliations they have with other hospitals for shared services, a combined system would be impressive. They would have more doctors, more support personnel and more economic and political clout in Minnesota than any competition.

At a time when everyone is saying, "Cut down on beds and contain costs," Platou and Van Hauer could find growth and challenge in building a super-system. Will they do it? They have been engaged in merger talk for more than three years. There are some retarding influences in this talk, particularly as it stretches over a period of years.

The unpaid trustees of each system may tire of the effort and attention required. Some give and take would be required of both organizations, particularly in how a merger would leave the power structures of the two organizations. Trustees seem to treat the organizations as their own turf when really it is a public trust. They should focus on a future, merged system that could benefit the public and the entire Upper Midwest. In spite of the greater promise of a merged system, the focus of discussion in 1975 remained on such questions as: Whose debt is larger? What might future expenditures be? Both systems can survive and prosper alone. Together they could become a truly great system of benefit to the entire Upper Midwest.

Both Platou and Van Hauer seem to want the merger to occur. Yet, neither manager has been quite able to get his board to take the leap into the future. And perhaps this is because neither manager has been quite able to admit that a future, more powerful board might really be in charge, and not the present two boards.

"The concept of a full-blown merger is going to take longer than we had conceived," Van Hauer said in December 1975. "We are going to proceed on an incremental basis, phasing in services." Eventually, he predicted, Health Central and Fairview would reach the point where they could consider longer steps, "with a minimum of wear and tear. There are too many distractions on each side. It is not logical yet to push on. We will operate under a shell that will serve as a useful front to continue on our cojoint activities." Initially this will be a shared services organization, Van Hauer said, although the two organizations hadn't been able to decide on a name. "We will off-load the whole field of activity in shared services—that's the purpose of it."[6]

And Platou commented at the time: "I don't think the consolidation is going to take place—not this year."[8] But he confirmed what Van Hauer said. "We are going to take the affiliate and managed facilities and form a management corporation to handle them and bring others in. This doesn't touch our boards. It is a vehicle to bring us together. The question now is—who is going to run it? This generates a spirit. The philosophy of it is more exciting than the organization form."[7]

There are other indications that before the hospital systems in this area shake down there will be more active participants in the game. There seems little doubt that both the Catholic hospitals in the area and the University of Minnesota will take positive steps to secure the advantages of hospital systems to perpetuate their own philosophies and institutional objectives.

One large system for the Detroit area seems a possibility. The Detroit Medical Center, Henry Ford Hospital and Peoples Community Hospital Authority would tie together all types of care and a variety of sites to a medical school, Wayne State.

There is little doubt that the Henry Ford Hospital is oriented to growth in the metropolitan area and elsewhere. Each of the satellite ambulatory care facilities will very likely become parts of satellite hospital complexes. At the West Bloomfield Clinic, for example, the hospital has said it will build a satellite when it is needed; the state certificate of need agency has said it will not approve a project until 1980 or after. Ford Hospital must go in this direction if for no other reason than to preserve the financial integrity of its base specialty center and its tremendous capital investment in downtown Detroit.

There is competition and some differences between hospitals in the Peoples Community service areas, Dr. Karl Klicka said. The proprietary chains "have economies of scale, very good control, and limited services. They only do the things they can show a profit on. We only need about a two percent return on investment; they need six or seven percent. They pay taxes and we don't. These are two ways we can beat them."[8]

As Jacques Cousin of the Detroit Medical Center suggested, the city is in ferment. It is rapidly becoming an area dominated by hospital systems in various states of development. Local systems are developing side-by-side, reaching out and forming a multiplicity of alliances including ties to Catholic-sponsored systems that have a regional and national base. The near-term future seems likely to be characterized by aggressive system-building efforts and competition among systems. The Henry Ford Hospital system is expanding to the west and north. Peoples Community Hospital Authority is expanding to the south and southwest. And the Detroit Medical Center is striving to become the major medical center and educational complex for the region. In the long-term, more alliances and consolidations seem likely.

In the Carolinas, a large geographically dispersed system could develop by joining the Charlotte and Greenville systems with Carolinas Health and Hospitals Services and other organizations, perhaps one of the four medical schools located in the Carolinas.

The local and immediate growth of the Charlotte-Mecklenburg system will depend on the ability to sell the plan to the county government and the community. Two local hospitals (Mercy and Presbyterian) approve of the plan, Zack Thomas said, and so does the eight-county Health Systems Agency set up under Public Law 93-641. The initial phase of development may cost over $30 million, according to first estimates by Thomas.[9] Growth also could occur in other ways. If the CMHA charter were revised, there would be an opportunity to extend the system's reach into surrounding counties through lease and contract arrangements with needy hospitals and communities without health care facilities.

CHHS represents an extension of shared service concepts into total hospital management. Developments in the future could conceivably include CHHS working with medical schools and medical societies to recruit physicians and other health professionals for rural areas. There also might be joint ventures developed with other hospital systems or medical centers that have the capability for supplying a wider range of professional and clinical suport services for the managed hospitals. CHHS needs working relationships with one or more institutions that have expertise in every area of hospital operations. Although CHHS needs closer clinical ties with other organizations, it is not blocked from expansion by political boundaries.

The growth outlook for some systems is not bullish, but could change. Peoples Community, Charlotte-Mecklenburg, North Broward and Greenville Hospital System are tied down by geographical limits imposed by law. They can expand to meet population needs; but once population groups cross county lines, their mandate becomes confused. State laws can be changed, however. These public systems may do quite a lot to advance the concept of regional government and regional service areas. Each of the authority-type hospital systems is located in a growing population area where existing hospitals could be tied into their system.

Some of the central differences between for-profit and not-for-profit systems have been highlighted in previous chapters.

In Central Appalachia, for example, the not-for-profit Appalachian Regional Hospitals is working toward a comprehensive system of care to meet overwhelming needs in a poor area of the nation. In the process, ARH has been walking on the edge of a knife, not knowing when reimbursement formulas will cause it to retrench in its efforts to provide for people in desperate need of basic medical and health care.

The for-profit systems, such as HCA and Hospital Affiliates, have concentrated on high-volume, high-payoff services in relatively affluent, middle-sized towns. Meanwhile, the for-profits have stayed away from the tremendous financial drain that comes from free care, charity patients, medical education and services that have a low profit margin.

In Texas, the Memorial Hospital System based in Houston is one of the nation's best examples of a highly-developed and vertically-integrated system that provides a full range of comprehensive services. It is geographically dispersed—a response to population shifts, population growth and the development of highways in the metropolitan area. In the future, it seems quite possible that this system will continue to develop through shared services and contract management linkages made to long-term care facilities, suburban outpatient clinics, and rural community hospitals.

NATIONAL HOSPITAL SYSTEMS

The typical national, multistate, and multiregional hospital systems would be very large corporations with effective management control over billions of dollars in assets and hundreds of millions of dollars in annual revenues. Corporate headquarters would be located in large banking centers, such as New York City, Atlanta, Chicago, St. Louis and Los Angeles. But all of the organizations would have offices in the Washington, D. C. area too, because of that region's proximity to members of the Congress and government agencies.

Corporate organizations for the large national hospital systems will be structured in much the same way as any other business with only a few differences. Attorneys, accountants, financial experts and others will keep close tabs on legislation, regulations and reimbursement policies. These experts will be in daily contact with policymakers in order to give shape and form to government programs and policies. Corporate officers will be salaried.

Local and regional arms of the large hospital systems will operate a variety of institutions in their service areas. They will also own or manage under contract other services, such as visiting nurse groups, halfway houses, health education programs, industrial health programs and a variety of services for senior citizens. The ties between the units of care and service will be primarily economic in the beginning. As the systems mature, however, strong referral relationships will develop between physicians in the hospital system. Local and regional arms of the larger systems will be dominated by efficiency early in their history. Later they will take on comprehensive characteristics; medical expertise will be used at specific points of need within the system.

American Hospital Supply Corporation, a multinational company with headquarters in Evanston, Illinois, is something of an industrial model of a nationwide hospital system. Organized in 1922 by Foster G. McGaw, AHS went public in 1951 and now has employees throughout the world. The company has 47 manufacturing plants and turns out over 13,000 different products ranging from kidney dialysis equipment to syringes. AHS's more than 110,000 customers are primarily hospitals, nursing homes and laboratories. "We used to talk products," said Karl D. Bays, chairman of the board and chief executive officer. "Now we talk products and services. We used to talk hospitals. Now we talk the entire range of health care."[10]

This industrial systems model has nine organizational groups: hospital, science specialties, medical specialties, dental, pharmaceutical, dietary, capital goods, services and international. AHS's Services Group was organized in the early 1970s and by 1974 it was providing more than 1,000 hospitals a variety of specialty services. These included "computer-assisted information systems that cover everything from cost control and accounting to dietary and menu planning, contract management of such hospital departments as housekeeping and laundry, and internal hospital communication services—everything from rental TV sets to training films to nurse-call systems. And a professional planning and consulting service offers hospitals services ranging from interior design to demographic studies and regional facilities planning."[11]

The company's contract management efforts are handled by a division named Red Top, Inc. The health care delivery planning, project management and consulting is handled by a division called American Health Facilities. Speaking of all its Service Group enterprises, the company said: "These services help hospitals effect a number of operating efficiencies, which increase their ability to contain costs and also set free more professional personnel to concentrate on patient care. The market for health care support services is expected to grow at a 15 to 20 percent rate."[12]

Diversification, expansion and growth are the characteristics of such corporate giants as American Hospital Supply. The company would not have to take many new or different steps to become a nationwide hospital system. It could begin through contract management of total hospitals, and then buy hospitals near all of its U.S. manufacturing sites to use as test facilities for its products and services. These hospitals could also become the base organizations for health maintenance organizations serving AHS employees who would be covered through a self-insurance program.

PHYSICIANS, ADMINISTRATORS AND TRUSTEES

Physicians will find many advantages in hospital systems as compared to single, autonomous hospitals.

Systems managers recognize that the practice of medicine is a local affair. At the same time they are sensitive to the need for quality medical practice to avoid liability claims. These managers want to keep the institution the favored place to develop new programs. They want to avoid overinvesting in losing services.

Physicians in contract managed hospitals seem to like the attention they receive. Fairness in considering their requests, getting capital for necessary equipment, obtaining a good administrator and helping the local hospital maintain a respectable image all work in favor of physicians' interests. Physicians with contracts for pathology, radiology and other such services find systems to be a bit tougher to bargain with, but not unfair.

Systems also will work with physicians. They will build office buildings and contract with physicians to provide services in doctor-owned facilities. Systems managers also help recruit physicians and can give assurances that a viable hospital will be available. All in all, systems seem more flexible in their relationships with physicians. Administrators seem more than willing to work with physicians on any basis which they prefer. If doctors prefer group practice and prepayment or loose solo practice with access to specialists either through hospital affiliations or other means, administrators will accommodate their interest so long as it doesn't threaten the survival of the institution. Ideological commitments to one form of medical practice or another doesn't seem to be a characteristic of any known systems except Kaiser and Henry Ford Hospital. Making the hospital attractive to doctors seems to be a universal characteristic, for without a committed medical staff hospitals can fail. On the other hand, an administrator has sufficient clout to keep the medical staff from railroading the board into losing programs.

Systems can effectively develop regional patterns of organizational control without artificially forcing doctors into the corporate practice of medicine. Doctors can, if they wish, link together and find systems willing to accommodate them. They can also stay in solo practice with assurance that systems will be responsive to their needs.

Systems provide physicians access to a full range of services; a financial base that can afford a spectrum of technological devices, if they are likely to pay off; back up so they can have time off and take vacations; malpractice coverage for practice within the hospital; and a buffer zone to deal with third-party agencies and government.

Many systems have links to medical schools and this provides doctors with an opportunity for clinical appointments, continuing education and consultative backup. Systems are more likely to employ doctors in the corporate structure to deal with peer review, recruitment, and continuing education. Even in rural-based systems, the incompetent doctor is more likely to be caught up, for there are fewer places to hide.

Doctors also have the advantage of dealing with a knowledgeable group of managers. And typically, a systems board is made up of the best representatives from a number of boards. The future looks bright for a hospital administrator in a system who wants to be more than either a caretaker responding to every whim of the medical staff or a secretary to a board that has little regard for the cost implications of its actions. Public programs and expectations make such a person obsolete anyway and not tolerable to systems.

Administrators will have more power. At the same time they will find that the system has other experts and competent managers looking on their operations. There will be little room for sloppy work. Mistakes will be caught and the administrator held accountable. For the competent and strong manager, peer review can be exciting and healthy.

For those preferring plant management, a systems job will be more satisfying professionally. Fewer people will represent the system in national and regional policy forums, although each administrator will be expected to have strong ties to local groups that can be mobilized when needed.

Transfers will occur more often within systems. Some managers will move up to regional and national levels of responsibility. Chief executive officers at the national level will be recruited for the strengths in financial and political areas rather than their specific expertise in running a local hospital. On the whole this approach will represent broader opportunities since few hospital administrators could aspire to lead a billion dollar corporation under today's system of autonomous hospitals.

Given the nature of the practice of medicine, the local hospital administrator will remain a very important figure—with more power and increased accountability.

The new administrators coming out of graduate school with joint degrees in health administration and majors in more traditional business fields— accounting, finance, policy and marketing—will find ample opportunities to become both plant managers and corporate officials. Others trained in management specialties without health administration will also find their skills rewarded in systems. In the long run, however, the industry will also require individuals with a sensitivity to personal health problems, public accountability and consumer demands.

Local boards of trustees are under heavy fire. They are increasingly being asked to account for the fiscal policies and medical services of their hospitals. Planning and regulatory agencies place heavy demands on hospitals—often demanding expertise not available in the single unit hospital. In systems, such expertise is available. And the collective political clout can be marshalled in favor of a single institution. When survival is at stake, these advantages can strongly outweigh the desire a community and board have for complete autonomy.

While no one is ever willing to surrender autonomy easily, trustees are likely to be on the winning side of systems development. In the past, wealthy hospitals could expand services and enrich programs and count upon Blue Cross to reimburse their cost, often at the expense of subscribers in the area. This approach to hospital development is changing. In return for giving up some autonomy, local boards obtain expertise vital to the survival of their hospital and the economic viability of the community.

Fortunately for the local boards, systems are developing without sufficient equity capital to fully own all of the member hospitals. Equity often must come from local residents being served by the system. These facts apply even to for-profit chains which through equity and debt can acquire ownership of local facilities. By retaining local ownership of capital, a community can retain considerable power over the direction of the enterprise.

Systems cannot operate as capricious absentee landlords. They must carefully organize and cater to the needs of local people and involve them in the decision process. Even when systems own the assets of the local hospital, they need to cultivate local residents to maintain goodwill. They need to promote community understanding in order to obtain capital donations and keep the favor of physicians.

STATE AND REGIONAL ASSOCIATIONS

Local, state and regional hospital associations will very likely evolve rapidly in the future as hospital systems develop more sophisticated management and more political power.

These groups have grown up primarily for fund-raising and public relations. Their efforts have been expanded modestly in recent years to include shared services and buffer roles to help hospitals deal with governmental programs, such as Comprehensive Health Planning, Regional Medical Programs, and more recently, Professional Standards Review Organization, and Health Systems Agencies.

As hospital systems develop, they generate their own internal shared service capacity for serving their own hospitals as well as other hospitals. Systems' shared services, such as a management engineering study, should have a much better chance to be implemented than an engineering study that only carries a recommendation from an association. Within a system, the central managers can ensure that information is used.

Systems create energy and forward motion by virtue of the things they have to do to support their hospitals. As they create volume, for example, in terms of electronic data processing, systems managers and their member institutions will begin to develop strong competitive positions with local and state associations that are providing the same services. The councils and associations don't want to be put in a position of competing with members. Therefore, the outlook for local and regional associations is primarily to retain their position as a *collective* voice for all hospitals, thereby going back to their original roles as political and public relations organizations.

Many of the same things that are happening within local and regional associations are having an impact on state associations. Government has long been forcing the development of regional groups and associations within states through such laws as Hill-Burton, Medicaid, Regional Medical Programs, Comprehensive Health Planning, Professional Standards Review Organizations, and Public Law 93-641. As administrators in individual hospitals see the regional patterns developing, they tend to think along the same lines.

For example, in New Jersey the state hospital association sees regional communities of interest developing among hospitals within the boundary lines of the four Health Systems Agencies designated for the state. The New Jersey Hospital Association has developed a wide range of shared services that are currently being marketed in New Jersey, Delaware, Pennsylvania and Maryland. At one time, the association even had a contract to provide engineering services for a hospital in Canada. In addition, the state assocation has on two occasions contracted to manage All Souls Hospital in Morristown, first to satisfy a court order that refused to allow All Souls to be closed, and more recently to manage the facility during a merger negotiation with a stronger institution, Morristown Memorial.

The New Jersey Hospital Association is trying to meet the needs of its member institutions for strong centralized management services. The association's primary competitive argument is one of a willingness to leave the individual institution a great amount of autonomy in how to use association services and recommendations. Hospital systems, on the other hand, insist on more control. And control seems to be the key to effectiveness.[13]

In Indiana, the Indiana Hospital Association has enlarged its organization along Health Systems Agency lines, opening and staffing district offices to help its member deal with the HSAs.[14] The American Hospital Association said in early 1976 that it could see this approach as a "national trend."[15]

According to whether the state is densely populated or not, there is every possibility that other state assocations will reorganize on the basis of the regional, geographical interest of their members in order to cope more effecitvely with the regional control and regulation patters being established by state and federal governments. There is also the possibility that associations will retard the development of systems in this way by continuing to offer shared services that seem to reduce the need for individual hospitals to link together into regional systems configurations. "The associations offer answers, but they have no power to implement their own recommendations," said a system manager. "We do," he added, "and therein lies the difference. This is not to say that we don't meet local needs. In the long run, it is only the truly effective organization that can survive."[16]

NATIONAL ASSOCIATIONS

The national associations, like the state associations, are responding to the regionalizing effects of federal programs and to the development of systems.

The American Hospital Association has developed Regional Advisory Boards that have increasingly strong input into association policies and programs. Just as the state associations are putting staff and offices into the HSA regions, the national associations have full-time staff in every U.S. census division. Systems managers are represented at every level of AHA policymaking. At the same time, the association has considerably beefed up its Washington staff in order to deal with the multitude of legislative and regulatory issues facing hospitals.

The Catholic Hospital Association has long had its national offices in Saint Louis, Missouri, because of strong Catholic influences in the region. The first Catholic-sponsored program in hospital administration was established at Saint Louis University. But in early 1976, the CHA announced that it was opening a Washington legislative office in order to maintain closer contact with members of the Congress and the federal bureaucracy.

The American Protestant Hospital Association, now headquartered in Chicago, may either have to go out of business or more closely define its constituency and begin to represent that constituency forcefully in Washington, perhaps even moving its office to the nation's capitol.

The General Conference of the Seventh-day Adventist Church has its national headquarters in a Washington, D.C., suburb, close to the power centers of national politics.

The Federation of American Hospitals, representative of the proprietary, investor-owned chains, is fundamentally a systems trade group. The FAH initially established its national headquarters in Little Rock, Arkansas, but opened a second office in Washington in 1971 and designated it as national headquarters. The FAH has become a potent political force in Washington, and several of the states.

The Blue Cross Association is a system response linking together the efforts of seventy-four plans in the United States and Puerto Rico, five affiliate plans in Canada, and one in Jamaica. The BCA is the strongest organization of its type in the United States. National Blue Cross reached an enrollment of 82.4 million in 1974. This membership includes the 5.9 million government employees and their dependents covered through the Federal Employees Health Benefits Program. Blue Cross plans also have 7.6 million Medicare beneficiaries covered for additional benefits, and are the fiscal intermediary for 25.5 million persons under Medicare and Medicaid.

Systems have more economic and political power than autonomous hospitals and will be able to bargain and negotiate more effectively with Blue Cross. As systems grow and develop across various plan jurisdictions, they will be able to expect most favored treatment from the "best" prepayment plan.[16] Systems will not tolerate wasteful competition between plans; and plans will not tolerate wasteful competition among systems.

Kaiser already operates its own prepayment plan. As large hospital systems develop, they will consider setting up organizations for the same purpose, usually beginning with a health maintenance organization.

One multistate not-for-profit hospital system that was facing difficulties negotiating through a state Blue Cross plan went directly to the Social Security Administration in Maryland to get a rapid resolution to its problem. An obvious alternative for the large hospital system is to deal directly with the government if it encounters difficulties in dealing with Blue Cross.

Several systems have chosen to develop benefit packages for their own employees that are then marketed by a Blue Cross plan. In these instances, the plans are paid for administrative services while the systems themselves have gone at risk.

Other systems have developed captive insurance companies, initially as a response to the malpractice crisis, but with an eye toward the future when they might develop their own prepayment plan for people served by the system. Three of the major systems already have growing HMOs, and others say they are planning to develop this prepayment system. A larger, and natural next step would be to reincorporate the marketing and financing aspects of prepayment currently performed by Blue Cross into a more fully integrated hospital system. BCA has consistently argued for the need for stronger management within hospitals. Systems can provide stronger management, but they also may provide stronger competition for Blue Cross plans.

INFLUENCE OF SOCIAL FORCES

Many social forces are dictating increased systems development. Economies of scale, cost containment, quality control and accessibility can be achieved along with increased provider power to keep a strong pluralistic system from becoming an arm of government. Simultaneously, government can implement and achieve public policy goals more easily through systems of health services that are backed up by strong managers.

Not every hospital will be a member of a system. But those hospitals that remain strong will benefit from systems innovations and retain their autonomy because strong systems have the power to demand a pluralistic arrangement for medical services. This is within the American tradition, not outside it. The value of retaining citizen involvement and religious dedication as part of the health care system will, we believe, benefit our country. The loss of some autonomy by autonomous hospitals will be more than compensated for by the achievements of systems. Providers can reorder their own house without the total loss of autonomy associated with a nationalized governmental system.

What will hospital systems mean to communities and consumers in the future? Generally, they are creating new opportunities.

The administrator has an opportunity to become the key individual for developing a preventive medicine program and a health care system with a community focus. Working through boards of trustees, an administrator can link together the care elements of a hospital with the workplace.

Across the United States, administrators may see their organizations evolve from hospital systems to health care systems with a broader view of what contributes to illness and what promotes health. This view will consider such forces as genetics, lifestyle and behavior, nutrition, education, the workplace, the physical environment and the absence or presence of disease.

The movement toward hospital systems is really a management revolution, led by a handful of people who are rapidly picking up followers. Hospital systems don't necessarily represent a Promised Land, but they do offer hospitals a way to survive, grow, prosper and continue to provide services to people.

NOTES

1. Personal communications to the authors.
2. Personal communication to the authors.
3. Telephone interview with Aladino A. Gavazzi, March 18, 1976.
4. Telephone interview with the Rev. Paul F. Medeck, January 30, 1976.
5. Telephone interview with C.N. Platou, December 4, 1975.
6. Telephone interview with Carl S. Klicka, M.D., December 10, 1975.
7. Interview with R.Z. Thomas, Jr., Chicago, August 18, 1975.
8. E. Darby, "Serving all Facets of Health Care," *Commerce* (November 1974), pp. 14-16, 104.
9. Ibid.
10. American Hospital Supply Corporation 1974 Annual Report.
11-16. Personal communications to the authors.

INDEX

297

About the Authors

Professor of Health Administration at Duke University, and former Director of Studies in Hospital and Health Services Administration, Northwestern University, Montague Brown is the recipient of the 1976 Dean Conley Award of the American College of Hospital Administrators for the most outstanding article of the year published in a health field journal. He served as a Senior Researcher at the National Center for Health Services Research in 1975-1976.

A writer, researcher and journalist, Howard L. Lewis has published numerous magazine articles on medicine, science, space and health care. He has won awards for his writing from the American Heart Association, the American Dental Association and the American Business Press.